Chiropractic Manipulative Skills

TO
My loving, supportive and totally unselfish wife, Annabel
and
My dear little daughter Sophia, whose determined knocks on my
office door will no longer have to be ignored.

CHIROPRACTIC MANIPULATIVE SKILLS

Edited by David Byfield BSc, DC

Program Director
International Managed Health Care

and

Technique Instructor, Division of Chiropractic Sciences
Canadian Memorial Chiropractic College
Toronto
Canada

With a Foreword by
A Grice MSc, DC, FCCS
Professor, Canadian Memorial
Chiropractic College, Toronto, Canada

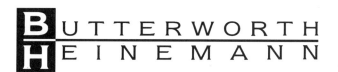

BUTTERWORTH
HEINEMANN

Butterworth-Heinemann
Linacre House, Jordan Hill, Oxford OX2 8DP
225 Wildwood Avenue, Woburn, MA 01801-2041
A division of Reed Educational and Professional Publishing Ltd

℞ A member of the Reed Elsevier plc group

OXFORD AUCKLAND BOSTON
JOHANNESBURG MELBOURNE NEW DELHI

First published 1996
Reprinted 2000

British Library Cataloguing in Publication Data
Chiropractic Manipulative Skills:
Fundamentals of Clinical Practice
  I. Byfield, David
  615.534

ISBN 0 7506 0968 0

Library of Congress Cataloguing in Publication Data
Chiropractic manipulative skills/Edited by David Byfield.
  p.   cm.
  Includes bibliographical references and index.
  ISBN 0 7506 0968 0
  1. Spinal adjustment. I. Byfield, David.
  [DNLM: 1. Chiropractic – methods. WB 905.9 C541]
  RZ265.S64C48
  615.5'34–dc20

                                                    95–30545
                                                    CIP

Printed in Great Britain by The Bath Press, Bath

Contents

Foreword

Up until the presentation of this text two important areas in developing spinal manipulative skills have been neglected. This text presents an organized, thoughtful and sequential approach to teaching and learning the complex psychomotor skill of adjusting and a biomechanical approach to postural efficiency in its delivery. Recent research has confirmed that the chiropractic dynamic adjustment is the most effective treatment for lower back pain, however, research has also shown that the practitioner suffers from the forces and postures used in its practice, resulting in high levels of occupationally induced back pain for the practitioner.

Learning the art and skill of adjusting requires practice and dedication. It's ultimate perfection should not depend on our innate abilities or sacrifice of our personal structure but rather it should be based on knowledgeable perfection of the nuances of the various adjustive procedures resulting in efficiency and precision of application.

Dr Byfield presents a systematic sequential evaluation of the doctor's and patient's positioning, along with control of the line of drive that will produce an adjustive thrust with maximum efficiency, minimal force and strain for both the patient and the doctor.

Imagery along with practice, based on knowledge can enhance our performance. This text, by juxta positioning the written material and the use of serial photo- graphs, allows student and practitioner alike to visualize each procedure in a step-by-step manner thus enhancing the overall performance.

The contributing authors broaden the teaching scope to include educational, biomechanical and physiological aspects of psychomotor learning, making this an appropriate teaching text for the student and teacher of spinal manipulation. The elegant simplicity of presentation and the systematic sequential steps to learning each of the psychomotor skills makes this text a must for the student/teacher/ practitioner who wishes to refine the art of spinal manipulation and protect their own anatomy, for success and longevity in practice.

I have no doubt that it will become a standard in our institutions since it thoroughly presents the basic principles of balance, control and efficiency which can lead to a degree of perfection in all areas of spinal manipulation. Discussions of theory and bias are avoided while the concepts are presented with humility and a generous use of appropriate references with suggested readings to broaden our knowledge and expertise.

A. Grice MSc DC FCCS

Acknowledgements

I thank David Antrobus DC and his company Atlas Clinical Ltd, Unit 51, Britannia Way, Lichfield WS14 9UY, UK (Tel & Fax 0543 255107) for supplying the table and other equipment used in the production of this book. The table that appears throughout this text is a highly developed piece of technical wizardry which in my opinion constitutes a foundation for the skilled performance of many chiropractic manipulative skills. The equipment provides comfort for both the patient and practitioner and yields clinical adaptability.

I also thank David for his extremely helpful attitude, enthusiasm and keen sense of spatial orientation when behind the camera during the long and tedious photographic sessions. Thanks also to David's father Harvey for his undivided attention and ability to move the very heavy table on numerous occasions to get the right angle.

I acknowledge Michael Kondracki MSc, DC as the model and thank him for his valuable suggestions during the numerous photo sessions.

I thank also my photographer, Mr John Dodds, Bournemouth, England and his staff for their patience, advice and professional manner during the actual photo sessions and the postproduction period.

I acknowledge Dr Peter McCarthy for his chapter and reviewing the manuscript before submission, Mr David O'Neill, the librarian at the Anglo-European College of Chiropractic and his staff for their assistance in retrieving reference material and my other two contributors, Kim Humphreys BSc, DC and Michael Kondracki for their long awaited, yet fine quality work.

Finally, I sincerely thank Adrian Grice DC, Howard Vernon DC, Ronald Gitelman DC, Len Faye, DC, Zoltan Szaraz DC and Lyman Johnson DC for giving me the opportunity and environment to learn from the best. I can only hope that they will appreciate my attempt to acknowledge their pioneering efforts.

A special thanks goes out to Ron King DC for encouraging me to undertake a teaching career.

Last but not least I extend a thankyou to Mr Tim Brown, my assistant editor for his understanding and ability to accept just about every excuse for my delay in submitting the final manuscript on time and to my editor, Caroline Makepeace for her belief and conviction that the project would succeed.

Contributors

David Byfield, BSc, DC
Program Director
International Managed Health Care

Technique Instructor
Division of Chiropractic Sciences
Canadian Memorial Chiropractic College
Toronto, Ontario, Canada

Kim Humphreys, BSc, DC, PhD
Head of Academic Affairs and Post Graduate Education
Anglo-European College of Chiropractic
Bournemouth, England

Michael Kondracki, MSc, DC
Senior Lecturer, Department of Chiropractic Clinical Sciences
Anglo-European College of Chiropractic
Bournemouth, England

Peter W. McCarthy, PhD
Senior Lecturer, Department of Chiropractic Sciences
Anglo-European College of Chiropractic
Bournemouth, England

Introduction

David Byfield

Chiropractic manipulative techniques are a complex interaction of numerous practised psychomotor skills. They constitute the foundation of chiropractic clinical therapeutics, and are an integral part of the management protocol for the treatment of musculoskeletal dysfunction. Manipulation formulates the art of the chiropractic profession, a talent and judgement that develops and matures with time and experience. Many years of practice are invested before any significant level of proficiency, clinical competence or *finesse* is attained (Paris, 1983). Learning good skills in manipulative practice not only benefits the patient, who receives a skilful manual thrust without pain, but is equally important to the practitioner to avoid needless injury and maintain a long professional life. Chiropractic manipulation is delivered in this fashion and above all, with finesse. *Manipulative finesse* is an extremely important factor to engender into the protomanipulator, particularly at the undergraduate level. Manual therapy, once dominated and practised primarily by those who were perceived to have sufficient muscular strength, is emerging as an elegant style characterized by smooth, controlled, and purposeful movements adaptable for all physical derivations and capabilities.

Furthermore, it should be reinforced that manipulation is a *full-time obligation*; one which requires a great deal of time and energy to acquire, master, and maintain the necessary clinical skills (Cassidy *et al.*, 1992). Skilled manipulation may appear quite simple to the uninformed observer. However, control of the adjustive thrust alone necessitates lengthy practice sessions and skill development in order that the practitioner be exact with respect to the magnitude, speed, and force of this thrust (Grice, 1980). Manipulation demands a long training programme and a professional commitment from those who undertake this life-work (Lewit, 1986). There is simply no room for unskilled, incompetent, amateurish, heavy-handed or clumsy clinicians in any health profession. No realistic, or for that matter, acceptable substitute exists for hard work and regular practice to assimilate the wealth of practical dexterity needed to perform skilled manipulation. The age old proverb *'knowledge without practice makes but half the artist'* goes without saying.

A curriculum which caters for an integrated approach to skills learning, including the vast amount of basic science and clinical knowledge to prepare the student for clinical training, cannot be ignored. This intensive psychomotor development, which is strengthened by an in-depth functional and diagnostic approach to the neuromusculoskeletal system, is the hallmark of chiropractic manipulative sciences. Many chiropractic colleges throughout the world today are restructuring and establishing stricter educational standards and developing a more flexible curriculum which justifies a full 4- or 5-year programme to fulfil their teaching objectives (Chapman-Smith, 1987, 1992, 1993). Competency-based education seems to be evolving as a dominant teaching strategy within chiropractic institutions, which revolves around professional activities and prepares clinicians for the realities of daily practice (Jamison, 1993). Furthermore, the importance of enhancing critical thinking and problem solving to develop confidence and establish sound clinical judgement 'as opposed to unsubstantiated or anecdotal belief systems' has been stressed (Mootz and Cohen, 1992).

The effectiveness of spinal manipulation for the treatment of musculoskeletal dysfunction, particularly low back pain, can no longer be justifiably questioned in light of more recent documentation (Manga *et al.*, 1993). Chronic back pain disability presents an entirely different picture for which there is very little substantiating evidence. Nonetheless, chiropractic management may play a significant role in multidisciplinary approach to this complicated issue. Many have heralded the important role of the therapist as a vital component of treatment interaction (Basmajian, 1993). A knowledgeable and confident clinician who comes into 'close contact' with the patient is likely to achieve at least 30–50% success no matter what treatment is actually given (Basmajian, 1993). This certainly supports the concept of a confident light touch and skilled hands during the care of a patient. Treatment effectiveness may also rest on the confidence of the clinician in obtaining total relaxation with the minimum amount of applied force (Curtis, 1988). The potency of a manipulative thrust has to be realized early in undergraduate training and not taken lightly or abused. This task remains within the domain of each educational institution.

Skills should be taught with understanding and reasoning, not merely by aimless repetition. Nonetheless, no one doubts that structured practice is the key ingredient toward the learning of complex motor skills (Lee *et al.*, 1991) and furthermore, placing manipulative skills and procedures in their intended clinical perspective should also enhance the learning and performance of these skills. Continuity, consistency and positive reinforcement combined with a strong biomechanical rationale and model are prominent features of this formula. The

rate and quality of skill acquisition will no doubt be significantly affected by individual variables, which in a flexible and open exchange would be well tolerated. Important diagnostic skills and indicators plus an intelligent approach to the relative and absolute contraindications to spinal manipulative therapy should be presented simultaneously. Clinical relevance, expectations of ability, criteria for skill performance, and treatment outcome measures are all factors to be considered during manipulative skills learning strategies.

What is the best strategy? Probably one in which clear learning aims and performance objectives have been consolidated into a concise institutional plan. Typically, manipulative techniques are taught through initial visual demonstration followed by practice sessions involving two or three partners. Direct personal feedback and individual instruction are somewhat limited due, in part, to the usually large class sizes in chiropractic colleges and the unpredictable student/tutor ratio. This does not provide an optimal environment for demonstration and learning of very complex skills. Many of the performance subtleties are overlooked and misinterpreted, which could lead to habitual motor behaviour and substandard performance. The final product or the manipulative procedure is often quickly demonstrated and students are expected to work *backwards* from this point instead of working *towards* it. Moreover, this type of teaching method does not exploit the potential for conceptualization of the physical procedure to play its full part (Stig *et al.*, 1989). Describing and illustrating the *whole* manipulative procedure, including a clinical example first, and then breaking the procedure down into its component parts or individual skills and rebuilding the whole could represent a very potent teaching strategy. This constitutes the basic theme of this book. Mentally imaging the spine and understanding the positive biomechanical/therapeutic outcome of a particular manipulative procedure has been shown to be a very effective way of teaching new manipulative techniques (Josefowitz *et al.*, 1986). Another study established that individually, mental practice and physical practice were equally effective methods used to acquire complex manipulative skills (Stig *et al.*, 1989). These studies indicate that there are more creative strategies for learning complex psychomotor skills besides the traditional demonstration method. A combination of many schemes appears promising whilst therapeutic intent and biomechanical rationale could also improve assimilation and performance. In a well known bestseller *The Inner Game of Tennis*, Timothy Gallwey (1974) has stated that 'images are better than words'. Developing an ability to visualize specific aspects of the necessary functional anatomy would be advantageous. Therefore, the role of the skills instructor is to create an environment in which communication is heightened and learning may be experienced as a direct result of the instructor's own motivational characteristics and enthusiasm.

The process of learning detailed psychomotor skills is both complex and difficult. Student perception, professional responsibility and motivational issues are only a few of the barriers encountered in the classroom. There is no substitute for hard work and repetition guided by clear performance objectives. Learning psychomotor skills has been described as directly dependent on the environment in which the skill is learned and the inherent skill learning capacity of the student (Good, 1993b). For example, a method of teaching which was perceived as more 'enjoyable' has been shown to be just as effective as more traditional procedures of teaching thrusting skills in the classroom (Good, 1993a). Whatever the instructor's style or methods, a balance should be attained to include a focused perspective and clearly defined performance criteria. Knowledge of results and internal proprioceptive feedback may be critical in the successful performance of psychomotor skills (Good, 1993b). In terms of reinforcement, considerable uncertainty exists about which approach is optimal in practical situations (Watts, 1990). However, it does appear that the effectiveness of any approach seems to depend upon the task itself, the

conditions under which practice occurs, the present level of skill of the student and a variety of student characteristics (Watts, 1990). Optimal results are achieved through continuous reinforcement in the initial learning stages to infrequent and sporadic feedback as learning advances and skills are attained (Watts, 1990). This may stimulate a complete reconsideration of the number of instructors and other resource implications required during the peak levels of skills learning. Chapter 1 of this book formulates key concepts of student learning derived from contemporary educational research and presents several basic principles that may be incorporated into more effective psychomotor skills learning, including appropriate clinical examples, clearly identified tasks and step-by-step practice methods taught in light of individual subcomponents as part of the clinical whole. Therefore, the ultimate educational goal is clinical competence and a confident performance in a real clinical setting (Newble, 1992).

The ability to learn the balance, control and coordination for the deft application of a dynamic thrust is an enormous task in such a relatively short period of time. The majority of physical practice involves learning these skills on a cooperative and relatively young cohort who are generally not ill. This represents an unrealistic situation considering patient age, attitude and initial apprehension encountered in a real clinical setting. This scenario is confounded by the student's impatience and sense of frustration when little progress is made. These learning plateaux are considered a common phenomenon in the acquisition of complex psychomotor skills (Good, 1993b). Inappropriate skills may result in an attempt to achieve the first 'joint crack' before the applicable neuromuscular reflexes are firmly established. Contrary to a well misunderstood concept, a joint crack does not represent, according to some, a viable means of performance feedback or treatment success (Helig, 1981; Plaugher, 1993) and furthermore, this attitude should be wholly discouraged and redirected into more clinically relevant issues such as patient care management. Notwithstanding, tissue noises and joint cracks are considered a trivial event and occur as natural and even habitual phenomena (Maigne, 1972; Nade, 1992). Therefore, it seems that it is the enthusiasm and creativity of the instructor investing time, patience, encouragement and, above all, rational attitudes which will direct these eager hands through these uncertain times. Colleges have a duty to prepare their students to be flexible and perform comfortably within the confines of clinical uncertainty (Cooperstein, 1990). For those who do not cope well with this incertitude, a career based upon the dogma and persuasion of the 'technique gurus' is a likely and unfortunate conclusion (Cooperstein, 1990).

It is not the intent of this book to promote or endorse any specific chiropractic systems technique. However, it is the aim to address some very basic motor skills necessary to perform a selection of the more common 'diversified' manipulative procedures used today in chiropractic practice. Recently, it has been stated that the majority of chiropractors – 91.1% in the USA (Chapman-Smith, 1993) and 51.1% in Europe (Pedersen *et al.*, 1993) – use diversified adjustive techniques, making it the most common form of full spine manipulation. 'The diversified approach attempts to apply the most ideal technique within the context of the reality of the clinical picture' and is based upon sound neurobiomechanical–orthopaedic principles (Gitelman and Fligg, 1992), the foundation of the biomechanical model (Fligg, 1985). Diversified techniques provide tremendous clinical flexibility, adaptability and variety as each procedure can be employed as either a mobilization or an adjustment/manipulation depending upon the specific biomechanical indications. This versatile scheme begins to prepare the student for fundamental decision making and problem solving skills required for clinical practice.

Surprisingly, the chiropractic profession as a whole has contributed very little to the peer reviewed literature describing these short and long lever diversified procedures, and there is presently no published research comparing the effectiveness of different chiropractic techniques (Bartol, 1993; Bergmann, 1993). Even less has been published concerning manipulative methods that use specific contacts on short levers (Bergmann, 1992). This scenario exists even though the chiropractic profession has practised manipulative therapy for almost a century. The basis of a well designed study would be a simple and straightforward definition and classification of chiropractic manipulative techniques which need to be fully described in detail before any comparisons can be made between these therapeutic methods (Moritz, 1979). The extensive knowledge base and reputable body of research that has accumulated over the last decade provides a favourable climate for the science of chiropractic to begin now, in earnest, to investigate the art of chiropractic seriously (Bergmann, 1993).

The foundation and principle nature of this textbook is *simplicity*. The aim is not to describe an endless number of manipulative permutations, their diagnostic indicators or therapeutic outcomes. There are many fine, high quality textbooks that have been written recently for this purpose. Furthermore, this would be an almost impossible task, particularly when over 500 individual diversified technique procedures have been identified (Bartol, 1992). The complex process of learning to make clinical decisions incorporates many elements and at some vital yet unknown point, an integration exercise takes place. The psychomotor skills required to perform numerous diagnostic and therapeutic actions are an integral component of this task and should be given at least equal time. It is considered a natural advantage to learn to crawl before one can walk and similarly, attempting to perform a Mozart concerto before mastering the basic scales would be ridiculous and futile.

The main objective of this text is to build a base for the purposeful balance and control necessary for efficient execution of spinal manipulation. Specifically, this will include: (i) fundamental and concise movement of both long and short levers to isolate a specific spinal motion segment or region; (ii) postural skills and weight distribution for both the doctor and the patient; (iii) concepts of tissue 'slack', tissue tension sense, joint tension and joint preload; (iv) minimum force and energy expenditure; (v) hand skills; (vi) basic side posture positional skills; (vii) accurate anatomical landmark location (Appendix I); and (viii) basic high-velocity low amplitude thrusting skills. This will be presented in the light of current teaching and learning strategies most applicable to the acquisition of complex psychomotor skills. Important background information including specific biomechanical issues relative to the spine and pelvis and a detailed description of the neurophysiology of how a skill is actually performed supplement the text. A list of the 'cardinal or golden rules' presented throughout the text (Appendix II) and a recommended 'learning sequence' of skills and manipulative procedures completes the book (Appendix III). The heart of the text is a detailed, step by step description of 20 manipulative procedures covering all regions of the spine and pelvis. The purpose of this exercise is to establish a fundamental framework of specific motor skills and movement patterns associated with spinal manipulative therapy. Each manipulative procedure will constitute a sequence of steps or *building blocks* made up of smaller reflex movement patterns which when performed together will produce a *smooth* coordinated whole manipulative action. The ultimate aim is to perform the manipulation in a graceful flowing action from beginning to end. Concise movements to locate the point of counter-rotation, control leg drop, stabilize the upper body, shift and control body weight and essential pivoting procedures are explained in detail. Common mistakes and exaggerated movements encountered while learning these manipulative procedures have also been included to deter unwanted habits forming during the early stages.

The skills chapters are presented in a *split-page format* (text on the left and figure on the right), to provide the reader with direct visual reinforcement and feedback of each step or 'block' described in the text. This type of layout is designed to be 'user friendly', thereby saving valuable time often wasted searching laboriously through several pages of text for the appropriate figure. This style is akin to a slow play, frame by frame video with an accompanying script. The speed at which the 'frames' are played is determined by the level of the reader's skill. Fast-forward and rewind facilities are also features of this type of presentation depending upon where the reader would like to review or concentrate the learning encounter.

I contend that this group of skills functions as a substrate for more complex and advanced treatment procedures that should be introduced later during vocational development. Each of the manipulative procedures is presented from the moment the patient is positioned on the table through a series of steps, up to and including intersegmental isolation and the localization and application of joint preload. All procedures process both long and short lever movement using all ranges of joint motion followed by a light oscillatory 'mock thrust' to begin to learn and appreciate tissue tension and joint preload. *The application of a full specific thrust has been purposefully discouraged throughout the manipulative procedures sections of the text.* This strategy has been adopted because the skills required to control thrust speed and depth are undoubtedly underdeveloped at this stage. Consequently, the specific movements and exercises to begin thrust skill development have been presented separately in Chapter 6. At which point a student should begin to deliver a thrust and under what conditions is still the subject of considerable debate. This lack of skill should not be underestimated and encouraged prematurely. Chapter 1 addresses this educational argument and presents some viable teaching options for consideration. Of utmost importance is that the student should begin to comprehend the number of intricate movement patterns and skills that are required *to prepare both patient and practitioner alike* for completion of a manipulative treatment procedure. Learning the concepts of mechanical advantage, light touch and minimal force are essential features of early skills training and a basic requirement for developing manipulative/adjustive procedures of the highest quality.

The manipulative procedures in this book are identified by a specific anatomical landmark on the spine or pelvis (i.e. spinous process, transverse process, PSIS, etc.). This represents the targetted lesion or the short lever through which the doctor directs the externally applied therapeutic leverage or thrust. This differs significantly, but also complements, a previously documented model for the categorization and standardization of chiropractic treatment procedures. This is based upon the 'method of delivery' (i.e. short lever, long lever, manual thrust and combinations thereof), rather than by a *named technique* (Bartol, 1993). This more descriptive method is a substantial step towards unifying manual treatment procedures and eliminating the inherent confusion which underpins the use of traditional terminology. Conventional diversified terms are used throughout the text for cross referencing.

This book does proclaim that a degree of segmental specificity is attainable even though many in the profession still question this assumption. As a focus for discussion, 'specificity of contact may not be necessary for specific correction of the true subluxation' (Haas, 1992) implies that the biological system and its complex multi-segmental neuroanatomical connections may tolerate segmental inaccuracy. This may explain why poor manipulative skills achieve favourable clinical results. Hopefully, this does not encourage or bolster an attitude of complacency and undermine the complexity and sophistication of our diagnostic and therapeutic skills. It can be said that applying a manipulative force in one region will undoubtedly cause some observable effects above and below this point. Experimentally, this concept has been supported with reference to at least which side of the spine should be adjusted in relation to measured dysfunctional findings (Nansel *et al.* 1989, 1993). Regardless of the outcome of this debate, therapeutic procedures should always be applied in the best interest of the patient.

There are some who contend that texts of this nature simply function as *aides-mémoire* and that there is no substitute for observing and learning from a skilled and experienced practitioner. The 'apprentice system' has its own merits, but a one-to-one teacher/student interaction is an unrealistic option partly due to resource restrictions in most learning institutions. A sensible balance has to be reached. This text goes beyond this view and fills a much needed gap to provide a structured base from which to begin the long and difficult undertaking of manipulative skills training.

This book is designed primarily for undergraduate education. However, it can easily be adapted for postgraduate purposes for those who wish to review and improve their manipulative skills. The essence of this text is control and smooth deliberate actions which should not be regarded as priority of the undergraduate domain. Observing the ease and efficiency of a top ranked tennis player or professional golfer is the end result of many hours and years of dedication and repetition in order to master the skills and yet, they still practise and continue to look for ways to perfect their swing. We have a professional responsibility and obligation to maintain a very high standard of practice and patient care which includes skilfully applied manipulation.

References

Bartol, K.M. (1992) Algorithm for the categorization of chiropractic technique procedures. *Chiropractic Technique*, **4**, 8–14

Bartol, K.M. (1993) The use of the generic nomenclature of chiropractic treatment procedures in chiropractic publications. *Journal of Chiropractic Education*, June, 29–34

Basmajian, J.V. (1993) Introduction: a plea for research and validation. In *Rational Manual Therapies* (eds. J.V. Basmajian and R. Nyberg). Williams and Wilkins, London, pp. 1–5

Bergmann, T.F. (1992) Short lever, specific contact articular chiropractic technique. *Journal of Manipulative and Physiological Therapeutics*, **15**, 591–595

Bergmann, T.F. (1993) Editorial: various forms of chiropractic technique. *Chiropractic Technique*, **5**, 53–55

Cassidy, J.D., Kirkaldy-Willis, W.H. and Thiel, H.W. (1992) Manipulation. In *Managing Low Back Pain*, 3rd edn. (eds. W.H. Kirkaldy-Willis and C.V. Burton). Churchill Livingstone, London, pp. 283–296

Chapman-Smith, D. (1987) Manipulation – professional standards of training and practice. *Chiropractic Report*, **1**, 2–4

Chapman-Smith, D. (1992) The chiropractic world – major current developments. *Chiropractic Report*, **6**, 2–3

Chapman-Smith, D. (1993) The chiropractic profession. *Chiropractic Report*, **7**, 3

Cooperstein, R. (1990) Brand name techniques and the confidence gap. *Journal of Chiropractic Education*, December, 89–93

Curtis, P. (1988) Spinal manipulation: does it work? *Occupational Medicine*, **3**, 31–44

Fligg, D.B. (1985) Biomechanical model. *Journal of the Canadian Chiropractic Association*, **29**, 152–153

Gallwey, W.T. (1974) Reflections on the mental side of tennis. In *The Inner Game of Tennis*. Bantam Books, Toronto, pp. 3–9

Gitelman, R. and Fligg, B. (1992) Diversified technique. In *Principles and Practice of Chiropractic*, 2nd edn. (ed. S. Haldeman). Appleton and Lange, San Mateo, California, pp. 483–501

Good, C.J. (1993a) An evaluation with the affective domain of teaching methods in manipulative technique laboratory: chirobics vs conventional thrusting exercises. *Journal of Chiropractic Education*, June, 19–28

Good, C.J. (1993b) Aspects of learning issues relevant to the chiropractic adjustment. *Journal of Chiropractic Education*, September, 59–68

Grice, A.S. (1980) A biomechanical approach to cervical and dorsal adjusting. In *Modern Developments in the Principles and Practice of Chiropractic*, 1st edn. (ed. S. Haldeman). Appleton-Century-Crofts, New York, pp. 331–358

Haas, M. (1992) Improving the reliability of palpation. In *Proceedings of the Eleventh International Conference on Back Pain and Manipulative Sciences* (Toronto, 1992). Canadian Memorial Chiropractic College and Consortium of Chiropractic Research

Helig, D. (1981) The thrust technique. *Journal of the American Osteopathic Association*, **81**, 244–248

Jamison, J.R. (1993) Competency-based professional standards: a fundamental consideration. *Journal of Manipulative and Physiological Therapeutics*, **16**, 498–504

Josefowitz, N., Stermac, L., Grice, A. *et al.* (1986) Cognitive processes in learning chiropractic skills: the role of imagery. *Journal of the Canadian Chiropractic Association*, **30**, 195–199

Lee, T.D., Swanson, L.R. and Hall, A.L. (1991) What is repeated in a repetition? Effects of practice conditions on motor skill acquisition. *Physical Therapy*, **71**, 150–156

Lewit, K. (1986) Manipulation – reflex therapy and/or restitution of impaired locomotor function. *Manual Medicine*, **2**, 99–100

Maigne, R. (1972) Localization of manipulation of the spine. In *Orthopaedic Medicine: A New Approach to Vertebral Manipulations* (ed. W.T. Liberson). Charles C. Thomas, Springfield, Illinois, pp. 131–136

Manga, P., Angus, D.E., Papadopoulos, C. *et al.* (1993) *The Effectiveness and Cost-effectiveness of Chiropractic Management of Low-back Pain*. Pran Manga and Associates, University of Ottawa, Canada

Mootz, R.D. and Cohen, P.A. (1992) Chiropractic clinical teaching. *Journal of Manipulative and Physiological Therapeutics*, **15**, 471–476

Moritz, U. (1979) Evaluation of manipulation and other manual therapy. *Scandinavian Journal of Rehabilitative Medicine*, **11**, 173–179

Nade, S. (1992) Clicks, clunks, creaks and crepitus. *Current Orthopaedics*, **6**, 60–64

Nansel, D.D., Cremata, E., Carlson, J. *et al.* (1989) Effect of unilateral spinal adjustments on goniometrically-assessed cervical lateral–flexion end-range asymmetries in otherwise asymptomatic subjects. *Journal of Manipulative and Physiological Therapeutics*, **12**, 419–427

Nansel, D., Szlazak, M. and Gaulin, G. (1993) Side-specific effects of upper cervical adjustments with respect to the amelioration of passive cervical rotational end-range asymmetries. In *Proceedings of the 1993 International Conference on Spinal Manipulation* (Montreal, 1993). Foundation for Chiropractic Education and Research, Arlington, p. 94

Newble, D.I. (1992) Assessing clinical competence at the undergraduate level. *Medical Education*, **26**, 504–511

Paris, S.V. (1983) Spinal manipulative therapy. *Clinical Orthopaedics and Related Research*, **179**, 55–61

Pedersen, P., Kleberg, P. and Walker, K. (1993) A pilot survey of patients and chiropractors in European chiropractic practices: socio-demographic, anamnestic and management procedures. *European Journal of Chiropractic*, **41**, 5–19

Plaugher, G. (1993) Clinical anatomy and biomechanics of the spine. In *Textbook of Clinical Chiropractic: A Specific Biomechanical Approach* (ed. G. Plaugher; assoc. ed. M.A. Lopes). Williams and Wilkins, London, pp. 12–51

Stig, L-C., Christensen, H.W., Byfield, D. and Sasnow, M. (1989) Comparison of the effectiveness of physical practice and mental practice in the learning of chiropractic adjustive skills. *European Journal of Chiropractic*, **37**, 70–76

Watts, N.T. (1990) The events of learning and functions of teaching. In *Textbook of Clinical Teaching*. Churchill Livingstone, London, pp. 24–27

Chapter

1

Educational aspects of the teaching and learning of skills

Kim Humphreys

Introduction

Chiropractic education has undergone an exceptional evolution in terms of curriculum design and development in the past three decades (Weise, 1993). With the increasing maturation of the colleges as institutions of higher learning has come the pursuit of excellence in terms of teaching and learning. The contemporary model of chiropractic education devotes considerable time to the teaching and learning of psychomotor skills relevant to clinical practice. Certainly the majority of effort and resources is concentrated on helping students to develop manipulative or adjustive skills to a competent level compatible with entry into chiropractic practice.

This is undoubtedly a difficult task. The colleges are asked to take students who are extreme novices of the nuances of manipulative skills and in a relatively short period of time, pronounce them 'safe' to treat the general public who may attend them for help. This is no small feat, and credit is justly given to the faculty of the colleges for achieving this goal.

Just as the previous decades produced meteoric leaps in the quality of chiropractic education, today presents the challenge of trying to enhance students' educational experiences. Quality research in higher and medical education is increasing at a rapid rate. Much work has centred on studying student learning in various curricula. Substantial research in the fields of

cognitive and instructional psychology as well as medical education has now identified ways in which students may acquire knowledge through learning and studying which will better prepare them for effective clinical thinking (Newble and Entwistle, 1986; Coles, 1985, 1989; Balla, 1990).

As exciting as this may sound, research does not presently extend to the learning of psychomotor skills relevant to chiropractic practice. Little has been devoted to uncovering how students go about the learning of the complex psychomotor skills needed to perform manipulations let alone how best to teach them. Perhaps this is the gauntlet to be thrown down to those interested and involved in the teaching f chiropractic technique. The time has come for qualitative and quantitative research to help students better attain the necessary skills so crucial to chiropractic practice.

The purpose of this chapter is to identify knowledge about psychomotor skills gleaned from various research disciplines which may be applicable to the teaching and learning of chiropractic manipulative techniques. Many chapters could possibly be written about important ideas and theories extrapolated from other disciplines which may be relevant to chiropractic psychomotor skills. The emphasis of this chapter will be on key concepts of student learning derived from contemporary research in medical and higher education as well as relevant constructs from work in the field of motor skills acquisition. The first part of the chapter will discuss what I believe to be the ethos or framework within which chiropractic psychomotor skills should be taught. The importance of this context will purposely be emphasized because it is either ignored or given only lip-service in most chiropractic colleges. It is also in keeping with contemporary curricular thinking in other health professions such as medicine, dentistry, nursing and physiotherapy (Newble, 1992; Feil, 1992; Doheny, 1993). The rest of the chapter will identify selected research which may be adapted to the teaching and learning of motor or psychomotor skills in chiropractic.

The Context of Learning

The purpose of undergraduate chiropractic education is to prepare students to enter the profession as primary health care practitioners. The context of the curriculum therefore is to provide students with a meaningful and clinically relevant education which closely resembles modern day chiropractic practice. In educational terms, the goal is to attain clinical competence, defined as 'the mastery of a body of relevant knowledge and the acquisition of a range of relevant skills, which would include interpersonal, clinical and technical components' (Newble, 1992; p.504). Mastery will of course differ from student to graduate to experienced clinician and refers to an expected level of achievement depending on training and experience.

The crucial point about the importance of the undergraduate learning context lies in the fact that clinical competence is an integration and interrelation of knowledge and skills (Hart and Harden, 1987; Bender *et al.*, 1990; Newble, 1992). For chiropractic education, psychomotor skills and especially the teaching and learning of manipulative techniques forms a considerable part of the whole and it is the integration of these skills with the relevant knowledge component which should be emphasized, demonstrated and practised. Graduates who are clinically competent should feel comfortable with private practice albeit with entry level clinical skills.

Recently however, increasing concern has been expressed by other health professions about the way in which their graduates are trained to meet the demands of modern clinical practice (Coles, 1990a, 1990b). In particular it has been argued that patients do not present in textbook fashion, which is the way students are taught in traditional curricula. Concern has also been expressed in other health professions about the current inordinate emphasis on acquiring cognitive and psychosocial skills with little attention paid to a holistic integration of psychomotor skills into the curriculum (Doheny, 1993).

Certainly these observations are also true of most modern chiropractic curricula. The teaching of psychomotor skills, particularly manipulative techniques, tends to be in isolation from the other subjects which students are learning. Students in technique classes are taught the necessary steps to position fellow students (set-up) for the delivery of the adjustive thrust. In later years, students may practise the various manipulative procedures from patient and practitioner positioning and other skills to completion of the manipulative thrust. Little if any time, however, is spent on allowing students to integrate these skills by practising the entire clinical procedure from history taking, physical examination, diagnosis, through to the appropriate selection and performance of the selected adjustive skills. Time concerns are important but even shortened versions equivalent to a regular patient visit and treatment session are not regularly practised or rehearsed. It is expected that students upon entering the clinical attachment in their final years will be able to make the appropriate transition from technique learned in isolation to its appropriate integration as a meaningful part of the whole clinical setting. In addition, the variety of possible clinical scenarios may compound this difficulty.

Rather than dwell on the problems associated with the learning of adjustive techniques outside of their clinical context, what does cognitive psychology and educational research suggest about more appropriate ways of learning psychomotor skills in chiropractic college?

The future graduate will have to continuously retrieve from memory the necessary knowledge and skills and then appropriately apply them to successfully complete his or her clinical duties. Chiropractors like other health professionals need to know a lot to function effectively in practice. It is now known that merely gathering information does not ensure that it will be recalled or used properly when dealing with patients (Coles, 1987). Work by Tulving and Thomson (1973) has shown that a learner's ability to recall information is very much dependent on the way in which it was acquired. Information processing theories support this idea as well as the importance of the setting in which the information was learned (Klatsky, 1980; Anderson, 1981). When students learn, not only do they store information which is being presented in whatever form, they also store information related to the setting in which it was presented (Coles, 1987).

Unfortunately when the students or graduates find themselves in a clinical situation necessitating recall of information, it may be distanced in time, space and nature from the original situation in which it was learned. Problems may arise for students trying to recall and appropriately apply previously learned information which is different from the setting or context in which it was learned. Mayer (1979) has called the ability to retrieve and apply information learned in one setting to another novel yet related situation the 'far transfer of knowledge'. In terms of the teaching of psychomotor skills, techniques taught in a repetitious, non-clinical, setting foreign to their eventual intended application must create both clinical and physical dilemmas for students when they are required to demonstrate clinical competencies.

Craik and Tulving (1975) have suggested the need to incorporate added information about possible retrieval scenarios which may help to facilitate easier access to knowledge stored in memory or provide a clearer route of access to stored memory (Broadbent, 1975).

In more simplistic terms, the knowledge to be acquired should be presented in a manner which reflects the way in which it should be used. This again reinforces the importance of the context of learning – the clinical setting. The reader may be wondering what this has to do with learning psychomotor skills? Firstly, clinical competence is a combination of relevant knowledge and relevant skills which interact with various attitudinal aspects (interpersonal, clinical and technical) to solve a clinical problem (Newble, 1992). Secondly, there should be no reason to suggest that complex psychomotor skills such as manipulative techniques are simply acquired involuntarily without the interaction of cognitive processes. Therefore it would seem reasonable that a concerted effort should be made to teach adjustive skills focused on their ultimate application in the context of the whole clinical process.

Elaborated Learning and its Facilitation

We now know that effective learning is closely related to what students actually do when confronted with their learning tasks and seems to be little influenced by any generalized form of instruction on study skills (Becher and Kogan, 1980; Hartley, 1986; Coles, 1990b). Recent research has also identified the kind of knowledge necessary for effective clinical practice. Much of this information came from studies seeking to identify differences between expert and novice clinicians as they approached similar diagnostic conditions.

It has been known for some time that diagnostic errors are not the result of a lack of medical knowledge; rather, it is a failure to access properly relevant knowledge stored in memory (Bordage and Allen, 1982; Bordage *et al.*, 1984; Allen and Bordage, 1987). The 'knowledge-based' model of clinical thinking arose from this work and suggests that the major determinant of diagnostic thinking is the organization and availability of *relevant* knowledge in memory (Bordage *et al.*, 1990).

Expert clinicians are such because they have developed rich networks of knowledge which are linked together by abstract relationships. Their rich network of knowledge has built in many possible cues which may trigger multiple access routes to the stored information. Problems associated with inappropriate or failure of recall are less likely to happen because of the expansive, interconnected knowledge network. In addition, problems associated with the 'far transfer of knowledge' (knowledge gained in one situation being retrieved and used in another related yet novel situation) are also less likely to occur because of the multiple links and cues which have built up with the clinician's cognitive structure (Mayer, 1979).

The process of creating the rich cognitive network of interconnecting information has been termed 'elaborated learning' (Coles, 1985; 1990a; 1990b). Essentially it involves the relating of theory to practice. It is now known that exposing students to theory in the early years of study does not necessitate its use or better understanding in the later or clinical years. It is more important to look at *the way* in which students acquire their knowledge; in particular helping students to see how one piece of knowledge relates to another and in turn linking theory to the eventual realities of clinical practice.

A common analogy used to describe the elaborated learning process is to compare it to the putting together of a jigsaw puzzle (Coles, 1990b). On the puzzle box is a picture. This may represent anything from concepts or process to clinical examples or practical situations and represents the learning context. The puzzle pieces inside the box are the more theoretical or abstract ideas relating to the concepts under study. The learning task of the student is to make the links between the different theoretical pieces in the puzzle and to see how these relationships connect to form the overall picture. By so doing, the student is able to develop cognitive structures which relate not only small items of information but also on a grander scale create complex knowledge networks. The analogy may be extended

to a three- or multidimensional puzzle. Students who elaborate their knowledge in this way are more likely to see the relevance of the information they are learning and to remember and apply it more judiciously (Coles, 1985; 1987; 1990a).

Tutors may help students to elaborate their knowledge when teaching the psychomotor skills by applying a few basic principles. First, the student must be given an appropriate analogy or example or be put into the picture of how the skill to be learned is eventually to be used. It must be remembered that students will at some time be expected to make the 'far transfer of knowledge' so a few examples or scenarios or some variations to the original concept may be needed. I like to call the method of teaching whereby relevant clinical examples introduce the practical material to be learned 'CLINICAL FRAMEWORKING' and initial studies have shown it to be helpful (Humphreys, 1990).

Second, the background information relating to the new skills is offered. In this case, the student must have clear access to all the necessary components of the skill such as a visual demonstration, mental imagery, tutor supervision and STEP-BY-STEP-PRACTICE. These points find expression as a common theme which will be elaborated throughout this book.

Third, students *must set goals* for themselves regarding their skill acquisition. This requires students with consultation to set reasonable performance criteria in keeping with the overall goals of the psychomotor skills class as well as addressing their particular strengths and weaknesses. They should be reasonably challenging but attainable and may include items such as improvement in speed, force, posture, pretension and patient set-up. Effective methods of quantifying their progress such as mechanical models, videos, in-depth performance criteria as well as a host of other possible tools are needed not only to give students accurate feedback but also to reinforce in the minds of students that their efforts are taken seriously and matched by reliable assessment measures. Performance goals should be written down and ideally discussed with a tutor. They may also be discussed and checked by fellow students who will act as the student's patient during practical classes. Valuable feedback may be given by those on the 'receiving end' of the student learning the new skill. The discussion and writing down help to consolidate the gains and areas still for improvement.

Fourth, the learner must have a clear idea of his/her task. That task is to make sense of the whole skill being taught in light of its components (puzzle pieces) and how they fit into the overall picture or clinical example. In other words *they are to relate theory to practice*. Students may be given coursework or assignments such as creating different case scenarios, alternative applications of the skill including indications and contraindications. They should also be encouraged to look out for examples during their clinical observations or treatment encounters with clinicians and fellow students.

Thus far, the discussion has centred on the importance of the *clinical context* in teaching psychomotor skills in chiropractic colleges. The most appropriate way for students to go about acquiring their knowledge, 'elaborated learning', has also been presented because it forms the foundation for developing clinical competence. Suggestions about practical ways in which 'clinical frameworking' may be incorporated into the teaching to facilitate the elaborated learning process have also been discussed.

The next part of the chapter will focus on research into motor skills derived from various fields of study which not only provide useful information for teaching and learning psychomotor skills but may act as a springboard for further research in *chiropractic education*.

Acquisition, Retention and Transferability of Motor Skills

Considerable attention has been directed towards the study of factors which may influence how motor skills are learned, stored in kinesthetic memory and general-ized to other motor skills of similar characteristics. In motor skills research, the terms acquisition, retention and transferability are commonly used to describe the fundamental features of learning skills which have been investigated.

Skills Acquisition

Acquisition is the learning and practice phase where students first receive information about the new skill. It may encompass a number of different teaching techniques such as mental imagery, visualization, demonstration and practice. In chiropractic education manual techniques usually involve the use of skilled models (tutors) who introduce the tasks to be learned via demonstrations. The nature of the motor task to be learned and the stage of the learner predicate the underlying processes which lead to the acquisition of the skill. Additionally, practice and feedback are two potent learning variables which enhance the acquisition of new motor skills (Poole, 1991). The following discussion will concentrate on the more important features of skills acquisition research and the possible implications for the teaching and learning of psychomotor skills in chiropractic.

Mental Imagery in Learning Chiropractic Techniques

Chiropractic manipulative techniques are complex psychomotor skills. Traditionally they have been taught by visual demonstration followed by practice under tutor supervision with feedback. A cognitive process used in psychology, behavioural counselling and sports science has been studied for the possible enhancement of learning motor skills. Imagery rehearsal, mental imagery or mental practice involves the creation of mental pictures or images of the motor skill to be learned or changed (Josefowitz *et al.*, 1986). The visual and kinesthetic images of the motor skill are then rehearsed in the mind.

Research has shown that if mental imagery is introduced prior to practising a new motor task, it is more effective than no practice at all (Feltz and Landers, 1983). Other studies (Wrisberg and Ragsdale, 1979; Ryan and Simons, 1982) showed that learning motor skills which have a high cognitive content are benefited as much by mental imagery as physical practice and certainly both are better than no practice. Not surprisingly, earlier work demonstrated that prior experience with mental practice improved subsequent motor skills learning with mental imagery (Phipps, 1969; Corbin, 1967; Suinn, 1983).

Recently Kohl *et al.* (1992) studied alternating actual and imagery practice. They found that actual practice and alternating actual practice with imagery produced similar results. However both of these groups were much better than the imagery group or the practice and rest group. They suggest that alternating actual and imagery practice might facilitate motor learning.

According to Cautela and McCullough (1980) the effectiveness of mental imagery is influenced by relaxation, clarity or vividness of image and controllability of the visual and kinesthetic forms. For these reasons, it is advised that students undergoing instruction in mental imagery need to be as relaxed and free from tension and anxiety as possible because they can influence the effectiveness of the process (Lang, 1977).

There have been two studies on the use of mental practice in learning chiropractic psychomotor skills. Both studies have shown that mental imagery may be a useful adjunct to learning the complex motor skills taught in chiropractic colleges (Josefowitz *et al.*, 1986; Stig *et al.*, 1989). Further investigations comparing different practice protocols are necessary to elucidate better ways of learning motor skills as well as maximizing the effects of actual practice and mental imagery.

The Effect of Practice on Skills Acquisition

Practice is fundamental to the development of expertise in any motor skill. To learn a psychomotor skill, especially one as complex as manual manipulation, requires a considerable amount of practice

(Stig *et al.*, 1989). However, the questions to be asked are: what types of practice and what sort of practice schedules are most beneficial in acquiring them? Unfortunately only extrapolation from research into motor skills from other disciplines is possible at this time.

Considerable work has been done in many fields on the importance of practice in developing motor skills. It is necessary to explain some of the more common terms used in current motor skills research. Two common protocols for the practice of motor or psychomotor skills are referred to in the literature as block and random practice. Block practice involves the repetitive performance of a specific motor task. Random practice does not imply chance. It is the performance of a number of different motor tasks during the same practice session. Block practice therefore is the performance of one specific task; random practice schedules rehearse a number of different motor tasks. Other common terms in the literature are massed practice and distributed practice. Massed practice is essentially block practice and is defined as the repetition of large numbers of trials of the same task within a particular practice session (Good, 1993a). Distributed practice, on the other hand involves variations in time intervals for practising learning tasks. The variations in time intervals are flexible and may encompass increased time between practice trials within a session or the spreading out of practice trials to cover a number of practice sessions (Newell, 1981; Good, 1993a).

In chiropractic technique classes, the predominant form of practice is the block or repetitive form (Josephowitz *et al.*, 1986; Stig *et al.*, 1989) and massed practice (Good, 1993a). Recent research, however, has shown that *repetitive performance* during practice tends to *inhibit cognitive processes* which are actually key elements of practice itself (Lee *et al.*, 1991). In addition, when compared to *random practice* where more tasks or variations of the same task are introduced, the random schedule of practice facilitates *greater skill performance as well* as better retention of the skill in the long term (Bortoli *et al.*, 1992). The possible implications for teaching chiropractic technique may be that random practice should be utilized and possibly interspersed with the more traditional block style practice sessions.

Utilization of Models During Skill Acquisition

Contemporary educational techniques would suggest that watching a skilled model perform a motor task prior to attempting to practise the new skill facilitates learning. Work by Lirgg and Feltz (1991) studied subjects divided into four groups who observed models (demonstrators) ranging from expert teacher to unskilled peers perform the Bachmann ladder task. Their results suggested that the skilled model group were more proficient after watching the model than the other groups and again after practice. In addition this group reported higher efficacy beliefs than the other groups. However an important finding was that students who were unfamiliar with the model regarded the skill as more salient than the status of the model (demonstrator).

Conflicting results come from the work of Pollock and Lee (1992). In their study of subjects learning a computer tracking task, observation of skilled and unskilled models prior to practice and again after practice showed marked learning in both groups with no differences between them after training trials.

It is obvious that the learning tasks are quite different in the two studies. However in light of previous work, skilled models are probably the most desirable but unskilled models may have their yet to be determined place in helping students to acquire psychomotor skills. Some of the possible benefits of students watching fellow unskilled students perform various adjustive set-ups may be that the learners are put more at ease realizing they are in a similar skill acquisition position. It may also give them a benchmark by which to judge their strengths and weaknesses. However, there is much work to be done

in this area especially to identify what presentation schedules by skilled and unskilled models are most advantageous for the acquisition and retention of new motor skills.

Motor Skills Retention

Retention is a measure of how well the new skill has been learned after a varying period of rest from the acquisition phase. In motor skills research, retention tests may be given to the learner immediately following a practice session, or hours, days or even weeks later. In chiropractic colleges, similar to other institutions of higher learning, assessments and examinations constitute the major form of evaluating students' retention as a result of their learning.

Chiropractic students similar to others learning psychomotor skills, receive two important types of information or feedback which aid them in their learning process. Intrinsic or internal feedback (Singer, 1975) describes the information a learner receives from his/her body after performing a motor task while knowledge of results (KR) refers to the feedback given to students by tutors or instructors on their performance (Schmidt, 1982).

Recently, considerable work has been done to identify the effects of KR on the retention of motor tasks. Del Rey and Shewokis (1993) looked at the interaction of summary KR on the order of presentation of practice tasks. They found that the advantage of summary KR was determined by the type of practice and when the feedback was given. In particular, for random practice, KR is most effective if it is given in the later practice sessions whereas KR was more effective if given after each practice trial when using block practice schedules. The effectiveness for each of the practice protocols was measured by tests of retention and transferability to other related tasks.

Although much is still to be learned with regard to the order of KR, there now seems to be some evidence that overall, KR given in a random fashion helps students to perform better on retention tests than KR given on a regular block-like schedule (Good, 1993b). It is thought that students would have to concentrate more on their learning tasks because of the uncertainty of when the next feedback would be given (Good, 1993b).

The amount of feedback is also an important issue. Most likely there is a limit to which feedback is useful even when using repetitive or block type of practice. Vander-Linden *et al.* (1993) studied three groups of subjects learning a motor task. The groups received concurrent feedback (feedback during and after each attempt), 100% feedback (after each attempt), and 50% feedback (after every second attempt). The results indicated that on immediate and delayed (48 hours) retention tests, subjects in the concurrent group demonstrated more error than either the 50% or 100% group and in fact the 50% group fared better than both the concurrent and 100% group. Vander-Linden *et al.* (1993) concluded that feedback to the learners about their learning task performance is *best given after the task is accomplished and most likely at a lower frequency* than after each practice. In fact their results showed that too much feedback had a tendency to inhibit some learners from completing their tasks.

These results help to confirm earlier work by Winstein and Schmidt (1990) who hypothesized that too frequent KR resulted in too frequent modifications or changes to the learning process (termed 'maladaptive short-term corrections').

Perhaps the message to students should be that feedback is useful, but only if given judiciously. Research evidence suggests that random feedback is most likely the best to use. This would allow students the opportunity to explore more fully their own intrinsic or internal feedback which should place them in a better position to take on board the intermittent yet timely feedback from tutors (KR).

Transferability of Motor Skills

The transferability of a newly acquired motor skill refers to the capacity of how well the learner is able to demonstrate a novel but related skill without the benefit of practice. The inference is that the acquisition of one skill must confer by the processes used during acquisition some sort of common core of motor learning or generalization which is available to the learner when presented with another similar task (Schmidt, 1975; Fleishman, 1972, 1978; Kerr and Boucher, 1992).

Schmidt (1975) proposed the *schema theory* which suggests that some parts of the learning of motor skills may be generalized. When the learner is acquiring the skill, he or she develops schema (rules) which are based on feedback related to a knowledge of the outcomes of the movement as well as sensory feedback (visual, tactile, kinesthetic, etc.). The important part is that the developed schema may be used to help the learner with variations or novel situations related to that skill.

The relevance to chiropractic education may be that certain skills or parts of skills have some sort of 'cross reactivity' with others. Therefore when learning new skills, components of previously learned tasks may facilitate new learning. This cross reactivity or 'facilitation' due to similarity of learned structure in memory may also facilitate the learning or applications of novel skills when students are faced with a different situation to that in which they first learned them (far transfer of knowledge). The end result may be that students are able to learn in a better way by being more able to apply their learning appropriately in differing situations and conditions as well as learning at a quicker pace. Again, caution must be given because at this point in time, research is speculative with respect to its applicability to chiropractic psychomotor skills education.

However, keeping the above in mind, Paillard (1982) suggested that the rules necessary to perform a particular motor function are present within an individual who has learned a skill. These rules (kinetic formulae) may be added to learning other skills. They were envisaged as *building blocks* which could be added to or modified to give to the learner an increasing or varied repertoire of movements. By extrapolation of this concept, individuals who possess more building blocks or more elaborate kinetic formulae in their movement repertoire than other learners should be more advantaged when learning a related motor skill.

In the early days of motor skills research, it was thought that there was some general motor ability or coordination factor. However, since the work of Henry and Rogers (1960) and Henry (1968), today most researchers feel that motor tasks have a large degree of specificity for that particular skill.

Recently Elliot and Jaeger (1988), Proteau *et al.* (1987), and Proteau *et al.* (1992) have attempted to elucidate the important relationships between significant sources of information on learning a complex motor task requiring high levels of visual input. By manipulating some of the variables, especially vision, they were able to identify what effects this had on subjects who had already learned a complex aiming skill. Their results suggest that when learning a particular motor skill, instead of sensory feedback becoming less important for movement control as the task is thought to become more 'open looped' (Proteau *et al.*, 1987), in fact there seems to be an increase in the dependency of the sensory input(s).

Perhaps the importance of this work is an understanding that a complex skill such as the adjustment requires students to come to terms with all sorts of sensory information about how it is to be performed. They may use visual and mental imagery as well as information about their own body position (kinaesthetic), touch (tactile) and motor input to perform the skill. Students may also have prioritized sensory input based on personality and previous learning experiences such that some information is considered primary (such as vision or kinaesthetic) while other information is secondary or reinforcing. Students who have constructed such a hierarchy of sensory information may then pay more attention to the primary information and less to the 'secondary' sensory inputs when learning a particular motor task. Additionally, when perfecting through practice a complex psychomotor skill perhaps such as an adjustment, students may concentrate even more on the primary sensory input while the secondary input may cause confusion or inhibition in the pursuit of better skill performance.

These notions find some support from the previously mentioned studies of Elliot and Jaeger (1988) and Proteau *et al.* (1987; 1992). They found when learning a task, rather than seeing a shift away from one or more important sources of sensory information or a gradual diminishing of the necessity of the information, there is a relative specificity for this information which is needed to perform it to the level at which it has been learned.

The study by Proteau *et al.* (1992) showed that when subjects had learned a task without a particular sensory input (in this case vision), the subsequent introduction of vision actually interfered with the performance of the skill. Learners had difficulty trying to cope with the new sensory information which had not been incorporated into the original sensorimotor programming. It took a while before the subjects were able to reorient themselves and to incorporate the new sensory component. Proteau *et al.* concluded that when learning a specific motor task which involves a number of important sensory components, *the learner determines the relationships between these components*. The task is then stored as an integrated sensorimotor representation. Also if a significant source of sensory information is added after a long practice period, the major control for the motor task will occur from one of the important sensory components present when the task was first learned.

These results are very exciting because a number of their conclusions may have important implications for the teaching and learning of chiropractic manual skills. *There may be concerns about the teaching of adjustive techniques in a sequential order*, with the components practised for long periods of time before another *component* is introduced. Perhaps a useful analogy would be the enhanced effect of cross-training to athletes who are attempting to improve their physical performance whether it be in triathlon, marathon or other sporting endeavours. The principles of cross-training may be useful in helping students to gain greater expertise in the performance of different adjustive techniques. Possible problems related to a dogmatic, sequential ordering of the technique class could be seen in the following example.

Students learn the thrusting portion of manipulation on models or tables during the first year. During the second year, students learn how to position a patient for the adjustment then later learn how to take the hand contacts to tension. In the third year the students may then be allowed under supervision to complete the adjustment from set-up to administration of a complete thrust. Each of the components of the manipulative techniques from years 1 to 3 probably involves different sensorimotor parts, and probably different controlling sources of information. Therefore, students probably have different types of sensorimotor representations of adjustive skills in their repertoires. When another major sensory component is added, it may interfere with their representation to date and it may take considerable time to incorporate or modify the new information into their integrated stores. If you consider that this is done a number of times during their studies, serious hurdles for students may be created as they attempt to come to grips with the learning of very complex psychomotor skills.

In light of this research, perhaps a way forward would be to develop full body models which as far as possible are a facsimile of the tension and viscoelastic properties of the human body. Such models could then be positioned like patients and students could be taught the whole adjustive technique from set-up to completion of a thrust on the model. In this way, major components of the adjustment could still be added sequentially over shorter periods of time; however, the benefit is that the *entire procedure could be practised time and again*. Students would have the advantage of acquiring an integrated sensorimotor representation of the adjustive techniques which would be a good representation of what they need in clinical practice.

Conclusions

The purpose of this chapter is to give the reader a flavour for current concepts in the teaching and learning of psychomotor skills derived from research in the fields of education, cognitive psychology, movement and sport science.

A number of issues have been raised regarding the teaching and learning of psychomotor skills by chiropractic students. I have tried to address some concerns regarding the importance of keeping the end-goal, the clinical context, constantly in the minds of students as they are learning the skills. If students have a better idea of what, when, how and where the skills are to be appropriately applied, it seems logical that it would facilitate a greater integration of the motor with the cognitive skills. To this end I have introduced the concept of clinical frameworking as an important goal towards which both students and tutors should aim.

Presently, very little is known about the way in which skills should be presented to chiropractic students to enhance their acquisition and mastery. Much needs to be done to see how different approaches work, such as: presentation of skills; when is the best time to give feedback; what types of practice schedules reinforce skills better than others, to name just a few. Currently, with little evidence to go on, caution might be the best approach. Students learn in different ways and no single approach will be sufficient for all. Therefore a mix of approaches to teaching the skills would, I suggest, be the way forward until more solid evidence is available on which to base some conclusions.

It is hoped that the work presented here will serve as a basis for discussion and possibly the motivation for some to investigate the many unresearched areas of the teaching and learning of psychomotor skills relevant to chiropractic practice.

References

Allen, T. and Bordage, G. (1987) Diagnostic errors in emergency medicine: a consequence of inadequate knowledge, faulty data interpretation or case type? *Annals of Emergency Medicine*, **16**, 506

Anderson, J.R. (1981) *Cognitive Psychology and its Implications*. W.H. Freeman, San Francisco

Balla, J.I. (1990) Insights into some aspects of clinical education – 1. clinical practice. *Postgraduate Medical Journal*. **66**, 212–217

Becher, T. and Kogan, M. (1980) *Process and Structure in Higher Education*. Heinemann, London

Bender, W., Hiemstra, R.J., Scherpbier, A.J.J.A. and Zwiestra, R.P. (eds.) (1990) *Teaching and Assessing Clinical Competence*. BoekWerk Publications, Groningen

Bordage, G. and Allen, T. (1982) The etiology of diagnostic errors: process or content? *Proceedings of the Twenty-first Annual Conference on Research in Medical Education of the American Association of Medical Colleges*, New Orleans, pp. 185–190

Bordage, G., Grant, J. and Marsden, P. (1990) Quantitative assessment of diagnostic ability. *Medical Education*, **24**, 413–425

Bordage, G., Villeneuve, M. and Leclere, H. (1984) Etiologie des erreurs diagnostiques chez les etudiants en debut de formation clinique. *Revue d'Education Medicale*, **3**, 101–107

Bortoli, L., Robazza, C., Durigon, V. and Carra, C. (1992) Effects of contextual interference on learning technical sports skills. *Perceptual and Motor Skills*, October; **75**, 555–562

Broadbent, D.E. (1975) Cognitive psychology and education. *British Journal of Educational Psychology*, **56**, 309–321

Cautela, J.R. and McCullough, L. (1980) Covert conditioning: a learning theory perspective on imagery. *The Power of Human Imagination: New Methods in Psychotherapy*, Chapter 8 (eds. J.L. Singer and K.S. Pope). Plenum Press, New York

Coles, C.R. (1985). *A Study of the Relationships between Curriculum and Learning in Undergraduate Medical Education*. PhD thesis, University of Southampton

Coles, C.R. (1987) The actual effects of examinations on medical student learning. *Assessment and Evaluation in Higher Education*. Vol. 12. No. 3, pp. 209–219.

Coles, C.R. (1989) The role of context in elaborated learning. In: Balla, J.I., Gibson, M. and Chang, A.M. (eds.). *Learning in Medical School: A Model for the Clinical Professions*. Hong Kong University Press, Hong Kong, pp. 41–57.

Coles, C.R. (1990a) Elaborated learning in undergraduate medical education. *Medical Education*, **24**, 14–22

Coles, C.R. (1990b) Helping students with learning difficulties in medical and health-care education. *Medical Education*, **24**, 300–312

Corbin, C.B. (1967) Effects of mental practice on skill development after controlled practice. *Research Quarterly*, **38**, 534–538

Craik, F.I.M. and Tulving, E. (1975) Depth of processing and its retention of words in episodic memory. *Journal of Experimental Psychology*. **104**, 268–294.

Del Rey, P. and Shewokis, P. (1993) Appropriate summary KR for learning timing tasks under conditions of high and low contextual interference. *Acta Psychologica* (*Amsterdam*) May, **83**, 1–12

Doheny, M.O. (1993) Mental practice: an alternative approach to teaching motor skills. *Journal of Nursing Education*, June; **32**, 260–264.

Elliot, D. and Jaeger, M. (1988) Practice and the visual control of manual aiming movements. *Journal of Human Movement Studies*, **14**, 279–291.

Feil, P. (1992) An assessment of the application of psychomotor learning theory constructs in preclinical laboratory instruction. *Journal of Dental Education*, **56**, 178–182

Feltz, D.L. and Landers, D.M. (1983) The effects of mental practice on motor skill learning and performance: a meta analysis. *Journal of Sport Psychology*, **5**, 25–27

Fleishman, E.A. (1972) On the relation between abilities, learning and human performance. *American Psychologist*, **27**, 1017–1032

Fleishman, E.A. (1978) Relating individual differences to the dimensions of human tasks. *Ergonomics*, **21**, 1007–1019

Good, C.J. (1993a) An evaluation within the affective domain of teaching methods in manipulative technique laboratory: chirobics vs. conventional thrusting exercises. *Journal of Chiropractic Education*, September, Vol. 7, No. 1, 19–28

Good, C.J. (1993b) Aspects of learning issues relevant to the chiropractic adjustment. *Journal of Chiropractic Education*, June, Vol. 7, No. 2, 59–68

Hart, I.R. and Harden, R.H. (eds.) (1987) *Further Developments in Assessing Clinical Competence*. Can Heal Publications, Montreal

Hartley, J. (1986) Improving study-skills. *British Educational Research Journal*, **12**, 111–123

Henry, F.M. (1968) Specificity vs. generality in learning motor skills. *Classical Studies on Physical Activity* (eds. R.C. Brown and G.S. Kenyon). Prentice-Hall, Englewood Cliffs, NJ, pp. 331–340

Henry, F.M. and Rogers, D.E. (1960) Increased response latency for complicated movements and a 'memory drum' theory of neuromotor reaction. *Research Quarterly*, **31**, 448–458

Humphreys, B.K. (1990) Problem identification and possible solutions to learning difficulties encountered by students at the Anglo-European College of Chiropractic. *Journal of Chiropractic Education*, **4**, 61

Josefowitz, N., Stermac, L., Grice, A. *et al.* (1986) Cognitive imagery in learning chiropractic skills: the role of imagery. *Journal of the Canadian Chiropractic Association*, **30**, 195–199

Kerr, R. and Boucher, J.L. (1992) Knowledge and motor performance. *Perceptual and Motor Skills*, **74**, 1195–1202

Klatsky, R.L. (1980) *Human Memory: Structure and Processes* (2nd edition). W.H. Freeman, San Francisco

Kohl, R.M., Ellis, S.D. and Roenker, D.L. (1992) Alternating actual and imagery practice: preliminary theoretical considerations. *Research Quarterly of Exercise and Sport*, **63**, 162–170

Lang, P.J. (1977) Imagery in therapy: an information processing analysis of fear. *Behaviour Therapy*, **8**, 862–886

Lee, T.D., Swanson, L.R. and Hall, A.L. (1991) What is repeated in a repetition? Effects of practice conditions on motor skill acquisition. *Physical Therapy*, February; **71**, 150–156

Lirgg, C.D. and Feltz, D.L. (1991) Teacher versus peer models revisited: effects on motor performance and self-efficacy. *Research Quarterly of Exercise and Sport*, **62**, 217–224

Mayer, R.E. (1979) Can advance organisers influence meaningful learning? *Review of Educational Research*, **49**, 371–383

Newble, D.I. (1992) Assessing clinical competence at the undergraduate level. Medical Education Booklet No. 25. *Medical Education*, **26**, 504–511

Newble, D.I. and Entwistle, N.J. (1986) Learning styles and approaches: implications for medical education. *Medical Education*, **20**, 162–175

Newell, K.M. (1981) Skill learning. In *Human Skills*. John Wiley, Chichester

Paillard, J. (1982) Apraxia and the neurophysiology of motor control. *Philosophical Transactions of the Royal Society of London*, **B298**, 111–134

Phipps, S.J. (1969) Effects of mental practice on the acquisition of motor skills of varied difficulty. *Research Quarterly*, **40**, 773–778

Pollock, B.J. and Lee, T.D. (1992) Effects of the model's skill level on observational motor learning. *Research Quarterly of Exercise and Sport*, **63**, 25–29

Poole, J.L. (1991) Application of motor learning principles in occupational therapy. *American Journal of Occupational Therapy*, June: **45**, 531–537

Proteau, L., Marteniuk, R.G., Girouard, Y. *et al.* (1987) On the type of information used to control and learn an aiming movement after moderate and extensive training. *Human Movement Science*, **6**, 181–199

Proteau, L., Marteniuk, R.G. and Levesque, L. (1992) A sensorimotor basis for motor learning: evidence indicating specificity of practice. *Quarterly Journal of Experimental Psychology*, **44A**, 557–575

Ryan, E.D. and Simons, J. (1982) Cognitive demand, imagery and frequency of mental rehearsal as factors influencing acquisition of motor skills. *Journal of Sport Psychology*, **3**, 35–45

Schmidt, R.A. (1975) A schema theory of discrete motor skill learning. *Psychological Review*, **82**, 225–260

Singer, R.N. (1975) *Motor Learning and Human Performance*. Macmillan, New York

Stig, L.C., Christensen, H.W., Byfield, D. *et al.* (1989) Comparison of the effectiveness of physical practice and mental practice in the learning of chiropractic adjustive skills. *European Journal of Chiropractic*, **37**, 70–76

Suinn, R. (1983) Imagery and sports. In: *Imagery – Current Theory, Research and Application*, Chapter 16 (ed. A.A. Sheikh). John Wiley, New York

Tulving, E. and Thomson, D.M. (1973) Encoding specificity and retrieval processes in episodic memory. *Psychological Review*, **80**, 352–373

Vander-Linden, D.W., Cauraugh, J.H. and Greene, T.A. (1993) The effect of frequency of kinetic feedback on learning an isometric force production task in non-disabled subjects. *Physical Therapy*, February, **73**, 79–87

Winstein, C.J. and Schmidt, R.A. (1990) Reduced frequency of knowledge of results enhances motor skill learning. *Journal of Experimental Psychology* (Learning, Memory, Cognition), **16**, 677–691

Wrisberg, C.A. and Ragsdale, M.R. (1979) Cognitive demand and practical level: factors in the mental rehearsal of motor skills. *Journal of Human Movement Studies*, **5**, 201–208

Further Reading

Adams, J.A., Gopher, D. and Lintern, G. (1977) Effects of visual and proprioceptive feedback on motor learning. *Journal of Motor Behaviour*, **9**, 11–22

Klein, R.M. (1979) Automatic and strategic processes in skilled performance. *Psychology of Motor Behaviour and Sport – 1978* (eds. G.C. Roberts and K.M. Newell). Human Kinetics, Champaign, IL, pp. 270–287

Proteau, L. and Cournoyer, J. (1990) Vision of the stylus in a manual aiming task: the effects of practice. *Quarterly Journal of Experimental Psychology*, **42A**, 811–828

Wright, D.L. and Shea, C.H. (1991) Contextual dependencies in motor skills. *Memory and Cognition*, **19**, 361–370

Wrisberg, C.A. and Liu, Z. (1991) The effect of contextual variety on the practice, retention and transfer of an applied motor skill. *Research Quarterly of Exercise and Sport*, **62**, 406–412

Chapter

2

Some biomechanical considerations in manipulative skills training

Michael Kondracki

The application of the laws of mechanics to the study of human systems and tissues is relatively new. As with all new sciences biomechanics has entered a 'wunderkind' phase and is now expected, quite unrealistically, to provide the solution to all manner of complex biomedical problems. This is certainly the case in most clinical sciences and especially true regarding the study of the human spine. Knowledge of the limitations of experimental methodologies and theoretical considerations is prerequisite to the interpretation of biomechanical data. Since there are a number of excellent texts covering the fundamentals of biomechanics, this chapter will not attempt to introduce the basic concepts of this science. For an introductory review of biomechanical knowledge the reader is referred to the relevant chapters in *Clinical Anatomy of the Lumbar Spine* (Bogduk and Twomey, 1991) and *Clinical Biomechanics of the Spine* (White and Panjabi, 1990). This chapter focuses on some topics in spinal biomechanics that I feel are relevant to students of chiropractic, graduate or undergraduate alike. This will by no means be an exhaustive appraisal of the state of spinal biomechanics but rather a brief review of controversial areas of research intended to stimulate thought and debate. The views expressed and the topics covered here are, of course, a personal selection of issues the author regards as pertinent to the study of 'spinal health' and skills training.

Spinal Forces

A useful illustration of research controversy is found among those attempting to model the forces within the spine, in particular the lumbar spine. A very readable reassessment of spinal modelling is provided by Richard Aspden in his review paper (Aspden, 1992). The author first deals with the way that forces within the spine are traditionally estimated. As he points out, most models of the spine assume the bony skeleton to be a simple lever with the muscles providing *externally* applied forces. Since the spine is both curved and flexible and capable of changing shape during motion, thus varying its response to applied forces with posture, this lever model, he argues, is a gross oversimplification.

Traditionally the sum of the forward bending moments created by the weight of the trunk, and any weight being lifted, are balanced by the forces generated by the erector spinae. The compressive force on the L/S joint is then taken to be the sum of the erector force plus the compressive components of the other loads. This, however, can result in highly unrealistic magnitudes of compression, especially during lifting. These forces, as calculated using a simple lever model, can be in the order of 10 kN. This is paradoxical since vertebral failure strengths are no greater than 8 kN. On the other hand Nicolai Bogduk, in a review paper on the lumbar disc (1991), claims that compression forces of this magnitude can be attained during lifting. A study by Swedish workers on high-level powerlifters using the lever model of Schultz (Schultz and Andersson, 1981) calculated a compressive load on the L3 segment of 36.4 kN in one subject (Granhed *et al.*, 1987). Considering the spine as an arch and not a lever will, Aspden maintains, go a long way towards reconciling the contradictory data generated when modelling the spine. 'The principal difference between an arch and a lever is that an arch is a curved structure which, if constructed properly, is intrinsically stable, whereas a lever needs to be externally supported.' Thus the forces calculated for an arch are less than those for a lever since there is no requirement for an externally applied balancing moment.

A major contributor to the axial compressive forces required to maintain stability in the spine are the longitudinal ligaments. These ligaments pre-strain the spine throughout the whole range of flexion and extension, reducing tensile forces which may damage the annular fibres. These tissues are viscoelastic and will therefore increase their stiffness when loaded rapidly. As the spine is curved the ligaments will generate more force; additionally, the greater the curvature of an arch the less axial force is required to produce equilibrium. The combination of these two effects will de-stress the active muscle and reduce the energy required to maintain a certain posture.

The observation noted by Goel *et al.* (1985) that extension of cadaveric whole lumbar spine specimens produced the most stable loading mode, may, in part, be explained by the increase in lumbar curvature. In the traditional lumbar spine model the closeness of the erector muscles to the vertebral column has proved problematic. The perpendicular distance between the action line of the muscles and the axis of the joint has been considered so short that it has seemed almost impossible for the erectors to produce the extensor moment required for equilibrium. Aspden reminds us, however, that the spine is not a simple lever and that muscles do not contract in straight lines between their attachments. The curved nature of the spine and in particular the lumbar lordosis will deflect the line of

action of the erectors and generate larger moments than previously estimated. Aspden also highlights the role of the lumbar multifidus muscles. These elements, deep to the erector group, are complex finely innervated structures that are capable of precisely controlling the local curvature of the lumbar spine.

In respect of the factors mentioned above, this fine control of lumbar curvature can have very profound effects on the gross function of the entire spine. This fact may help explain why some chiropractors make great efforts to influence this muscle through adjustive procedures (Grice, 1979). The thoracolumbar fascia and the abdominal muscles together have been credited with the ability to apply an extensor moment to the spinous processes and thus supplement the mechanically disadvantaged erectors. This phenomenon has been dubbed the 'hydraulic amplifier' by Gracovetsky *et al.* (1985). Aspden, however, points out the work of Tesh *et al.* (1987), which demonstrates that the ratio of axial to circumferential tension is a mere 0.4. Aspden feels that the major function of the thoracolumbar fascia is in tightly constraining the erector muscles. During contraction of these muscles their cross-sectional area will increase; if this expansion is constrained by fascia the stiffness and strength of the muscle should increase, by up to 30%, rendering the spine able to support a greater load. This enhanced stiffness will also increase the resistance of the muscle to bending. In a similar way I propose that intra-abdominal pressure will increase stiffness of the lumbar spine to bending and thus provide additional stability during lifting.

Almost all of these biomechanical models of lifting, however, choose to ignore the influence of the pelvis. As chiropractors we are, of course, deeply interested in the mechanics of the pelvic ring and in particular the sacroiliac (SI) joints. A recent paper by Snijders *et al.* (1993) goes some way towards redressing the balance and deals, almost exclusively, with the role of the SI joints and the pelvic ring in the transfer of upper body loads to the legs. The first part of this publication looks at how the SI joints resist the very large shear loads imposed upon them. The flat nature of these joints make them well suited to the transfer of large bending moments but susceptible to shear forces which would tend to displace the sacrum inferiorly with respect to the iliac bones, bearing in mind that up to 60% of the body weight is supported by the sacrum. In a similar way to Aspden, these authors view the pelvis as an arched structure. They describe a mechanism whereby displacements of the sacrum are reduced to a minimum by a constant compressive force across the SI joints, the 'self-bracing' effect. This mechanism is dependent not only on joint compression but on friction forces within the joint, sacral wedge angle and the influence of muscles and ligaments. The authors also show that if the pelvis is treated as an arch the intrinsic stability and mechanical function of the SI joints do not depend on an intact 'pelvic ring'. They go on to suggest that by far the greatest factor in SI joint stability is the compressive forces acting across the joint surfaces (fig. 2.1). These forces, together with the propeller-like orientation of the sacral surfaces, will resist sacral slipping. Of greatest interest perhaps to chiropractors is the suggestion that forces generated within certain pelvic muscles, particularly the gluteus maximus and piriformis, can markedly increase the compressive forces across the joint and thus improve stability. By the same token it would seem logical that in order to manipulate or adjust these joints one should exploit the influence these muscles have on their related articulation. It is my opinion that the passive tension within these myofascial structures is probably of greater importance to adjustive skills than the final 'thrust' itself and therefore a working knowledge of the mechanical properties and effects of muscular tissues is essential to all manipulative clinicians. Snijders *et al.* (1993) also hypothesize that, through connections with the lumbodorsal fascia, other muscles such as the latissimus dorsi may work in synergy with the gluteus maximus, under certain loading conditions, to support the SI joints.

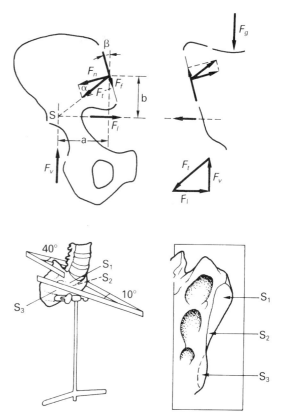

Fig 2.1 The self-bracing effect as proposed by Snijders *et al.* Force F_l can be increased by the action of certain muscles, ligaments and by the application of a trochanteric belt. The self-bracing mechanism is reinforced with increasing friction between the surfaces, force F_f, by enlarging the normal force F_n using muscle tension, the fibres of the gluteus maximus having the most effective direction. Note also the propeller-like orientation of the sacral auricular surface. (Adapted from Snijders *et al.*, 1993.)

These papers also support the use of trochanteric or pelvic belts for the treatment of injured SI joints. The effect of the belt is thought to enhance the 'self-bracing' forces around the joints and the line of action of the belt is compared to that of the piriformis muscle. The sacrotuberous ligament is also thought to play a central role in SI stability. In an earlier paper Vleeming *et al.* (1989) suggest that, through connections with the long head of biceps femoris, the straight leg raising (SLR) test can directly affect the SI joint. Thus pain elicited by the SLR test may reflect SI dysfunction rather than nerve root tethering. They further suggest that the stabilizing effect of gluteus maximus may be partly mediated through tension in the sacrotuberous ligament. This is hardly a surprising function of the ligament; however, the concept that through attachments with the lumbodorsal fascia, gluteus maximus and biceps femoris muscles this stabilizing function may be modified certainly provokes interest. The reductionist view that muscles and ligaments subserve entirely separate functions may well be outdated. Indeed Snijders and co-workers have compared the SI joint to a multidirectional force transducer, presuming the existence of mechanoreceptors in the surrounding ligaments. They point out the logic of having these two 'sensors' in the path of considerable force streams being transferred by the pelvis from the upper body to the legs. This view is also shared by Panjabi (1992) in his hypothesis of spinal stability. Panjabi, on the other hand, suggests that spinal ligaments will act more like strain gauges than force transducers. He submits that the large deformations that occur in these tissues around the neutral position will better stimulate receptor cells than the forces (stress) generated as a consequence of load. Panjabi sees the stability of the spine as a function of three subsystems (fig. 2.2) with the ligaments, disc and bony vertebrae as the passive subsystem: passive only in as much as they cannot directly alter or modify the forces and moments placed upon them but very much active as transducers in the vicinity of the neutral position, or neutral zone. The information generated by these sensors can then, Panjabi feels, be used via the neural subsystem to modify muscular responses to imposed loading (the active subsystem) and restore mechanical stability if it has been compromised.

Whatever the details, it is clear that both these researchers see articular stability as an active process rather than a passive or static resistance to imposed demands. Furthermore it seems likely that one can influence this mechanism externally through alterations to muscular tone and by indirect stimulation of mechanoreceptors, a possible effect of manipulation. The neuromusculoskeletal system and its ramifications are the natural domain of

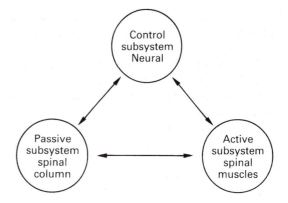

Fig 2.2 The spinal stability system as proposed by Panjabi. The passive subsystem comprises the vertebrae, facet joints, discs, spinal ligaments, joint capsules and the passive mechanical properties of skeletal muscle. The active subsystem includes all skeletal muscles and tendons surrounding the spinal column. The neural subsystem includes the various force and motion transducers found in ligaments, tendons and muscle together with the neural control centres. These subsystems are considered functionally interdependent in maintaining spinal stability. (Adapted from Panjabi, 1992, with permission.)

chiropractic and it behoves us to continually sharpen our skills in light of new knowledge. Chiropractic, like the human condition it studies, should be a dynamic science.

To Lordose or not to Lordose

For controversy, few topics of spinal mechanics can raise opinion more than spinal curvatures. The function and requirement for lumbar and cervical lordoses in particular can provoke much debate among bioengineers and chiropractors alike. The lumbar lordosis and its role in load bearing is just one such issue. The view that preservation of the lumbar lordosis is necessary for generating the forces required in lifting is not without its critics. Another researcher with extensive experience in lumbar spine mechanics, and disc injury in particular, is Mike Adams (Adams and Hutton, 1982, 1985). In a recent paper on the influence of hip and lumbar mobility on the generation of bending moments (Dolan and Adams, 1993), it was found that all subjects flattened or reversed their lumbar lordosis when lifting. Various bending and lifting activities were performed from putting on a sock to lifting a large 10 kg box. In all these activities all subjects flattened their lumbar spines even when lifting with knees flexed. Not surprisingly they found that a reduction in sagittal spinal mobility was indeed associated with higher bending stresses. This is important since Adams has shown previously that compressive forces on the lumbar discs can cause prolapse only when combined with bending moments (Adams and Hutton, 1985). Previous work (Adams and Dolan, 1991) had shown Adams that over much of its range the lumbar spine exhibits little resistance to bending, but towards the elastic limits of flexion and extension the resistance rises rapidly. Adams observed that this region of low bending moment formed a relatively constant proportion of the full range. This suggests that individuals with good flexibility can perform a much greater range of flexion/extension before generating high bending stresses within the spine. Similarly those individuals who possess stiff, inflexible musculoskeletal structures will generate high bending moments over a very short range of flexion/extension. What Adams alludes to here, I suspect, is what Manohar Panjabi refers to as the 'neutral and elastic zones'.

Chiropractic in the Neutral Zone

Recently Panjabi (1992) expressed concern over the methods employed in cadaveric studies, in particular the practice of preconditioning or prestressing spinal specimens before load–deformation measurements. This procedure has been used to reduce the viscoelastic effects and produce linear, or near-linear results. In life, however, spinal tissues exhibit highly non-linear behaviour. Indeed this non-linearity in load–deformation may well hold the key to the understanding of spinal dysfunction. Spinal, and many other, ligaments possess the ability to vary their stiffness throughout a range of movement. This viscoelastic behaviour allows greater

movement within and around the neutral position but progressively limits motion towards the end of the range. The region of relative ligamentous laxity around the neutral position has been termed the *neutral zone* (NZ) and that part of the range of motion associated with increasing ligament stiffness the *elastic zone* (EZ) (Panjabi, 1992) (fig. 2.3).

This biphasic nature of spinal motion allows minimum energy expenditure for movements around the neutral position, but provides opposition to potentially damaging movements at the end of range. Utilizing data from a previous study (Yamamoto *et al.*, 1989), Panjabi (1992) demonstrated a method of measuring the NZ *in vitro* and proposed that it represents an index of clinical instability. What Panjabi suggests is that although an individual's overall range of spinal motion may be within normal limits, an increase in the NZ would indicate instability. As Dolan and Adams (1993) point out, this 'region of low bending moment' (fig. 2.4), as they refer to it, is a fairly constant proportion of the range and therefore should not be expected to change under normal circumstances. For chiropractors, however, segmental instability is but one clinical entity that we may encounter. Closer to home is the spinal fixation,

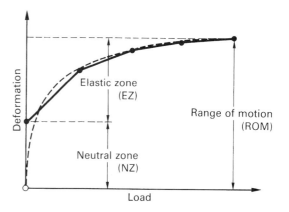

Fig 2.3 The load–deformation curve of a soft tissue or body joint showing the highly non-linear nature of these tissues. The region of high flexibility is the neutral zone and the region of high stiffness the elastic zone. The two zones together constitute the physiological range of motion of a joint. (Adapted from Panjabi, 1992, with permission.)

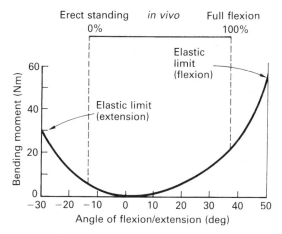

Fig 2.4 The bending moment acting on the lumbar spine across the full range of flexion and extension. Note how the bending moment increases rapidly towards the limits of motion, the elastic zone, and the region of low bending moment around the mid or neutral position, in other words the neutral zone. (Adapted from Dolan and Adams, 1993.)

subluxation, dysarthrosis or 'biomechanical dysfunction' that we locate in almost all of our patients. Call it what you will, what it represents is a perceived reduction in relative segmental motion. What I would like to suggest is that if segmental instability depicts one end of a spectrum of spinal motion disorders, then perhaps the subluxation/fixation represents the other end. Consequently, if an increase in the NZ characterizes instability, perhaps a reduction of this 'region of low bending moment' can characterize the spinal subluxation/fixation. In practical terms then, perhaps the perceived tissue resistance that we detect on segmental motion palpation is simply the commencement of the EZ sooner than anticipated, i.e. a fixation; in other words, a decrease in the NZ. This area of clinical biomechanics has been discussed by many chiropractors, notably Sandoz (1976) who proposed the passive range/elastic barrier concept of joint motion. Here he suggests that the chiropractic adjustment takes the joint through the 'elastic barrier' of resistance into the 'paraphysiological space'. After the adjustment takes place, Sandoz suggests the 'range of movement is slightly increased beyond the usual physiological limit'. This concept is, I believe, in concert with that of Panjabi's NZ. The elastic bar-

rier will be found shortly after the commencement of the EZ. Thus the EZ contains both the elastic barrier and the paraphysiological space and ends with the 'limit of anatomical integrity'. An adjustment, therefore, should be followed by a slight increase in the NZ. Until we can measure the NZ *in vivo*, however, the above statement remains a hypothesis.

In terms of manipulative skills the NZ can be useful in another respect. If we regard the NZ as the 'slack' that is taken up when we bring a joint to tension before an adjustive thrust, then knowledge of the various NZs for each vertebral level might be valuable to us. For example (see Table 2.1) the NZ for axial rotation of the C0–C1 segment is some 22% of the movement, in other words the first 22% of axial rotation at that level will be required to bring that joint to tension before an adjustive thrust can be gainfully applied. In contrast to that, the same manoeuvre at the C1–C2 articulation will require the first 76% of axial rotation in approaching tension. In the lumbar spine the situation is somewhat similar. The NZ takes up 39% of axial rotation at the L1–L2 segment compared to only 18% at the L4–L5 level. The range of motion (ROM), however, between the two spinal regions is very much different. The ROM at C1–C2 for axial rotation is nearly 40 degrees which is in stark contrast with the 2.3 degrees seen at L1–L2 for the same movement. This, however, is a rather simplistic interpretation of the data and life is rarely that simple. What Panjabi refers to in his papers are the NZs and EZs for all intervening soft tissues at individual functional spinal units (FSUs) in pure axial rotation or flexion/extension as determined by cadaveric experimentation. In manipulative procedures the situation is somewhat different. If we take axial rotation at C1–C2 as an example we note that the EZ is reached only after some 30 degrees of rotation between the segments. In the living subject, especially in high-risk groups, this would represent some risk to related vascular structures. Thus combined movements can be employed to bring the segment to tension at an earlier point. Introducing lateral flexion will pre-stretch

Table 2.1 Average neutral zones, in degrees, for the main rotatory motions for representative functional spinal units at different regions of the spine.

Region	Flexion/extension	Lateral bending	Axial rotation
C0–C1	1.1	1.6	1.5
C1–C2	3.2	1.2	29.6
C3–C6	4.9	4.0	3.8
L1–L2/L3–L4	1.5	1.6	0.7
L5–S1	3.0	1.8	0.4

Adapted from White and Panjabi 1990.

or pre-load the soft tissues before axial rotation is applied and, in effect, reduce the NZ. One should also bear in mind the sequential nature of the living spine. In life one can create stresses at certain segments of the spine by causing movement at points distant from the desired level. These stresses can again be used to reduce the NZ, bringing the EZ closer to 'home' and allowing us to perform an adjustment in a safer loading mode and with less force. One need only attempt a thumb-move at T1 without rotating the patient's head from neutral, to see what is meant by this. These stresses are there by virtue of the sequential attachment of soft tissues, both passive and active. This again shows the importance of muscle in spinal mechanics. If one ignores the role of these tissues and simply adjusts ad infinitum, then one will inevitably encounter the law of diminishing returns. If you truly wish to create change in the mechanical response of the spine then you must look to the muscular tissues. The active elements can be strengthened and toned for improved stability or the passive elements stretched and lengthened to restore motion.

Biomechanics and the Art of Motion Palpation

For students of chiropractic, some of the most difficult skills to master are those of motion palpation. Here we attempt to feel segmental motion and determine if it is abnormal or not. This would imply a knowledge of what constitutes normal segmental motion and naturally one would turn to the science of biomechanics for

the answer. Which way should the spinous of L4 rotate on sidebending? Will it change if the subject extends the lumbar spine at the same time? The answers to these sorts of questions rely heavily on a knowledge of the effects of coupling or combined movements within the spine and have been the subject of much research. The coupling patterns of the cervical spine, particularly the lower cervical spine, have been well established (Lysell, 1969; Panjabi *et al.*, 1986; Moroney *et al.*, 1988). Coupling in the lumbar spine, however, remains controversial especially as regards the association between axial rotation and lateral bending (Pope *et al.*, 1977; Stokes *et al.*, 1981). Some researchers report little or no such association in the lumbar spine (Rolander, 1966; Schultz *et al.*, 1979). Coupling patterns may be clinically important and indicate spinal dysfunction (Weitz, 1981; Pearcy *et al.*, 1984; Pearcy, 1985). On the other hand coupling characteristics may vary considerably within normal limits and might have a strong dependence on posture and other variables. Without this fundamental knowledge observation of coupling patterns *in vivo* have limited clinical significance. In an attempt to address this very question Panjabi and co-workers (Yamamoto *et al.*, 1989) applied axial torque and lateral bending moments, separately, to cadaveric whole lumbar spine (L1–S1) specimens. The three-dimensional intervertebral motions of each segment were recorded by stereophotogrammetry and the response to loading studied in five spinal postures (full extension and flexion, half extension and flexion and neutral positions). The authors applied an axial compressive pre-load of 100 N, to simulate *in vivo* loads, and horizontal forces, either anteriorly or posteriorly, to create the flexed or extended postures. In order to generate lateral bending and axial rotation, only physiological pure moments were applied, through the body of L1, along the relevant axes. This ensured that each intervertebral joint received the same magnitude of moment. The components of the moment vector, however, will vary at each joint as a function of the lumbar lordosis. The moments were applied in three load/unload cycles with a 30 second rest period to allow for creep. Vertebral motion was recorded only after the third load cycle. In other words the specimens were preconditioned in an effort to reduce their viscoelastic properties.

The findings of this study demonstrated that posture and intervertebral level are two very important factors in determining the magnitude and characteristics of both the main and coupled motions in the lumbar spine. This study again highlights the functional division between the lumbar and lumbosacral spine. In the neutral position, for example, left axial torque brought about contrasting effects between upper and lower lumbar levels. Upper lumbar segments were driven into right lateral bending, that is bending to the opposite side of axial rotation. At lower lumbar levels, however, the lateral bending was to the same side, with the L3/4 FSU acting as a transitional segment. The authors also noted a distinct lack of mechanical reciprocity in lumbar coupling. In other words, when left axial torque was applied to L4/5, for example, this produced left lateral bending. However, when left lateral bending was applied the coupling was with right, and not left, axial rotation. Although the distinction between lumbar and lumbosacral levels was not as clear, the findings of this study were in uncommon agreement with the *in vivo* findings of Pearcy and Tibrewal (1984). In their study the transitional segment for lateral bending direction appeared to be L4/5. The magnitudes of main and coupled motions, however, were remarkably similar. The only other major difference in findings between the two studies was in the associated sagittal

plane coupling with axial torque and lateral bending. In addition to lateral bending accompanying the main axial rotation and vice versa, Panjabi and co-workers found a second coupling effect. They noted, in the neutral posture, a sagittal plane rotation which tended towards flexion at all levels. Pearcy and Tibrewal (1984), on the other hand, found the opposite. They noted extension as the predominant sagittal plane coupled motion, with the exception of the lumbosacral segment which showed an equivocal response. Panjabi and colleagues suggested that this paradox could be explained if Pearcy's subjects were standing in a slightly flexed posture at the time of screening. This is, of course, speculation and the fundamental differences in the two studies make the interpretation of contrasting results difficult. In the Panjabi experiment the active or passive components of the spinal musculature could play no part in coupling effects. With the *in vivo* work of Pearcy and Tibrewal (1984), however, muscle influences were present but unquantifiable. Nevertheless, there was good agreement between findings, despite the obviously dissimilar methodologies, and the complementary nature of the two papers remains quite unique. It is interesting to note that in a later *in vivo* collaboration (Pearcy and Hindle, 1989) Pearcy's findings support those of Panjabi and co-workers. Using an electromagnetic position sensor, the 3Space Isotrak, Pearcy and Hindle showed a strong coupling of flexion with lateral bending.

Conclusion

This chapter has demonstrated the immense complexity of the human spine and the deficits in current knowledge. This is not intended to be viewed in a negative way but positively as an indication of the common ground that researcher and clinician alike must share. This chapter also demonstrates that what is known and verifiable concerning spinal function can be successfully applied to manipulative therapeutics.

Better knowledge and understanding of spinal structure and function will not directly improve manipulative skills. The skills of the early manipulator some 3000 years ago were probably as good, if not better, than those of manipulators today. What they lacked, however, was a rational basis upon which to assess the appropriateness or non-appropriateness of the application of their skills. Knowledge and understanding allow you to make the best use of your skills, to gain maximum efficacy from your therapeutic approach and, in short, make you a better practitioner in the long run. It would appear that an understanding of both traditional and contemporary bioengineering and bioclinical concepts may combine to enhance and reinforce the acquisition of basic manual skills during the early training years. This, no doubt, would be strengthened by a knowledgeable and committed teaching team who are willing to step beyond conservative restraints and integrate more innovative instructional methods into the curriculum.

References

Adams, M.A. and Dolan, P. (1991) A technique for quantifying bending moment acting on the lumbar spine in-vivo. *Journal of Biomechanics*, **24**, 117–126

Adams, M.A. and Hutton, W.C. (1982) Prolapsed intervertebral disc. A hyperflexion injury. *Spine*, **7**, 184–191

Adams, M.A. and Hutton, W.C. (1985) Gradual disc prolapse. *Spine*, **10**, 524–531

Aspden, R.M. (1992) Review of the functional anatomy of the spinal ligaments and the lumbar erector spinae muscles. *Clinical Anatomy*, **5**, 372–387

Bogduk, N. (1991) The lumbar disc and low back pain. *Neurosurgery Clinics of North America*, **2**, 791–806

Bogduk, N. and Twomey, L. (1991) *Clinical Anatomy of the Lumbar Spine*, 2nd edn. Churchill Livingstone, Edinburgh

Dolan, P. and Adams, M.A. (1993) Influence of lumbar and hip mobility on the bending stresses acting on the lumbar spine. *Clinical Biomechanics*, **8**, 185–192

Goel, V.K., Goyal, S., Clark, C. *et al.* (1985) Kinematics of the whole lumbar spine: effect of discectomy. *Spine*, **10**, 543–554

Gracovetsky, S., Farfan, H. and Helleur, C. (1985) The abdominal mechanism. *Spine*, **10**, 317–324

Granhed, H., Jonson, R. and Hansson, T. (1987) The loads on the lumbar spine during extreme weight lifting. *Spine*, **12**, 146–149

Grice, A. (1979) Radiographic, biomechanical and clinical factors in lumbar lateral flexion. *Journal of Manipulative and Physiological Therapeutics*, **2**, 26–34

Lysell, E. (1969) Motion in the cervical spine. *Acta Orthopaedica Scandinavica*, **123** (Suppl), 1–61

Moroney, S.P., Schultz, A.B., Miller, J.A.A. *et al.* (1988) Load-displacement properties of lower cervical spine motion segments. *Journal of Biomechanics*, **21**, 769–779

Panjabi, M.M. (1992) The stabilizing system of the spine. Part 1. Function, dysfunction, adaptation and enhancement. Part 2. Neutral zone and instability hypothesis. *Journal of Spinal Disorders*, **5**, 383–397

Panjabi, M.M., Summers, D.J., Pelker, R.R. *et al.* (1986) Three-dimensional load displacement curves of the cervical spine. *Journal of Orthopaedic Research*, **4**, 152–161

Pearcy, M. J. (1985) Stereo radiography of lumber spine motion. Acta Orthopaedica Scandinavica, 56 (Suppl 212)

Pearcy, M.J. and Hindle, R.J. (1989) New method for the non-invasive three-dimensional measurement of human back movement. *Clinical Biomechanics*, **4**, 73–79

Pearcy, M., Portek, I. and Shepherd, J. (1984) Three-dimensional X-ray analysis of normal movement in the lumbar spine. *Spine*, **9**, 294–297

Pearcy, M.J. and Tibrewal, S.B. (1984) Axial rotation and bending in the normal lumbar spine measured by three-dimensional radiography. *Spine*, **9**, 582–587

Pope, M.H., Wilder, D.G., Matteri, R.E. *et al.* (1977) Experimental measurements of vertebral motion under load. *Orthopaedic Clinics of North America*, **8**, 155–167

Rolander, S.D. (1966) Motion of the lumbar spine with special reference to the stabilizing effect of posterior fusion – an experimental study on autopsy specimens. *Acta Orthopaedica Scandinavica*, (Suppl 90)

Sandoz, R. (1976) Some physical mechanisms and effects of spinal adjustments. *Annals of the Swiss Chiropractors' Association*, **VI**, 91–141

Schultz, A.B. and Andersson G.B.J. (1981) Analysis of loads on the lumbar spine. *Spine*, **6**, 76–82

Schultz, A.B., Warwick, D.N., Berkson, M.H. *et al.* (1979) Mechanical properties of human lumbar spine motion segments. Part 1. Responses in flexion, extension, lateral bending and torsion. *Journal of Biomechanical Engineering*, **101**, 46–52

Snijders, C.J., Vleeming, A. and Stoeckart, R. (1993) Transfer of lumbosacral load to iliac bones and legs. *Clinical Biomechanics*, **8**, 285–301

Stokes, I.A.F., Wilder, D.G., Frymoyer, J.W. *et al.* (1981) Assessment of patients with low-back pain by biplanar radiographic measurement of intervertebral motion. *Spine*, **6**, 233–240

Tesh, K., Shaw-Dunn, J. and Evans, J.H. (1987) The abdominal muscles and vertebral stability. *Spine*, **12**, 501–508

Vleeming, A., Stoeckart, R. and Snijders, C.J. (1989) The sacrotuberous ligament: a conceptual approach to its dynamic role in stabilizing the sacroiliac joint. *Clinical Biomechanics*, **4**, 201–203

Weitz, E. (1981) The lateral bending sign. *Spine*, **6**, 388–397

White, A.A. and Panjabi, M.M. (1990) *Clinical Biomechanics of the Spine*, 2nd edn. Lippincott, Philadelphia

Yamamoto, I., Panjabi, M.M., Crisco, T. *et al.* (1989) Three-dimensional movements of the whole lumbar spine and lumbosacral joint. *Spine*, **14**, 1256–1260

3

The physiology of skill performance

Peter W. McCarthy

In any discipline involving a specific manual skill, the development of that skill is one of the most daunting prospects facing student and tutor alike. Some of the problems can be better appreciated, and even resolved, if one has a greater understanding of the underlying neurophysiological mechanisms. This chapter aims to address this by describing the mechanisms underlying a skilled movement, hopefully giving some insight into how skills may be acquired more easily and possibly even facilitate the process of acquisition.

Skilled Movement – The Basic Concepts

A skilled movement is essentially a smooth action. Smooth actions can be formed by combining a group of simple, natural movements to form a new or unusual one. A smooth movement becomes a skill as it is repeated to bring about a certain degree of adaptability and fine control. These characteristics would suggest that there is a degree of 'hard wiring' within the nervous system which can be activated to produce the skilled movement. Therefore, a skilled movement could also be described as a reflex (or series of reflexes). The reflexes which underlie a skill require stimuli which are not 'natural': this type of reflex is described as being 'conditioned'. The alternative is a reflex which is triggered by natural stimuli, usually termed unconditioned. The 'conditioning' which links the action to an unnatural stimulus (which will eventually act to initiate the skilled action) takes place throughout the training period. In addition to learning the stimulus, the training period is also used by the neuromuscular system to experiment in order to find the easiest, but not necessarily the best, way of performing the action. Simultaneously, the learning period allows those tissues, whose rate of use has changed, to be built up in response to the changing load put upon them. Such changes would include both the strength (protein production and neuromuscular coordination) and flexibility (elastin and collagen).

In order to give the reader some idea of the size of this problem from the perspective of the body, an outline of the requirements is needed. This will, at the same time, illustrate why it takes time to develop a skill. The achievement of a skilled 'smooth reflex' requires the coordination of several joint movements. Each joint movement consists of a coordinated series of muscle actions involving contraction of some muscles and relaxation of others: this will take a large amount of nervous activity to control. Furthermore, consideration must also be given to the supporting structures and tissues affected by the increased demand. This scenario will be examined in greater detail once the basics have been described.

The next sections will outline those features of each component required for the performance of any movement. Those tissues which produce the action, such as muscle and ligaments, will be described first, followed by neuromuscular integration. This will lead into the role of higher centres of the CNS in motor skill acquisition and performance.

Muscle and Associated Tissues

Types of Muscle Fibre

Striated (skeletal) is otherwise known as voluntary muscle. This can be subdivided into extra- and intra-fusal fibres. Contraction of these fibres is controlled by the activity of the two basic types of motoneurone: alpha for extrafusal and gamma for intrafusal fibres. The alpha-motoneurones have larger diameter axons and conduct their information to the muscle faster than the gamma-motoneurones. Intrafusal fibres are under control of the gamma-motoneurones. The non-muscular section of these fibres is innervated by muscle afferents (Ia, Ib and II stretch receptor afferents) involved with feedback of information concerning length and rate of change of length in the muscle. Gamma-motoneurone activity sets the length of these fibres which determines both the sensitivity and activity of the associated stretch receptor. Conversely, the alpha-motoneurone activity drives the contraction of the extrafusal fibres, which are the active contractile units. Extrafusal fibres can be subdivided into two groups, based on speed of twitch (contraction caused by a single action potential) development and cellular metabolic characteristics. Type I extrafusal fibres have slower twitch characteristics and are fatigue resistant; these fibres have importance in posture maintenance. Type II fibres have faster twitch production and probably have a significant role to play in developing speed of movement, such as in a manipulative thrust.

The proportion of type I to type II fibres in any muscle tends to be related to function, training and genetic predisposition. Muscles with a high proportion of type I fibres are found where prolonged contraction is necessary, for example postural muscles such as soleus. In contrast, a higher proportion of type II fibres are found where short bursts of rapid onset contraction are required. It is interesting to note that extensor digitorum longus along with certain facial muscles, such as orbicularis oris, have almost all type II fibres. The muscles of the upper arm (biceps) and some of the lower leg (gastrocnemius) have roughly equal proportions of type I and II. The absolute proportions in any muscle vary between individuals because of the genetic and training differences. However, there is a trend towards individuality, in that each person appears to have proportions of fibres skewed towards either type I or type II which are consistent throughout the muscles of his/her body (Bellemare *et al.*, 1983).

In any skill development, attention should be paid to the present use of the muscle, and therefore, to some degree the predominant fibre type. Although it is commonly believed that the initial fibre type proportions are important in determination of final ability, there is little evidence to support this. There may be a general link between muscle fibre type distribution and the ease with which a muscle or skill may be developed; anyway, some limited change does appear possible with training. Those factors which would play a role are general fitness, previous skill training demanding similar abilities and prior development of the respective parts of the body.

Intrinsic Properties

Joint stabilization is an important requirement, especially when considering repetitive movements, such as those asked for in certain manipulative procedures. There are numerous problems associated with poor development of the stabilizing elements, for example, inflamed ligaments/tendons and ensuing nerve root irritation which in the wrist leads to carpal tunnel syndrome. Muscles can stabilize joints and regulate motion through two mechanisms. Firstly, via the neuromuscular system including feedback loops and reflexes involving the spinal cord and higher centres (see Figures 3.1 and 3.2). However, this can take between 50 ms

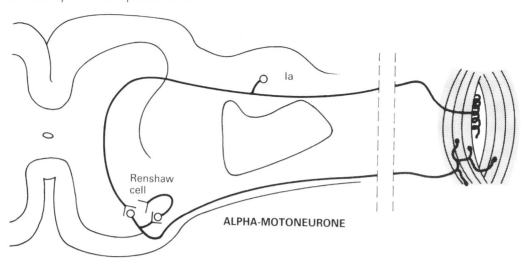

Fig 3.1 The components of a 'monosynaptic' or stretch reflex. Action potentials generated by stretching the spindle in the intrafusal fibres travel along the Ia primary afferent neurone into the spinal cord. The Ia fibre synapses onto an alpha-motoneurone in the ventral horn which is excited and eventually results in a muscle contraction. The motoneurone has a naturally high frequency of action potential firing, which is not necessary and potentially damaging to the muscle if sustained. Therefore, the activity of the motoneurone is suppressed soon after it is initiated, due to the presence of the recurrent collateral which stimulates the Renshaw cell (an inhibitory interneurone).

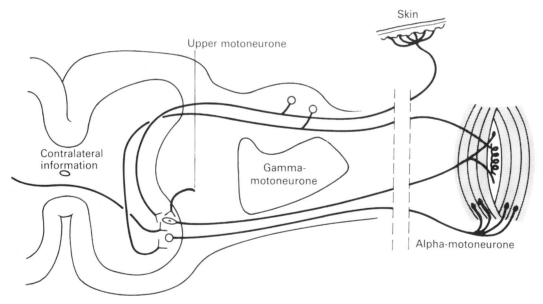

Fig 3.2 The components of a gamma loop, or reflex. Activity in the gamma-motoneurones determines the degree of activity in the intrafusal muscle fibres and thus the relative degree of stretch in the spindle (stretch receptor). The gamma-motoneurone is used to maintain the relative length of the intrafusal fibre in proportion to the extrafusal fibres, so that any unexpected stretch on the muscle can be compensated for rapidly. However, gamma-motoneurone activity can also be affected by descending, contralateral or cutaneous (skin afferent) stimulation.

and 100 ms to affect change and may produce unwanted oscillations in the movement. A second mechanism relates to the intrinsic properties of muscle (the force–length and force–velocity relationships) which include both the contractile and non-contractile (resistive, elastic) elements of the muscle. Added to this is the recently described effect of moment arm of the muscle across the joint (Young *et al.*, 1992). The moment arms tend to increase as the muscle is lengthened, which leads to an increase in its effective force and rate of onset in the direction of the joint's neutral point (balance point). If the agonist muscle lengthens, the antagonist muscles will tend to shorten, thus exerting less force. This results in the stabilization of the joint on co-activation of the agonist and antagonist muscles: this has been shown in the stabilization of such complex joints such as the ankle (Young *et al.*, 1992).

Ligaments and Joints

Ligaments, tendons and joint capsules come in various guises, the components being mainly collagen and elastin. Ligaments, which generally have much more collagen than elastin, tend to have a role of limiting movement and can be found spanning joints or wrapping around tendons. Tendons have more elastin than ligaments, in their role of dampening and storing force generated by the muscle. All of these tissues have a relatively poor blood supply, which is probably related to their slow adaptation and repair rates.

Synovial fluid is a proteoglycans/water mixture found inside joint spaces. It has many roles including: nutrition, hydration, shock absorption and lubrication. The synovial fluid also has the property of thixotropism; in other words if the solution was left undisturbed it would become a gel. Other structures such as ligaments and tendons may have this property, albeit to a lesser extent. It follows that joints should be eased back into use after a period of immobility. This is one factor which would support the use of 'warming-up' before exercise. Stiffness also occurs in recently traumatized muscles, tendons, ligaments and joints. However, this more than likely involves a different mechanism, namely the inflammatory response. The effects are particularly apparent in the morning when there is a general 'stiffness' in the damaged tissues. As the stiffness tends to disappear after a short period of movement or stretching, it again indicates the benefit of 'warming up'. The poorly coordinated use of the muscles during the initial stages

of any complex skill acquisition can also lead to trauma; as such, the benefits of preconditioning the muscle, 'warming up', may also have implications with respect to protecting the muscle against trauma.

Repetitive Injury and Skills Training

An important aspect of skill performance is practice by repetition; this can, however, potentially lead to damage. There are two periods in which the damage may manifest. The first is during the acquisition phase when the neuromuscular system is being adapted and built up. Simultaneously, tendons and ligaments are also adapting; however, these tissues take longer to strengthen which predisposes them to trauma. Secondly, after learning the skill there is repetitive strain injury (RSI) or recurrent microtrauma, which is damage more commonly found in people skilled in a task which has been repeated on a daily basis, continually over years. Overuse compounded by the increasing ability to override feedback regulatory mechanisms such as the stretch receptor (fig. 3.1) and golgi tendon organ mediated systems can create microtrauma. In normal use, the repair systems would be given ample opportunities to recover from this trauma. However, due to the continual use, sufficient time is not allowed for repair which ultimately leads to an RSI. Any type of trauma can reduce efficiency of the skill and even lead to abnormal performance as the body attempts to compensate for the damage. Such effects are compounded by the relatively slow response of the body to trauma to the tendonous and ligamentous tissues, during which an appreciable degree of disuse atrophy can occur in the associated muscles. In addition, scar tissue is less elastic, more collagenic, than the original tissue, therefore changing its properties and invariably limiting the range of future uses.

Care must be taken during the acquisition of new skills to incorporate acceptable training principles including adequate rest, flexibility, and cross-training strategies to reduce possible tissue damage and recurrent injury.

Neuromuscular Reflexes: Simple or Complex

Prior to any discussion of how a skilled movement works it is helpful to look at the basic building blocks, namely the components of a spinal reflex. Spinal reflexes come in many different forms, from the knee-jerk (patella reflex) to more complex ones such as those concerned with posture control. One way of keeping perspective is to consider each reflex as being a motor (efferent) response, initiated by some form of sensory (afferent) input. This is best illustrated by the simple monosynaptic stretch reflex as in Figure 3.1. Although an oversimplification, this reflex contains some of the important elements with which a basic understanding can be gained. In addition, the stretch reflex also forms the basis for the control of muscle length using what is known as the gamma loop (activity in gamma-motoneurones altering sensitivity of the stretch receptors, which change alpha-motoneurone activity, and therefore muscle length). The circuit is illustrated in Figure 3.2.

An important concept requires introduction at this point, namely *reciprocal inhibition*. Reciprocal inhibition is a way of preventing, or reducing interference from the antagonist muscles, e.g. the withdrawal reflexes outlined above. To perform this task, we have an important element of the spinal reflex, the inhibitory interneurone (illustrated in Figures 3.1 and 3.3). Inhibitory interneurones are a series of neurones found in the spinal cord grey matter which are involved with the integration, dissemination and regulation of information from sensory input and upper motoneurones onto the spinal motoneurone pool. A summary of the inputs onto a hypothetical inhibitory interneurone is illustrated in Figure 3.3. In the performance of a simple 'triceps flick', a recoil thrust which forms the basis of many manipulative procedures, for example, there is an extension driven by the triceps activity. This transiently suppresses the antagonist muscle, biceps, via activation of the interneurones which inactivate the alpha-motoneurones to that muscle. However, as the degree of extension increases it becomes evident that a braking action by the biceps is required to prevent hyperextension of the elbow and associated microtrauma. As the rate of movement increases along with the degree of extension (both of which occur rapidly) the biceps activity also increases to counter the inertia created by the triceps. The change in biceps activity is due to many factors, such as increasing activity in the biceps stretch receptors or decay of the interneuronal inhibitory drive onto the biceps motoneurone pool (both inhibition of the antagonist and the Renshaw cell driven inhibition of the agonist).

As intimated above, activity in the large alpha-motoneurones can be affected in various ways: firstly, direct stimulation by descending fibres (upper motor neurones); secondly, suppression of activity by the inhibitory interneurones: these are in turn affected by input from higher centres or by local sensory afferents (contralateral as well as ipsilateral, as can be seen in Figure 3.3). The third type of modulation comes from the Renshaw cells whose role is recurrent inhibition (regulation) of motoneurone firing frequency (fig. 3.1). An overview of the interactions within this system, and an indication of the reflexes which may be evoked are illustrated in Figures 3.2 and 3.3. It can be seen that the alpha-motoneurones are not limited to involvement with the ipsilateral side.

A series of 'cross-spinal' interactions form an important part of the coordination needed in everyday movement such as the initiation of walking. In this case extension of one side is synchronous with the flexion of the other. The 'hard-wired' nature of this becomes apparent when one attempts to walk without swinging the arms (or swinging them asynchronously with the leg movements). These connections exist between the different levels of the spinal cord to facilitate coordination of limb activity: this is probably of greater relevance to quadrupeds but still of importance to balance in bipeds. An example

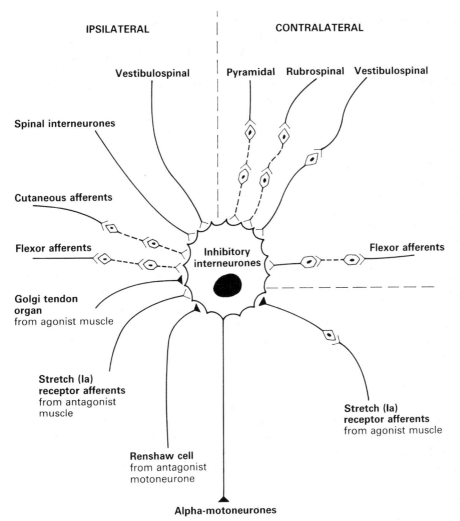

Fig 3.3 Sources of input which affects inhibitory interneurone activity. There are two types of inhibitory interneurone which have a direct output onto motoneurones, the Ia and the Ib. These have been represented as a single entity in this figure for ease of understanding an overview of the factors which can affect the motoneurone output. The activity in the interneurone can be increased (—<) or decreased (—◀) by the incoming signals, the integrated sum of this input determining the activity which in turn determines the degree of suppression of the motoneurone. Ia-inhibitory interneurones have output onto alpha-motoneurones and take input from flexor afferents, cutaneous afferents, stretch receptors, Renshaw cells and supraspinal centres. Ib-inhibitory interneurones have output onto alpha-motoneurones and take input from cutaneous afferents, golgi tendon organs and supraspinal centres.

of their use in humans can be seen in competitive running; note the pumping action of the arms to facilitate the leg muscle contractions: the greater the need the more forceful the arm movements. There is also a basic balance requirement for the performance of psychomotor skills, where the practitioner needs to have the correct postural balance derived from a clear postural awareness. This latter point relates to an aspect of learning which is difficult to explain to a student, yet

which is crucial to the successful performance of the technique and prevention of strain injuries.

A key factor in any skilled motor performance lies in the ability of the system to predict or anticipate an event and therefore prepare for it. Such anticipatory adjustments can be appreciated when walking with your eyes closed (or even in the dark) where footfalls, which are usually of minimal impact, become jarring collisions with the floor. The adjustments made in preparation for change, especially of balance and posture, are issued from the cerebellar–brainstem nuclei, require no conscious attention and can affect all muscles involved with maintenance of posture.

The majority of reflexes described so far are used to move limbs, and are reliant on spinal reflexes. However, following noxious stimulation, other reflexes such as those involving verbal motor control become apparent. This gives an opportunity to illustrate reflexes based in higher centres! These may be from the brainstem–midbrain, producing a sharp intake of breath due to respiratory muscle activation, or the thalamus-cerebral cortex to produce a simple word (expletive) or other forms of relatively coherent prose.

Although not an obvious part of skill performance, there are many reflexes which do not have a voluntary muscle component, but whose existence is worthy of mention. Such reflexes have their motor response through the autonomic nervous system via changes in secretion (such as salivation) or smooth muscle tone (in the case of pupil diameter). Similar pathways to the voluntary muscle mediated reflexes are used with the tendency for these to be initiated simultaneously: however, autonomic reflexes use motoneurone fibres which have lower conduction velocities. The speed of response to a stimulus does not necessarily indicate the level of importance of the reflex to survival. However, speed probably relates more to functional significance, for example the need for rapid conduction of messages in control of posture. As the conduction velocity of an axon is in proportion to its diameter (even in myelinated axons) it can be seen that speed is a luxury; where it is not required it is not used.

The existence of consciously driven movement is reliant upon reflexes. Such an interconnected, ready to use system reduces the amount of processing in the higher centres; which raises the question: 'what is the role of the higher centres?'. As such, the role of the higher centres must be addressed.

Higher Motor Centres

Sensory Input

Sensory messages from the body have various ways of ascending the spinal cord, depending on where they originate and what sensory modality they carry. They all tend to have synapses in the spinal cord at or near their level of entry, which act via interneurones to produce the reflex responses described above. The cell whose axon carries the information upwards, being second in the chain, is often referred to as the second order neurone. The axons carrying discriminative information (light touch, vibration and position sense) tend to ascend in the dorsal columns or lemniscal system (fig. 3.4). Information from crude touch, skin mechanoreceptors, nociceptive (pain) and temperature receptors ascends in the spinothalamic tracts. These systems also give off collaterals to brainstem and midbrain whose information contributes to arousal and awareness. Thalamocortical pathways allow the information to access the cerebral hemispheres. A further possibility is an ascent via the spinocerebellar tracks, where the information can be used in the assessment of 'correctness' with respect to the execution of motor activity, or the forward planning of new movements.

Motor Output

The interactions between those areas which have control over initiation, generation and performance of motor activity are outlined in Figure 3.5. The following text gives supplementary information.

Basal Ganglia

These are probably the most important areas with respect to the initiation and generation of pre-programmed movement. The major components are the putamen and caudate nucleus (neostriatum) and the globus pallidus. Other regions often associated with the basal ganglia are the subthalamic nucleus, striatum and the substantia nigra; the latter being 'famous'

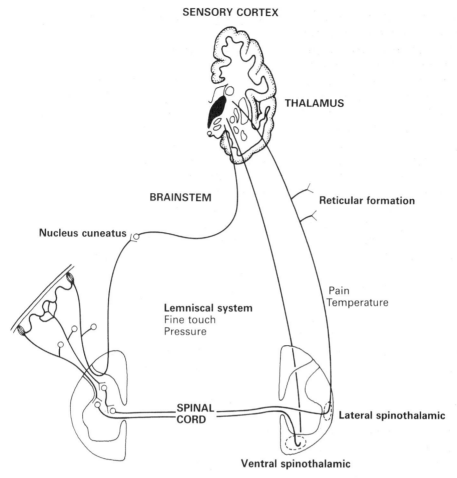

SENSORY CORTEX

THALAMUS

BRAINSTEM

Reticular formation

Nucleus cuneatus

Pain
Temperature

Lemniscal system
Fine touch
Pressure

SPINAL
CORD

Lateral spinothalamic

Ventral spinothalamic

Fig 3.4 Location of some important components of the sensory (afferent) system. Details of three possible pathways by which sensory information from somatic receptors may ascend to reach the centres involved with conscious awareness. The faster conducted information concerned with touch and pressure makes only a single synapse onto a second order neurone with an axon collateral which terminates in the thalamus. The synapse may be in either the spinal cord at the level of entry or the brainstem (nucleus cuneatus). Axons from the second order neurones in the spinal cord ascend in the ventral spinothalamic tracts. Those primary afferent axon collaterals to the nucleus cuneatus travel in the 'lateral funiculus' and from this region the second order axons travel with those from the ventral spinothalamic tracts. This final section is also known as the lemniscal system. The slower conducted signals from receptors of nociception and temperature tend to be polysynaptic at the level of entry into the spinal cord. As with the above pathways, the axon of the 'second' order neurone crosses over prior to ascending to the thalamus in the lateral spinothalamic tracts. The axons of this tract send collaterals into the reticular formation, an important factor in awareness and functions such as onset of sleep: it is difficult to sleep when you are in pain! Collaterals to the Raphe nucleus in the brainstem are important for the activation of descending systems which suppress the spinal activity due to active nociceptive afferents – endogenous pain relief.

because of the link between its degeneration and Parkinson's disease. Other diseases associated with damage (of a vascular nature) or degeneration in this area are hemiballismus, or more commonly ballisms (associated with damage to the globus pallidus/subthalamic nucleus) and choreiform movements, more commonly referred to as chorea

(associated with degeneration of the intrastriatal and cortical cholinergic and GABAergic neurones).

Cerebral Cortex

There are two main classes of cerebral cortex area which are involved with motor output. Firstly, those which form

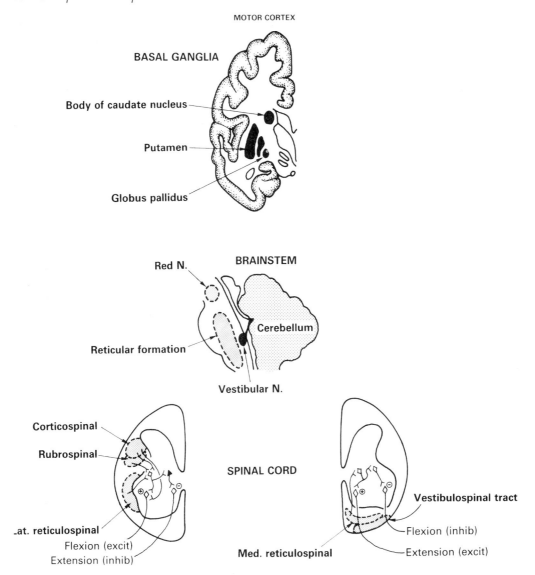

Fig 3.5 Location of the basic neurophysiological elements in the motor (efferent) system. This illustration gives some indication of the approximate location of the principal components of the motor system. Information descends from the motor cortex/basal ganglia complex through two main pathways, the pyramidal and extrapyramidal tracts: these are not shown, to maintain clarity. Pyramidal tracts contain axons which originate in the cerebral cortex and travel direct to spinal motoneurones. Extrapyramidal tracts contain all those motor systems outside the pyramidal tracts. This is an 'indirect' system concerned with postural control output from the basal ganglia, brainstem and cerebellum.

the primary motor cortex and lie adjacent to the primary sensory cortex. These areas are associated with precise movement; their outputs descend through the pyramidal tracts via the corticospinal tracts. Secondly, the other class of motor areas are referred to as the supplementary motor areas (such as the speech centres) which access the motor system via the primary motor cortex. The patterning of a movement in both the spatial positioning and the timing of individual contractions is thought to be derived from these centres.

Brainstem

The level of activity in this region tends to reflect the general state of awareness or arousal of the body. Those nuclei which relay the motor signals down through the 'extrapyramidal tracts' are found in this area. The major nuclei involved are: (1) the red nuclei, descending down the rubrospinal tracts; (2) the vestibular nuclei, descending in the vestibulospinal tracts to influence postural mechanisms by inhibiting flexors and exciting extensors; and (3) the reticular formation descending via the reticulospinal tracts modifies and helps to coordinate reflexes at the spinal level.

Cerebellum

The role of the cerebellum pertains to control and learning (via an estimation of correctness or comparison) of motor skills. By integrating information from proprioceptors, visual, auditory and vestibular systems with that from the cerebral cortex and the basal ganglia, the cerebellum can output corrections to all motor centres from the motor cortex down to the spinal cord. Without this system movements would be less smooth and controllable with noticeable pendular overshooting. There would also be a reduction in the anticipatory changes required to maintain balance and posture control.

Acquisition of New Reflexes

There are many types of reflex and furthermore the capacity to use them in a graded fashion. However, what happens if we are required to develop a totally new movement to a high level of proficiency? At this point, it is important to develop an appreciation of the changes required.

To reiterate, a skilled movement is essentially a smooth motor activity which may be 'unusual'. The activity can be the result of combining a group of simple, natural reflexes; however, occasionally other reflexes need to be inhibited or overridden temporarily. An example of this is found in the performance of somersaults with respect to the inhibition of the vestibular (righting) reflex. In addition, since acquired skills tend to be 'unnatural', the sensory trigger for the event tends to be a conditioned stimulus. Learning to adapt reflexes to unfamiliar stimuli is also a fac-

tor, which should increase in rapidity with practice. This follows from a recent study (Kerr and Boucher, 1992) where it would appear that performance in acquiring skills is related to previous learning of skills: these do not necessarily have to have been of the same type. This aspect will be described in greater detail in the following chapter.

Although it may appear that only a small number of movements, and therefore muscles, are used in any skilled task, a large part of the available musculature is probably involved to some degree. This becomes apparent even if one studies a skill involving relatively simple movements such as typing. Each key strike consists of a series of organized, discrete and precise finger movements. These are essentially under cortical control, but are facilitated by spinal reflexes. The position of the hands, and those of the arm and shoulder are also under spinal reflex control, however, this time under commands from the basal ganglia via the extrapyramidal tracts. As the system also requires a firm base to work from, this suggests a role for the muscles around the spinal column, the torso and the legs. The importance of this system can only be fully appreciated when it is impaired, as can be seen in patients who suffer from low back pain.

It is apparent that a great deal of muscle activity and coordination are required to organize the natural reflexes into a final coherent action. If the concept of feedback control is added (try typing without looking at the keys) then the complexity increases further. Feedback control is initially based upon visual feedback as the method of assessing correctness. With time and practice the reliance on visual feedback may be reduced and replaced by other forms of sensory feedback: in this example the replacement would be proprioceptive, as in the aptly named 'touch-typist'. This also illustrates the change in control emphasis, in that the cortex devolves some of the direct control of the movement while retaining the driving force or direction.

The changes in the higher centres are related to motor system programming and would need to include the setting up of programmes for muscle contractions with new spatial and temporal relationships. The conditioning stimuli for the prototype skill are developed from the start, while there is still a large degree of conscious control. Conscious control is obvious as it increases processing time which tends to slow down the performance. In addition, there is an incorporation of extraneous movements, which appear to serve no obvious purpose. These extra movements may even interfere with the objective of the prototype skill. However, as the skill becomes established the reflex pattern becomes more internal-feedback regulated and loses these aspects of conscious intervention. The role of the cortex instead becoming one of strategy determination. The final skilled movement is somehow stored in the CNS and can be totally recalled by a 'simple' trigger, which in some cases can be the advent of a conscious need or want.

As the skill becomes more established, there still appears to be sequential activation of the supplementary motor cortex followed by the motor cortex. This is probably related to the execution of previously learned patterns (Grafton *et al.*, 1992) which are somehow stored in the CNS and can be totally recalled by a 'simple' sensory trigger (probably via the supplementary motor cortex). The role of the cerebellum as a tutor of the motor cortex (Ito, 1972) may not be important for all types of motor learning. This hypothesis follows from two studies of brain blood flow, one of which showed no change in the cerebellum (Grafton *et al.*, 1992) whereas the other, a more automatic and less visual skill, showed changes in cerebellar blood flow which attenuated with practice (Friston *et al.*, 1991). It may be, therefore, that the cerebellum is more concerned with the consolidation of some learned skills than with their acquisition.

It has been suggested that a strategy of construction and facilitation of previously learned 'subskills' is adopted during the early stages of practice for a new motor skill (Eysenck and Frith, 1977). Such strategies are said to account for the rapid increase in skill performance during the early stages of acquisition. This is supported by recent evidence which showed increases in blood flow to the motor cortex and supplementary motor area with repeated trial during the first few attempts concomitant with the rapid increase in performance (Grafton *et al.*, 1992).

Practical Guidelines to Skill Acquisition

The acquisition of a new skill can be facilitated by following simple guidelines. 1) The final movements should be broken down into smaller and simpler reflexes and practised in sequence. 2) Feedback should be given on the performance. 3) The feedback should be of a modality which is appropriate to the skill and its trigger (in other words visuospatial, as in a video of the student's performance with a superimposed image of the tutor or ideal performance). 4) Any unwanted or confounding reflexes should be discouraged from the outset.

It is often said that the student's experience in any course of education to practitioner status in the manipulative arts is like learning to drive: once on the road the student really learns to drive! This is more true than most people would like to admit; however, acquisition of both forms of skill can be facilitated if the visuospatial feedback elements are taken more seriously before there has been some otherwise avoidable accident!

References

Bellemare, F., Woods, J.J., Johansson, R. *et al.* (1983) Motor-unit discharge rates in maximal voluntary contractions of three human muscles. *Journal of Neurophysiology*, **50**, 1380–1392

Eysenck, H.J. and Frith, C.D. (1977) *Reminiscence, Motivation and Personality*. Plenum Press: New York

Friston, K.J., Frith, C.D., Liddle, P.F. *et al.* (1991) The cerebellum in skill learning. *Journal of Cerebral Blood Flow Metabalism*, **11** (Suppl), S440

Grafton, S.T., Mazziotta, J.C., Presty, S. *et al.* (1992) Functional anatomy of human procedural learning determined with regional cerebral blood flow and PET. *Journal of Neuroscience*, **12**, 2542–2548

Kerr, R. and Boucher, J-L. (1992) Knowledge and motor performance. *Perceptual and Motor Skills*, **74**, 1195–1202

Ito, M. (1972) Neural design of the cerebellar motor control system. *Brain Research*, **40**, 81–102

Young, R.P., Scott, S.H. and Loeb, G.E. (1992) An intrinsic mechanism to stabilize posture-joint-angle-dependent moment arms of the feline ankle muscles. *Neuroscience Letters*, **145**, 137–140

Interesting Texts

Alexander, G.E., Delong, M.R. and Strick, P.L. (1986) Parallel organisation of functionally segregated circuits linking basal ganglia and cortex. *Ann Rev Neurosci*, **9**, 357–381
Feedback loops

Cohen, H. (1993) *Neuroscience for Rehabilitation*, J.B. Lippincott, Philadelphia
An easy-to-read, extensive text with a valuable annotated bibliography at the end of each chapter

Eccles, J.C. (1989) *Evolution of the Brain, Creation of the Self*. Routledge, London
An interesting read from the perspective of evolutionary significance of those areas of the nervous system important in skill performance

Gowitzke, B.A. and Milner, M. (1988) *Scientific Bases of Human Movement*, 3rd edn. Williams and Wilkins, Baltimore
A detailed and easy-to-read study of the topic. The many pictures add a more appropriate demesne to the written description of the topic

Rosenbaum, D.A. (1991) *Human Motor Control*. Academic Press, San Diego
A useful text which delves into the psychology of movement and motor learning using various tasks as examples

Chapter

4

Postural considerations for the practitioner

David Byfield

Introduction

Occupationally related injuries to the musculoskeletal system represent a growing health care and socioeconomic problem in most industrial countries. Hildebrandt (1987) established that age, physical fitness, relative muscle strength, previous back problems and work experience could constitute individual risk factors for back pain. He also identified heavy physical work, prolonged sitting postures, frequent lifting, rotating the trunk and pushing/pulling actions to be work-related risk factors. However, an association between any single vocational factor, such as heavy physical work or forceful movements, is difficult to make because these factors all occur together (Andersson, 1985). All these factors do increase the load on the spine regardless of their individual effects. It does appear that back injuries in the workplace are more the result of overexertion than a direct traumatic event (Andersson, 1992). Even though there is great difficulty associating the incidence of low back pain and specific risk factors, six physical work-related activities have been identified as occupational hazards. These include frequent bending, lifting, pushing and pulling, repetitive work and static work postures (Andersson, 1992). Pheasant (1993) has also identified prolonged work in a stooped posture as an ergonomic factor in back pain. It can be reasonably argued that these risk factors constitute a normal work day in a chiropractic office and therefore, it is not surprising that the type of job and the work environment have been closely linked with back pain (Diakow and Cassidy, 1984).

Occupational Injury and the Practitioner

Chiropractic daily practice involves the constant performance of manipulative therapy and other manual tasks in a variety of different working postures which subject the musculoskeletal system to potentially large repetitive mechanical loads. Many of these manipulative skills and techniques force practitioners to bend and twist the trunk (figs 4.1

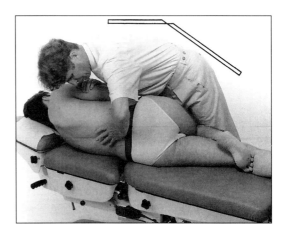

Fig 4.1

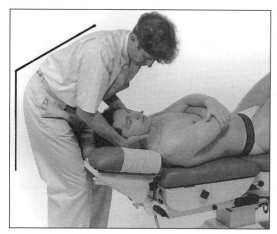

Fig 4.2

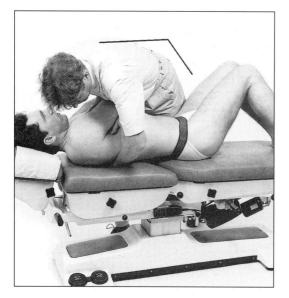

Fig 4.3

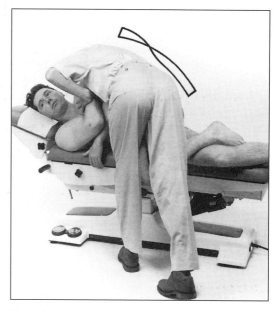

Fig 4.4

an increase in disc prolapse (Adams and Hutton, 1981) (fig. 4.4). The soft tissues of the upper back and shoulder girdle are particularly vulnerable to injury due to the high loads encountered as a result of repetitive manual thrusting and its use as a long lever (fig. 4.5). Issues such as keeping the legs straight or bent during forward flexion have different mechanical effects upon lumbosacral junction. Fortunately, the chiropractor is continually changing postures to meet the demands of clinical practice. A more mobile and varied work posture has been correlated with a lower incidence of

and 4.2), generate pushing and pulling actions and simultaneously reach and stretch around the patient (fig. 4.3). The constant lifting of patients, readjusting their body weight and position on the table prior to the thrust, represent professional risk factors for the chiropractor. The overall stress could substantially increase during mobilization procedures, which require the clinician to adopt awkward postures for extended periods of time. The majority of our manipulative techniques combine a degree of forward flexion and lateral bending plus a rotational component. This torquing activity has been identified as a physical risk factor and it has been argued that it is responsible for

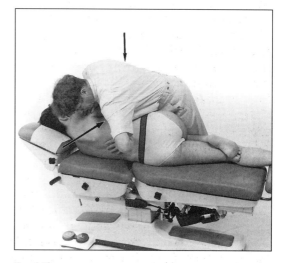

Fig 4.5

low back pain (Bendix, 1986) and probably reduces the mechanical effects of continual bending and twisting. The constant manual thrusting and a combination of fatigue, poor technique, inadequate skills and selection of inappropriate technique may contribute to an increased risk of musculoskeletal injury in the office. These occupational injuries are not confined to the spine. The continual mechanical stress applied to, for example, the shoulder girdle, elbow, and wrist joints during thrust delivery may result in repetitive injuries to the supportive soft tissues. This particular topic will be presented in more detail in chapters 5 and 6.

There are a number of mechanical and individual factors which have been identified as potential risk factors in occupational low back pain and which are of importance to the chiropractor. Age (35–55 years) and gender seem to be the only factors which have a direct influence on occupational back pain (Andersson, 1992). Smoking and lack of fitness have also been targetted as probable risk factors (Burton and Cassidy, 1992). Posture, muscle strength, physical fitness, spinal mobility, height, trunk strength, body build and obesity are considered of low importance and questionable (Andersson, 1992; Burton and Cassidy, 1992). It does appear that, due to the rather inconclusive effects of individual risk factors, the interaction of various occupational conditions that mechanically load the spine are of more importance than the person performing them. How the various movements are performed could also be a factor in this situation.

Mior and Diakow (1987) investigated the prevalence of back pain in a group of 500 chiropractors and found that the incidence of back pain was 87% overall with 74% complaining specifically of low back pain. This incidence represents the upper end of the scale reported for the general population and is higher than those figures reported for heavy physical work in industrial samples (Andersson, 1985). It also appears that the prevalence of low back pain in chiropractors is higher than among other health professionals. Diakow and Cassidy (1984) reported a 57% prevalence in Canadian dentists which was similar to the 52% incidence of low back pain in physiotherapists (Mior and Diakow, 1987). This high incidence of low back pain within the chiropractic profession may represent a biased sampling error in the study which did not identify those who entered the profession because they suffered back pain and were successfully treated by a chiropractor.

Reported differences between male and female practitioners have been compared. Males complain most often of lumbar pain while females complain most often of thoracic pain (Mior and Diakow, 1987). Shoulder pain was common in both groups but more prevalent in females. This might imply that chiropractors with a smaller stature could be placing greater physical stresses on their upper backs and shoulders in order to execute various manual techniques. It has been shown using an adjustment simulator that male chiropractors are able to produce higher forces than female chiropractors, (Adams and Wood, 1984). They suggested that this difference was probably due to a greater grip strength and heavier body weight shown by the males. This could also imply that male practitioners make more effective use of their body weight, which creates less strain on the upper body. The importance of improving upper body strength and more effective use of body weight cannot be overemphasized. This difference could also indicate the medium- to long-term effects of poor habitual skills and improper manipulation selection for the patient's needs and the doctor's abilities. Doctor positioning, table height and patient size have been isolated as possible aetiological factors (Mior and Diakow, 1987). Therefore, it is becoming more apparent that there are specific occupational hazards causing mechanical stress to the musculoskeletal system of those engaged in spinal manipulative therapy. How can we as a profession minimize these risks?

One method could be through a systematic review and breakdown of each of the common diversified techniques for each spinal region combined with a review of practitioner performance and assessment of the relevant skills. Clinical life can be mundane and routine. The constant use of the same manipulative techniques, day after day and year after year could contribute to time dependent chronic overuse syndromes. Practice growth and the increased demands on the chiropractor are directly proportional. Practitioners should strive to limit and control these inherent occupational short-comings. Clinicians alike should become aware of various techniques that produce the same treatment outcome, thereby reducing the effects of using the same manipulative procedure on each patient. In addition, learning to perform all manipulative procedures efficiently from both sides of the table could possibly reduce the effects of musculoskeletal fati-gue and the development of mechanical pain. Practitioners are creatures of rou-tine and tend to use those few techniques that produce clinical results. It may be more a question of habit than awareness of clinical outcome. However, it is clini-cally advantageous to master a wider range of manipulative skills that can be used interchangeably, producing similar clinical results. Varying patient postures, including sitting and standing will undoubtedly ease the accumulative effects of mechanical overload. Further to this, maintaining full body fitness, stretching during the day to relieve mus-cular tightness and improving upper body strength to help stabilize the shoulder girdle are other considerations. Another method may be the use of more sophisticated and specialized tables that are presently available. Tables that pro-vide comfort for both practitioner and patient and are vertically adjustable are particularly beneficial. The use of a multi-functional table extends our armamentar-ium and permits the use of many manipulative techniques. Stationary tables do not account for differences in patient thickness, which means that the practitioner is continually working at dif-ferent heights. This may upset postural balance and important weight distribu-tion over the targeted joint, compromis-ing the efficiency of the manipulative procedure and at the same time risking

injury to both patient and practitioner. This scenario is more apparent in multi-practitioner clinics using common tables. Therefore, using equipment to suit both the patient and practitioner completes this important triad.

Underestimating a clinical situation and controlling patient's movement are vital safety factors to follow. Repeatedly thrust-ing on a joint to get it 'to go' or 'crack' is not a reasonable approach. One, maybe two, dynamic thrusts followed by an immediate re-examination of the joint often proves a successful functional restoration without all the additional effort and the potential risks to the patient. The use of the high velocity low ampli-tude thrust is a very economical method of spinal manipulation. It is fast and efficient when performed skilfully when compared to the effort involved in mobilization procedures. The doctor has to make the clinical choice as to which therapeutic intervention is most applic-able for the patient and the manipulator. Judging the situation remains a conse-quence of experience and an awareness of the multidimensional nature of manip-ulative procedures. Practitioners have a mandate at least to maintain their skills if not continue to improve their perfor-mance and repeatability under a number of quite different clinical situations and patient types. On a final note, it is a well known anecdote that chiropractors tend to ignore their own mechanical problems not seeking help because of time restraints and lack of practitioner availability. This is our livelihood and our ability to meet the demands of daily practice depends on our own state of health. Maintaining a comfortable posture and balance mini-mizes energy expenditure and workloads. The use of adjustable height and motor-ized adjusting tables and improving pos-tural awareness may reduce the effects of our high occupational risk status.

The purpose of this chapter is to present an overview of a few basic aspects of the practitioner's working posture. It is by no means inclusive, the details being covered in the appropriate following chapters. Posture, in the narrowest sense, may be considered to be the upright, *well-*

balanced stance of the human subject in a 'normal' position (Basmajian, 1993). From a chiropractor's point of view, posture is vitally important in terms of efficient performance of a highly complex set of psychomotor skills, spinal manipulative therapy. The chain of events leading up to the delivery of an effective manipulative or mobilization force is somewhat dependent upon the doctor's control of his or her centre of gravity. The importance of recognizing clinical risk factors early is equally as important as instituting appropriate preventive measures to eliminate these hazards (Andersson, 1993). Emphasis will be placed upon the position of the suprasternal (jugular) notch relative to the anatomical contact point as the optimal position of the clinician's body weight for ideal control and efficiency of the dynamic thrust.

1) Standing at the head of the table with the legs straight and spine fully flexed with the patient's head unsupported held out in front increases the bending moment at the lumbosacral spine and could compromise the efficiency and control of the dynamic impulse thrust (fig. 4.6). The longer levers acting on the head and neck may create more twisting action and arm fatigue. There is increased flexion of the thoracic spine, placing more mechanical loads on the cervical extensors.

2) Figure 4.7 illustrates better practitioner posture and patient comfort prior to the manipulative thrust. The practitioner is using the mechanical advantage of the lower extremities, flexing the hips and knees in order to effectively distribute the body weight across several joints. There is less flexion angle at the lumbosacral and thoracic spines taking the stress off the spinal extensors reducing potential muscular fatigue. The clinician is also leaning against the head of the table supporting his own weight and is positioned at about 45 degrees ipsilateral to the mechanical lesion, shortening the manipulating lever. The position of the practitioner's suprasternal notch is over the cervical spine, placing the centre of gravity very close to the patient and maximizing the mechanical efficiency of the manipulator.

Cervical Spine

With recent attention to the complications of and the contraindications to spinal manipulative therapy of the cervical spine (Gatterman, 1991), the importance of modifying excessive rotational movements becomes clinically imperative. The manoeuvrability of the practitioner plays a key role in performing confident and safe manipulation of both the upper and lower cervical spine.

The following represents some basic aspects of practitioner posture and positioning with respect to manipulative therapy directed to the cervical spine. Common errors will be presented and suggestions of a more appropriate postural performance will be given.

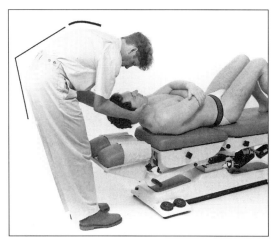

Fig 4.6

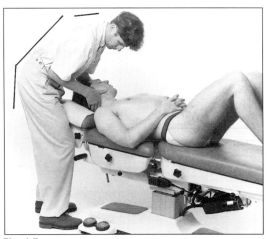

Fig 4.7

3) The practitioner's arms are held in close to the body with almost equal flexion occurring at both the shoulders and elbow joints to minimize any asymmetrical load on the joints and muscles of the upper extremity (fig. 4.8). Note the position of the doctor's suprasternal (jugular) notch (*) in relation to the area of the spine under tension (*). The weight of the patient's head is supported by the headpiece to reduce the carrying load on the arms and upper back.

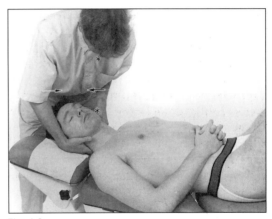

Fig 4.8

4) The sitting position for the practitioner reduces the load on the lumbar and thoracic spine by modifying the flexion angle of both areas of the spine (fig. 4.9). Care has to be taken to ensure that the stool used is mobile, can move from side to side and has an adjustable height to allow more flexibility with different patient types. The ability to position the jugular notch (*) over the contact point (*) is difficult, reducing the efficiency of the manipulative thrust and increasing the stress on the shoulders.

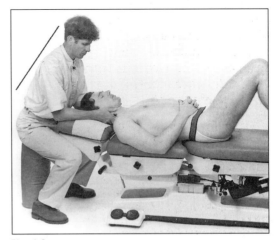

Fig 4.9

5) Standing cervical manipulative techniques have an advantage in limiting the loads on the spine by distributing forces through flexion of the hips, knees and ankles (fig. 4.10). Care has to be taken to use a stool for the patient that has an adjustable height in order to maximize hand and arm position for thrust delivery. Major disadvantages are reduced patient relaxation due to weight-bearing posture of the head, and potential reflex muscle guarding prior to manipulative thrust. If the patient is too high or low, the efficiency of the thrust is reduced.

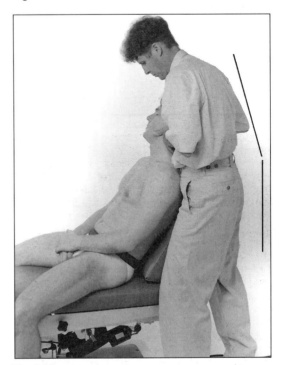

Fig 4.10

Thoracic Spine

Manipulation of the thoracic spine offers two main advantages. First, many of the more common procedures are performed while the patient is in the prone position and second, the mechanical stability of the rib cage helps to prevent excessive movement, improving specificity. The prone position is an advantage to the patient in that the area being manipulated is virtually fixed and the practitioner can use this relatively stationary position to control patient movement and maximize the mechanical effects of the manipulative thrust. The following represents some basic aspects of practitioner posture and positioning with respect to manipulative therapy directed to the thoracic spine. Common errors will be presented along with more appropriate postures and performance advice.

1) Figure 4.11 illustrates the correct position of the suprasternal notch (*) in line with the contact hands (*). The doctor's shoulders are relaxed and angled towards the table, keeping the elbows relatively flexed. The practitioner is leaning against the table in order to help support body weight and reduce the mechanical stress. There is very little flexion of the trunk.

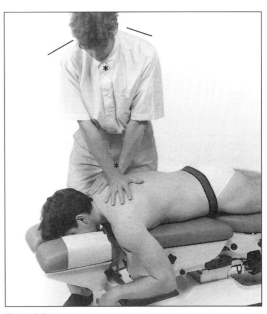

Fig 4.11

2) The practitioner is positioned at 45 degrees to both the table and patient in a fencer stance posture (fig. 4.12). The trunk, pelvis, hips and lower extremities are all positioned at 45 degrees to eliminate any potential torsional forces developing in any of the major joints of the body. Note that the arms are also symmetrically placed in order to maximize the manipulative thrust and minimize the stress on the practitioner relative to the jugular notch (*) and the centre of gravity.

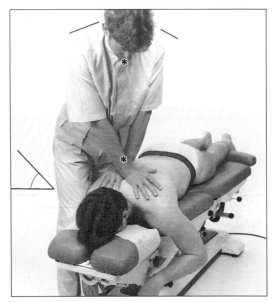

Fig 4.12

3) Figure 4.13 illustrates the overall effect of the body positioned at 45 degrees low fencer stance from the feet to the trunk and head with the suprasternal notch over contact hands positions. The centre of gravity is positioned for a weight distribution advantage. The hips and knees of the practitioner are flexed to assist the impulse body drop. The body weight is forward over the front leg effectively placing it over the patient and the table to maximize its use. The plantar flexion of the hind foot pushes the weight forward and adds spring to the lower extremities. The legs are in contact with the table to help support body weight.

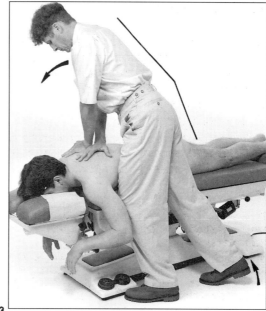

Fig 4.13

4) Figure 4.14 demonstrates the practitioner positioned back and away from the table losing the support of the table and advantage created by the position of the centre of gravity. This subsequently compromises the mechanical advantage of the doctor's body weight and body drop thrust. This posture places greater demands on the doctor in terms of overall work demand. Flexion angles are increased and there is more stress on the shoulders. Jugular notch and contact point have become uncoupled (*).

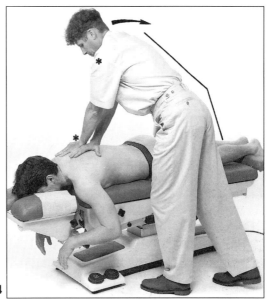

Fig 4.14

5) Techniques which require the practitioner to reach around the patient (fig. 4.15) require a great deal of trunk flexion thereby stressing the lumbo-pelvic region of the spine. However, if the practitioner maintains a 45 degree stance to the table, keeps the hips and knees flexed and leans over the patient positioning the centre of gravity close to the patient (*), the effects of the mechanical overload may be negated. Keeping the shoulders parallel to the table decreases the torque in the thoracolumbar spine. This also controls the twist in the arm.

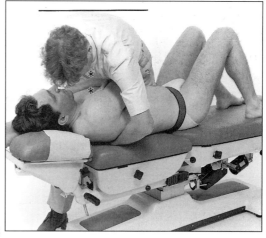

Fig 4.15

6) Manipulative techniques for the cervic-thoracic spine illustrate the use of correct positioning of the jugular notch (∗) and the targetted joint dysfunction (fig. 4.16). Flexion of both hips and knees while leaning against the table distributes the weight of the practitioner over the centre of the spine. This reduces mechanical stress even though it appears that trunk flexion is excessive. The shoulders are relaxed and level decreasing spinal twist and maximizing the thrust speed of the shoulder girdle.

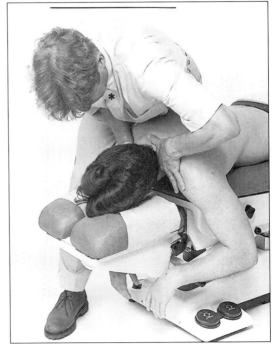

Fig 4.16

Lumbar/Pelvic

Manipulation of the lumbar spine in the treatment and management of acute and chronic low back pain has been well documented (Shekelle *et al.*, 1991). The high incidence of low back pain in the general population would suggest that chiropractors spend the majority of their clinical time treating low back pain. The high incidence of low back and sacroiliac pain reported in chiropractors could be due to the rigorous physical demands and skill required in order to perform side posture rotational diversified manipulative techniques. These techniques place increased demands on the practitioner to control his/her weight plus the weight and movement of the patient simultaneously. The patient is far less stable in the side lying position compared to the prone or supine postures. It is quite conceivable to suggest that improper skill performance can cause repetitive strain on various soft tissues and joints of the practitioner during the performance of side posture spinal manipulation.

The following represents some basic aspects of practitioner posture and positioning with respect to manipulative therapy directed to the lumbar/pelvic region. Common errors will be presented along with more appropriate postures and performance advice.

1) Figure 4.17 illustrates symmetrical positioning of the upper body during a side posture lumbar roll rotational manipulation. Note the position of the suprasternal notch (*) over the contact hand on the spine (*) and the square position of the shoulders. The contact hand arm and the arm supporting the patient's upper body are almost mirror images, reducing shoulder stress and torque in the upper back. Also note that there is very little torque in the patient's spine.

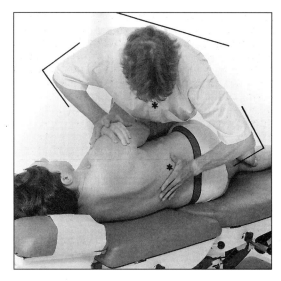

Fig 4.17

2) In contrast Figure 4.18 illustrates some of the common mistakes encountered during performance of this manipulation. Note the asymmetry of the shoulders, particularly the left side which is internally rotated, placing stress on both soft tissues of the upper back and torquing the arm. This position also exaggerates the angle at both the elbow and wrist, affecting the thrust efficiency and force localization. There is an increased flexion angle at the trunk plus twist in both the lumbar and thoracic spines. The centre of gravity is too low, which will increase load on the shoulders and lumbar spine. There is also greater twist in the patient's upper back. Patient relaxation and compliance may be compromised.

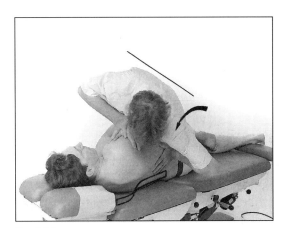

Fig 4.18

3) Figure 4.19 illustrates a poorly executed side posture lumbar roll as described previously. Note the twist in both the lumbar and thoracic spines and the exaggerated shoulder angle. There is also a torquing effect in the hips and lower extremities, increasing subsequent mechanical loads on these joints. The ability to perform an effective body drop in this position is questionable.

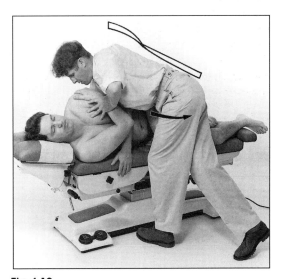

Fig 4.19

4) Overall symmetry with respect to the upper back and shoulders is illustrated in Figure 4.20 as compared to Figure 4.19. The practitioner is positioned at 45 degrees to the table and patient with equal distribution of weight and force through the whole body and with a well placed centre of gravity over the patient. The shoulder and pelvic girdle are relaxed. The trunk flexion angle is still excessive; however, by distributing body weight on the patient and the table the mechanical effects are reduced.

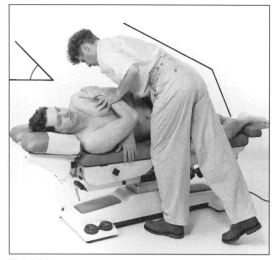

Fig 4.20

5) Controlling the patient's weight and movement on the table during side posture can be done by gently squeezing the patient's top leg (*) between the practitioner's legs, reducing excessive leg drop and stress on the hip lever (fig. 4.21). Stabilizing patient movement reduces the amount of effort required by the practitioner to maintain overall control during the application of the manipulative thrust. Also note the 45 degree position of the feet relative to the table and especially the left foot posture. This helps to place the weight forward towards the patient and table, helping to support the patient's position. The doctor's feet should only be hip distance apart.

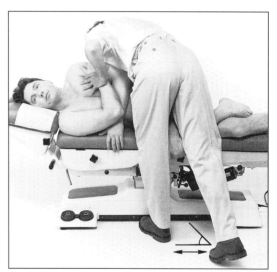

Fig 4.21

6) Figure 4.22 illustrates a wide foot placement which causes a large gap between the practitioner's legs. Patient movement is increased and control minimized. More effort is required to control patient movement detracting from the efficiency of the manipulation. The outward rotation of the right foot could place potential stress on the knee during the body drop.

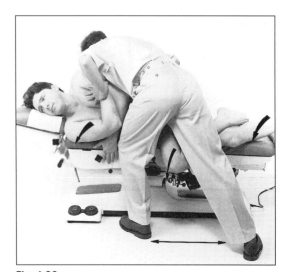

Fig 4.22

7) Other manipulative techniques which utilize different contact and basic arm and hand positions are illustrated in Figures 4.23–4.26. Figures 4.23 and 4.24 demonstrate arm positions close to the body of the practitioner which shorten the lever arm and improve mechanical advantage, subsequently reducing overall stress on the doctor. Figure 4.24 illustrates an excellent body position relative to the targetted joint (*) and symmetrical shoulders. Figure 4.25 shows a technique, although difficult to perform, which does reduce the flexion angle at the lumbosacral region. Figure 4.26 shows a sitting rotational manipulation which has advantages for the practitioner regarding body posture but patient movements are increased, reducing control, which may outweigh the benefits. This technique requires more work, does not localize thrust forces and may not be as clinically specific.

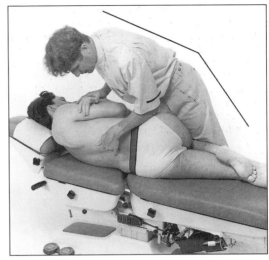

Fig 4.23

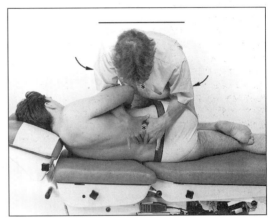

Fig 4.24

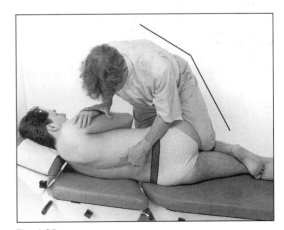

Fig 4.25

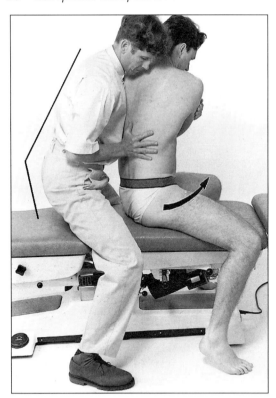

Fig 4.26

Conclusions

This chapter has presented an introduction to some of the more common postural and positional errors associated with manipulative skills and techniques of the spine and pelvis. The intent was to demonstrate good and bad positioning and at the same time present alternative postures which could minimize the overall mechanical effects to both the practitioner and patient. The more efficient posture and use of body weight adopted prior to the delivery of the dynamic thrust should enhance its efficiency and effects.

References

Adams, A.A. and Wood, J. (1984) Forces used in selected chiropractic adjustments of the low back: a preliminary study. *The Research Forum*, Palmer College of Chiropractic, **1**, 5–9

Adams, M.A. and Hutton, W.C. (1981) Relevance of torsion to the mechanical derangement of the lumbar spine. *Spine*, **6**, 241–248

Andersson, G.B.J. (1985) Epidemiology of low back pain. In *Empirical Approaches to the Validation of Spinal Manipulation* (eds A.A. Buerger and P.E. Greenman). Charles C. Thomas, Springfield, IL, pp. 53–70

Andersson, G.B.J. (1992) Factors important in the genesis and prevention of occupational back pain and disability. *Journal of Manipulative and Physiological Therapeutics*, **15**, 43–46

Andersson, G. (1993) Risk factors in the workplace. In *Proceedings of the 1993 World Chiropractic Congress* (London, 1993). World Federation of Chiropractic, Toronto

Basmajian, J.V. (1993) Functional anatomy of the spine and associated structures. In *Rational Manual Therapies* (eds. J.V. Basmajian and R. Nyberg). Williams and Wilkins, London, p. 49

Bendix, T. (1986) Sitting postures – a review of biomechanic and ergonomic aspects. *Manual Medicine*, **2**, 77–81

Burton, C.V. and Cassidy, J.D. (1992) Economics, epidemiology, and risk factors. In *Managing Low Back Pain*, 3rd edn. (eds W.H. Kirkaldy-Willis and C.V. Burton). Churchill Livingstone, London, pp. 1–6

Diakow, P.R. and Cassidy, J.D. (1984) Back pain in dentists. *Journal of Manipulative and Physiological Therapeutics*, **7**, 85–88

Gatterman, M.I. (1991) Standards of practice relative to complications of and contraindications to spinal manipulative therapy. *Journal of the Canadian Chiropractic Association*, **35**, 232–236

Hildebrandt, V.H. (1987) A review of epidemiological research on risk factors of low back pain. In: *Musculoskeletal Disorders at Work* (ed. P. Buckle). Taylor & Francis, London, pp. 9–16

Mior, S.A. and Diakow, P.R. (1987) Prevalence of back pain in chiropractors. *Journal of Manipulative and Physiological Therapeutics*, **6**, 305–309

Pheasant, S. (1993) Back injury at work: strategies for prevention. In *Proceedings of the 1993 World Chiropractic Congress* (London, 1993). World Federation of Chiropractic, Toronto

Shekelle, P.G., Adams, A.H., Chassin, M.R. *et al.* (1991) *The Appropriateness of Spinal Manipulation for Low-Back Pain: Project Overview and Literature Review*. RAND, Santa Monica, California. Monograph No. R-4025/1 – CCR/FCER

Chapter

5

Hand–arm–shoulder positional skills

David Byfield

Introduction

The application of spinal manipulative therapy is a 'hands on' affair. The hand/patient interface represents that all important unwritten communication between the doctor and the patient. This chiropractor–patient interaction has been described as the 'chiropractic healing encounter' (Vernon, 1991) and provides valuable information for the practitioner. Moreover, this contact also permits the patient to 'feel' the skill and confidence of the practitioner! The hands should be placed gently and comfortably over an irritated and painful area, as heavy pressure may undermine the patient's confidence and possibly jeopardize the therapeutic intent. Furthermore, any patient apprehension should be regarded as a strong indicator to modify or stop further manipulative intervention.

The hand is a highly sophisticated sensory device which not only probes the patient's reaction but helps the practitioner to gauge the amount of force, depth and speed which will be required to carry out a successful therapeutic event. Maintaining the proprioceptive feedback necessary to discriminate the point of physiological limits of the tissue should not be interrupted. Any methods to enhance this concept should be strongly developed. In addition, any excessive tension in the clinician's hands will automatically be perceived by the patient and affect the therapeutic outcome and compliance. The ability to communicate a sense of clinical skill and competence to the patient is a major com-

ponent of the art of chiropractic. It is the responsibility of those engaged in manipulative methods to develop the strength, flexibility and agility of the hands in order to meet clinical demands.

The hand is capable of great dexterity, assuming various different shapes and postures which are clinically useful. It also has the capacity to distort to accommodate the more inaccessible anatomical contact points. The hand is basically a tool. In order to get the best out of that tool, one has to learn to use it and understand its potential, thus making the task simpler and easier to carry out.

The first thing to learn is that the hand does not contribute to the force applied to the patient. It acts as a transfer point. Any excessive tension in the forearm or hand musculature will distort this contact and the effective transmission of the thrust. The hand is magnificently designed featuring small, padded areas which provide very effective buffers for the contact and manipulative thrust. If the contact on the patient is smaller, less force will be dissipated into surrounding tissue and subsequently less 'work' will be required overall. A soft contact cushions the transfer of energy making the event less painful for the patient at the thrust transfer point. Realizing these very basic concepts and the fact that the thrust force is generated from the whole body, through the shoulder, down the arm and across the hand through a chain of progressively shorter levers, should put this exercise into its clinical perspective. The forces produced by the body during an impulse thrust are substantial. If the hand is inaccurately placed, weak or inflexible, the soft tissues and joints of the hand and fingers may be vulnerable to injury. The forces transferred to the patient may be subsequently distorted and dissipated inefficiently into the neighbouring tissues. As previously discussed in Chapter 4, the soft tissues of the shoulder, elbow, and wrist are equally at risk due to faulty posture and inappropriate force transmission along the kinetic chain. For the force applied, there is an equal and opposite force transmitted back through the body. Undoubtedly, misuse of these forces over a period of time could possibly account for the high incidence of overuse injuries within the chiropractic profession and others practising manual therapy (Molumphy *et al.*, 1985; Mior and Diakow, 1987; Scholey and Hair, 1989). Transferring forces and mechanically loading joints along this chain at unnecessary and extreme ranges of motion may account for this potentially higher incidence. It is not uncommon to see undergraduates using various taping techniques or supports to protect injured peripheral joints. Inadequate physical and instructional rehabilitation at this stage of educational development may impair efficient psychomotor skill acquisition and reinforce inappropriate long-term practice methods.

The hand is the most important short lever contact point used during the application of spinal manipulative therapeutics. The development of good hand skills and dexterity is essential. The ability to establish a firm and confident contact on the patient's body without causing excessive pressure or force represents considerable practice to master. The hand is normally dextrous, flexible and capable of fine, intricate controlled movements, when properly trained.

The student, when initially introduced to manipulative skills, has the tendency to use the hand as a hammer, thinking that a bone on bone contact is better: 'I'll find that mamillary process if it's the last thing I do!' Students must appreciate that a firm but *gentle* contact is less painful and softer for the patient. A tense, distressed and uncomfortable patient will naturally resist a practitioner's best efforts. Think back to that time when sitting in a dental chair and recollect how hard your head is pushing back into the headrest, not to mention the vice grip on the handles of the chair itself. This type of scenario is counter-productive and should be rigorously discouraged. The student should concentrate on the feedback from the patient, actively visualize the structures and postures involved and learn to 'feel' the event. This degree of sensitivity is frustrating to learn but full appreciation of this feedback will guide many of the proceeding actions of the overall manipulative skill.

The human handshake can be regarded as a comparable analogy. A good, firm grip communicates many things about the other individual. A handshake has been known to make or break a business deal. It can express confidence and maturity and give the recipient a sense of security that this individual can be trusted. Such human interactions constitute a very important and basic aspect of chiropractic clinical methods and communication.

Postmanipulative reactions and complications are fortunately a clinical rarity, but emotive. There is no place in our profession for aggressive rotational manipulation of the cervical spine, excessive twisting movements of the lumbar spine or forceful adjustments of the thoracics. The apparent success of chiropractic treatment for low back pain seems to be a combination of pain reduction and, more interestingly, patient satisfaction (Vernon, 1991; Bolton, 1993). People will generally react favourably when treated with consideration and basic courtesy. This begins in a clinical context with an appreciation of *the meaning of light touch*. This chapter will present the skills associated with developing the basic hand postures used in spinal manipulative therapy. It is recommended that these skills be practised every day in order to develop proficiency, confidence and fine motor control of the hands. The angular relationship between the hand, arm and shoulder through the wrist and elbow will also be presented in light of the increasing number of occupational strain/sprain injuries at these specific peripheral joints.

The Chiropractic Manipulative Contact Hand

There are at least 12 areas on the hand that can be used to contact the skin surface and anatomical levers of the patient (Grecco, 1953; States, 1968; Christensen, 1984; Schafer and Faye, 1989) (fig. 5.1). These contact points are used with varying degrees of frequency depending on the specific manipulative technique. The

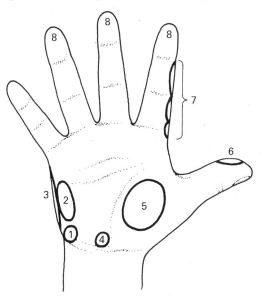

Fig 5.1 The various common contact points of the manipulator's hand: 1, pisiform; 2, hypothenar; 3, metacarpal; 4, calcaneal (heel); 5, thenar; 6, thumb; 7, interphalangeal; 8, finger tip (pad) or digital.

basic hand postures for diversified techniques will be presented. Practitioners develop a personal preference, but it is recommended that proficiency is gained in all hand skills.

Hand Postures and Skills

The operative words will be *gentle and slow, but firm*. The undergraduate should be able to perform the individual hand postures and contact points competently before applying these skills on a patient. The flexibility and dexterity necessary for

optimal use of the hand takes time to develop.

The Chiropractic Arch

The chiropractic arch is the most fundamental and basic of chiropractic hand postures. The arch places the hand in the most advantageous position in such a way that it exposes most of the more common contact points necessary when learning the basic manipulative techniques for each region of the spine and pelvis. The arched hand provides a buffer system between the doctor and patient. The chiropractic arch is a *natural posture for the hand* due to the anatomical and functional tendency of ulnar deviation in the resting position.

There are a series of steps as the undergraduate slowly develops the dexterity and fine motor control needed to acquire the necessary skills with his or her hands. Flexibility of the joints of the hand and fingers will assist the learning of the following skills. The student and graduate must realize that developing control and strength of the hand and finger muscles is mandatory and will enhance the learning of all skills. As an introduction to the basic manipulative hand skills, the following flexibility exercises are presented. It is recommended that they be practised daily in combination with all other skills. A general exercise programme covering full body flexibility, strength, and cardiovascular fitness is advised to meet the new physical demands required during the acquisition of manipulative skills. Improving muscular speed and coordination and at the same time increasing joint range of motion and stability through strength training will cause adaptive changes in the neuromuscular system. This will result in fuller activation of prime movers, better coordinated activation of the muscles supporting the prime movers, and an overall greater net force (Sale, 1988). *Speed, strength, coordination and finesse* are the core elements for the development of foundation manipulative pyschomotor skills. The importance of developing bilateral strength and flexibility will give the student and graduate the confidence to learn these skills equally on both sides of the body.

1) The ability to separate the thumb and index finger is necessary in order to manoeuvre the contact fingers around various anatomical locations. Therefore, the flexibility of the web of the hand should be maximized. This can be extended to the other fingers as well. Figure 5.2a illustrates the position of the fingers and thumb and Figure 5.2b shows the required flexibility using a slow developmental stretch (SDS) or proprioceptive neuromuscular facilitation (PNF) procedures. Remember, some people have natural flexibility and loose ligamentous holding elements. If you are tight jointed and less flexible, you have your work ahead of you, but with time and regular stretching flexibility will improve.

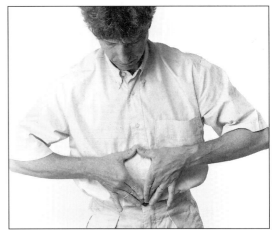

Fig 5.2a

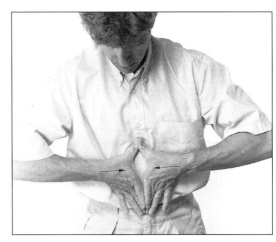

Fig 5.2b

2) The ability to gain both 90 degrees of flexion and extension at the wrist is necessary for many of the manipulative skills. Figure 5.3a demonstrates the flexibility required. Figures 5.3b and 5.3c illustrate the position to introduce both SDS and PNF to comfortably increase soft tissue extensibility and the range of motion of the wrist and forearm musculature. The elbow is kept relatively straight during this exercise.

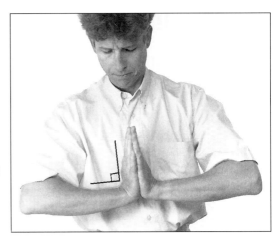

Fig 5.3a

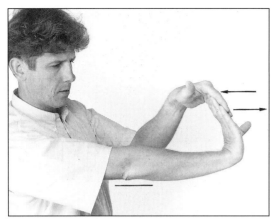

Fig 5.3b

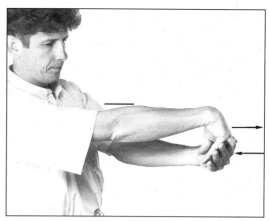

Fig 5.3c

3) Strength, as part of any fitness programme will accelerate the learning of these skills and reduce possible joint injury as a result of the demands placed upon the upper extremity during manipulative skills. Any number of methods to gradually increase strength and stabilize the wrist and hand can be used. Balance the exercise by using small hand weights for arms, forearm and finger strength for both flexor and extensor mechanisms (figs. 5.4a and b). Begin with wrist curls in both flexion and extension and then incorporate arm and shoulder repeats.

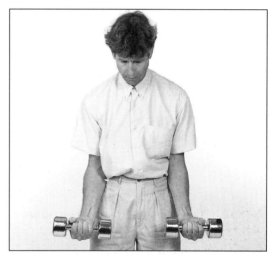

Fig 5.4a

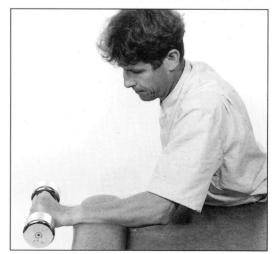

Fig 5.4b

4) Increasing the strength, flexibility and endurance of the shoulders and upper body would also be advantageous, particularly with respect to thrust skills. Stretching the arm extensors and shoulder girdle will improve the range of motion and efficiency of the shoulder mechanism (fig. 5.5a). A very low weight high repetition programme to tone the shoulder girdle is illustrated in Figure 5.5b.

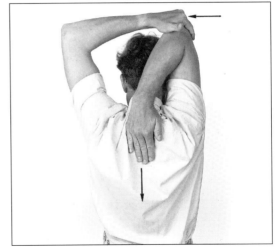

Fig 5.5a

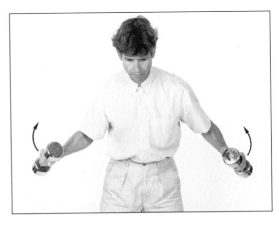

Fig 5.5b

5) Simple push-ups (fig. 5.6a) and the inclusion of a more structured fitness programme to improve overall body fitness including a swimming programme (fig. 5.6b) would help develop the strength and endurance necessary to learn the manipulative skills presented in this and future chapters.

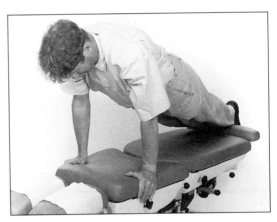

Fig 5.6a

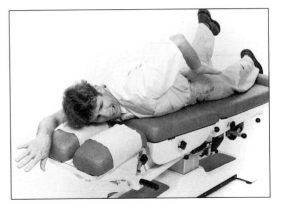

Fig 5.6b

Chiropractic Arch Hand Skills

The illustrations will include only the right hand for convenience and continuity in the text, but proficiency and performance demonstrating dexterity with both hands is a fundamental requirement.

1) The starting position is with the hand placed on a flat surface with the fingers and thumb spread slightly (fig. 5.7). There should be **no tension** in the hand while in this starting position. The hand should be slightly ulnar deviated in this position. This is a natural posture for the hand otherwise allow the hand to find its own natural resting position.

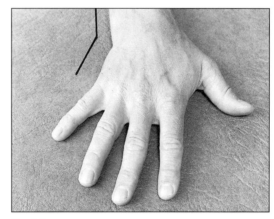

Fig 5.7

2) The next step is to lift and flex the metacarpophalangeal joints up from the surface to form a bridge or V shape with the hand so that the only areas in contact with the surface are the lateral aspects of the thumb, the fingertip pads and the calcaneal aspect of the palm (fig. 5.8). There should be no muscular tension in the hand or forearm.

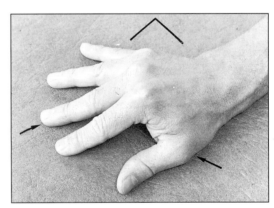

Fig 5.8

3) The hand is then SLOWLY SUPINATED while extending and slightly adducting the thumb (fig. 5.9a). The hand and forearm are completely relaxed. The only contact with the surface of the table is the hypothenar eminence, the pisiform and the four finger pads (*) (fig. 5.9b). The fingers are then spread a little wider apart to stabilize the weight through the hand. This bridge is similar to the one used by the professional snooker players.

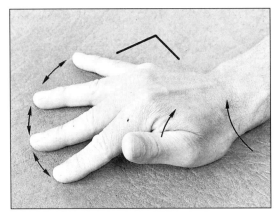

Fig 5.9a

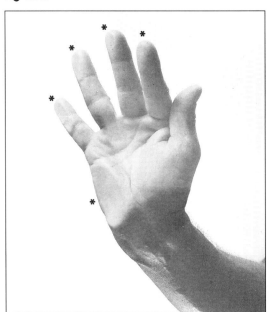

Fig 5.9b

4) Once this movement pattern has been rehearsed, it is important to learn how to begin to use the fingers to tighten up the underlying soft tissues (taking up the slack) in order to stabilize the contact hand over an anatomical contact point. This can be rehearsed by placing the hand on a small towel with the fingers spread wider apart, and running through steps 1–3 as described above. This time press the fingers *gently* into the towel and draw it up under the fingers to simulate tissue pull and at the same time slowly supinate the hand, drawing the towel in the opposite direction with the heel of the hand. The hand should finish in the bridge posture with the hypothenar eminence and pisiform in contact with the surface of the towel (fig. 5.10). There should be a mild amount of tension in the hand, mainly the flexors, in order to stabilize the contact. Tension should be felt equally throughout the hand and fingers with *no excessive muscular tension* in the forearm.

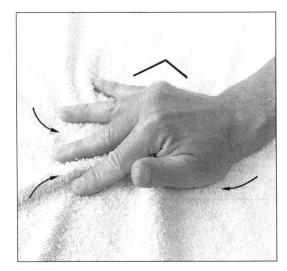

Fig 5.10

5) The position of the arm and forearm in relation to the wrist and basic hand contact is important. This will ensure better transfer of thrust force generated from muscle contraction in the shoulder girdle and central body to the arm, wrist and hand through the contact point.

With the hand in the basic bridge posture with a hypothenar contact the angle between the forearm and the hand should be about 100–110 degrees with the extensor muscle group in line with the hand, the elbow locked but not hyperextended and the shoulder relaxed, lowered and slightly adducted to the chest (fig. 5.11). Move the arm further forward and back to get a feel for the strain on the wrist and hand.

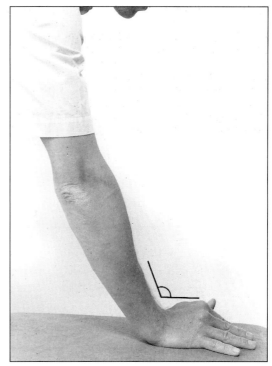

Fig 5.11

6) There are three common errors encountered when learning hand posture skills.

i) The student assumes that the *only real contact* is the pisiform. There is a tendency to lift all the fingers up from the surface of the table, hyperextending the wrist (fig. 5.12a). This limits the stability of the arch and flexes the arm excessively. The pisiform (*) is a bony contact and could feel much harder to the patient when applied during potentially painful clinical conditions (fig. 5.12b).

Hyperextending the wrist statically for a period of time with increased tension in the extensor muscle group could contribute to injury.

It is recommended that the combination pisiform/hypothenar contact be adopted instead of a pisiform alone (fig. 5.9b)

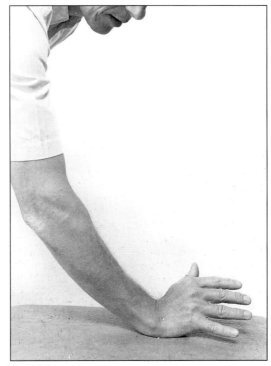

Fig 5.12a

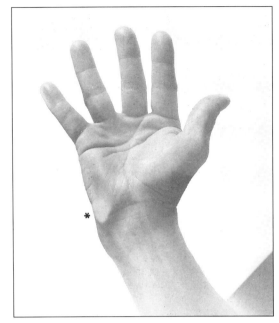

Fig 5.12b

ii) The student will often get the contact point correct but will not position the fingers in the inverted V bridge posture. This prevents the use of the hand to help take out the tissue slack under the hand contact and isolate contact point (fig. 5.13).

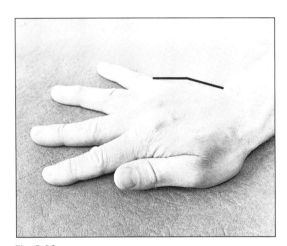

Fig 5.13

iii) Students tend to develop excessive and unnecessary tension in the muscles of the hand and fingers. The fingers should be relaxed sufficiently at all times in the arch posture so that they can be lifted with ease from the surface of the table. This will ensure only slight muscle contraction of the flexor muscles of the hand (fig. 5.14).

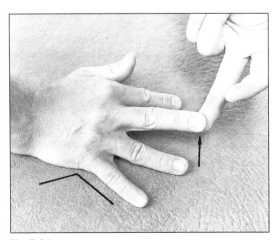

Fig 5.14

Variations of the Chiropractic Arch Hand Contact

The basic V-arched bridge posture of the hand (fig. 5.9a) provides the foundation for a number of other important hand configurations used during the application of other regional manipulative procedures. This hand posture provides the flexibility and the versatility necessary for the transition of manipulative forces between the doctor and the patient. The following variations describe three of the most important chiropractic arch derivatives.

Digital or Finger Tip/Goose-Neck Contact

1) With no supination or pronation of the hand or wrist, the hand is held over the edge of a table supporting the forearm with the elbow positioned at 90 degrees. The wrist is then dropped over the edge of the table maintaining the arch at the metacarpal joints (fig. 5.15). The hand posture is held firmly, but there is no excess tension in the muscles of the hand or arm. *There is a very small amount of ulnar deviation at the wrist.*

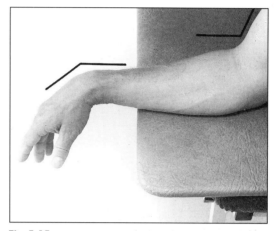

Fig 5.15

2) The middle finger is then reinforced by the index and ring fingers to stabilize and strengthen the arch and the middle finger and at the same time the wrist is flexed further, causing moderate tension in the flexor group of muscles of the forearm (fig. 5.16a). This focuses the force through the middle finger. The fingers should still be able to be moved, indicating minimal tension in the hand. This configuration is known as the 'goose-neck' posture and is used as a standard contact for many spinous process contact manipulative procedures in the lumbar spine. *Note* how the chiropractic arch is still maintained and the thumb is extended clear of the hand (fig. 5.16b). The finger pads provide a very good small but padded contact point. The 5th digit pinky extension is optional (*).

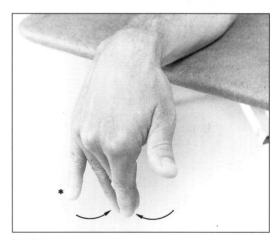

Fig 5.16a

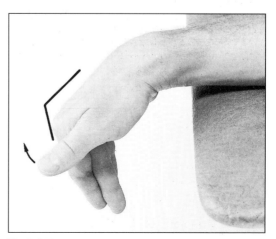

Fig 5.16b

3) There is one commonly encountered fault to be aware of when learning the goose-neck hand posture.

The wrist is not flexed to the desired 90 degrees, but still maintains the chiropractic arch (fig. 5.17). This compromises the mechanical advantage of the arched hand and the efficiency of the contact. The other problem is too little or too excessive tension in the forearm and hand.

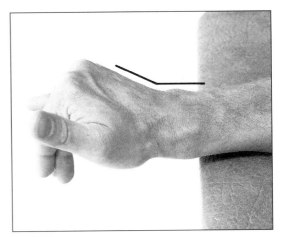

Fig 5.17

Index/Metacarpal/Interphalangeal Contact

The finesse and control associated with this particular contact is one of the most difficult to learn. This is in part due to the delicate and sensitive nature of the soft tissues of the cervical spine where this contact is most commonly used. The ability to maintain a firm, yet flexible and compliant contact with the tissue is the learning objective.

1) The starting position is the elbow at 90 degrees, the wrist held in the neutral position with the hand **totally** relaxed in ulnar deviation (fig. 5.18). There should be no flexion of the wrist (*). The wrist should feel floppy.

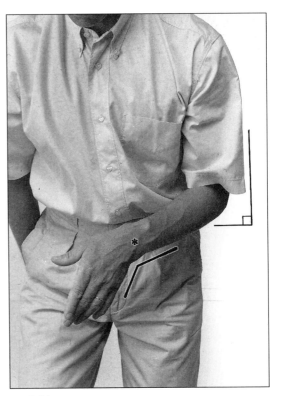

Fig 5.18

2) The hand is actively ulnar deviated, bringing the index finger almost perpendicular to the line of the forearm. This action exposes the actual interphalangeal contact points on the medial edge of the index finger (*). The thumb is simultaneously extended, making sure that the wrist remains neutral (fig. 5.19). The hand and fingers are still floppy and relaxed.

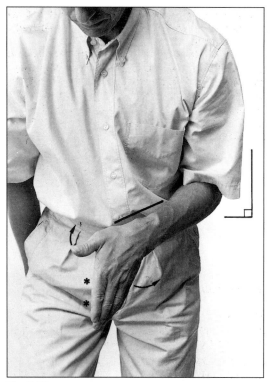

Fig 5.19

3) The final position for the completion of this skill brings the fingers together with slight flexion of the distal interphalangeal joints to support the index finger (the contact point). The fingers are firm, but not rigid (fig. 5.20). There should be a substantial amount of spring in the fingers, which are eventually used to cushion the contact on the sensitive cervical structures (*). **Forearm and hand are directly in line with a straight wrist**.

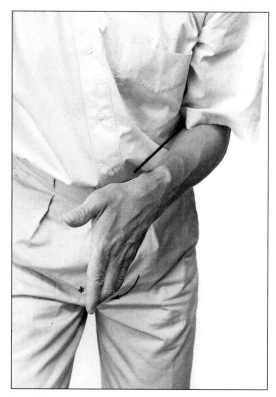

Fig 5.20

4) There are two major faults to be aware of when learning this contact.

i) During ulnar deviation of the hand the wrist has a tendency to flex excessively (fig. 5.21). The wrist is susceptible to injury during an impulse thrust in this position.

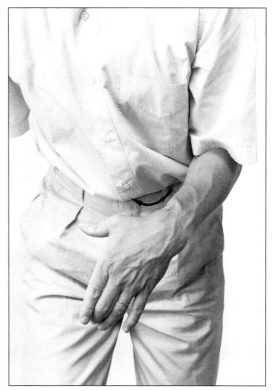

Fig 5.21

ii) The wrist is not ulnar deviated enough and consequently the metacarpal/interphalangeal contact point does not reach the perpendicular finishing position (fig. 5.22). In this posture the contact becomes too firm and broad, creating a push type thrust against sensitive structures of the spine.

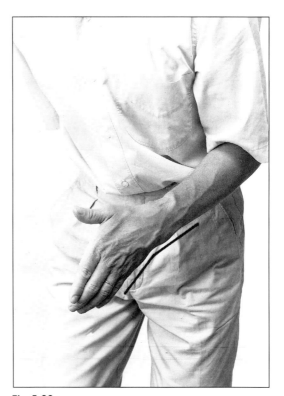

Fig 5.22

Thumb Contact

The thumb contact is used primarily in manipulative techniques associated with the cervicothoracic spine using the head as a lever and for rotary manipulation of the cervical spine. The thumb provides a particularly soft, fleshy contact for most spinous process contacts. As with the other contact skills, there are specific hand and arm movements which need to be rehearsed and learned before they can be applied in a clinical situation.

Remember, it is the slow and controlled movement patterns that are important. Keep in mind, the first metacarpophalangeal joint is vulnerable to injury and collapse when used in this fashion, reinforcing the need to strengthen the hand muscles overall and particularly the thenar eminence. Learning to brace the hand during the acquisition of these skills will protect the soft tissues.

1) The starting position is similar to the fingertip contact described in Figure 5.18 with the hand ulnar deviated in line with the forearm. The end of the table is grasped in a similar fashion to trapezius, with the hand arched and the fingers grasping the cushion (fig. 5.23). The shoulder is relaxed with no excess torsion keeping everything fairly symmetrical. **The elbow pivots around the wrist not the shoulder. The wrist, forearm and upper arm are kept in line and relaxed throughout this skill development. The arm is kept close to the body.**

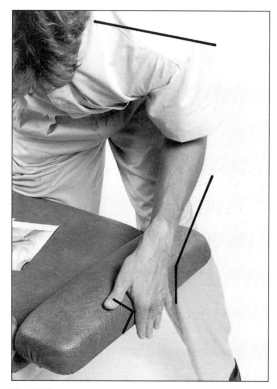

Fig 5.23

2) There are two learning faults to be aware of regarding thumb contact skills.

Insufficient ulnar deviation and flexion of the wrist without the pivot action of the arm and shoulder combine to distort the overall efficiency of the skill placing excess stress on the kinetic chain structures (fig. 5.24).

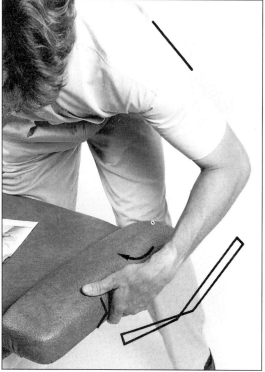

Fig 5.24

Metacarpal/Hypothenar Contact

The metacarpal/hypothenar contact is the fleshy lateral outside aspect of the hand which, although a minor contact point in terms of manipulative skills, provides a delicate yet firm surface. Although similar to other skills learned so far, the combination of these skills in various configurations is important in training the hands to consistently perform various fine and controlled movements.

1) The basic hand bridge is supinated perpendicular to the table from the prone position until the extreme lateral edge of the hypothenar eminence and the metacarpal aspect of the hand is in contact with the surface of table (fig. 5.25). The hand is relaxed.

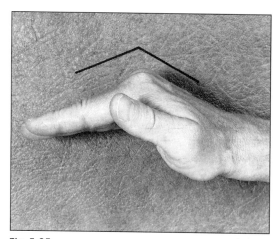

Fig 5.25

2) The wrist is then radially deviated slowly bringing the proximal aspect of the lateral edge of the hypothenar eminence into contact with the table to make the actual contact point firm. The wrist remains slightly flexed (fig. 5.26a). There will be some muscular contraction of the flexors and abductors of the hypothenar eminence so that the 5th digit remains flat on the contact and the contact point is firm (*) (fig. 5.26b).

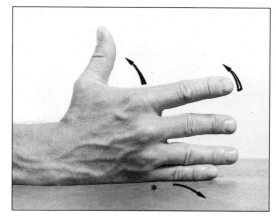

Fig 5.26a

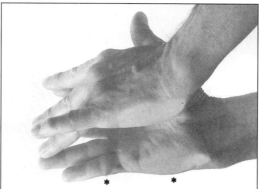

Fig 5.26b

3) There is only one minor error to be aware of during the learning of this hand skill.

There is a tendency to deviate the hand radially beyond what is necessary. This hardens the contact and causes excessive muscle contraction in the forearm, stressing the wrist (fig. 5.27) which also destabilizes the contact point.

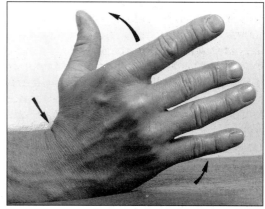

Fig 5.27

Thenar Contact

This contact has considerable clinical use as an acceptable alternative to the hypothenar/pisiform contact. The only problem is that the thenar contact is not as natural a hand position. It is also a slightly larger muscle mass, which may dissipate some of the thrust force. However, due to its muscle bulk, the thenar eminence offers considerable comfort for the patient and at the same time provides a specific contact point. There are two types of thenar contact, prone and supine. The prone contact is generally used for lower thoracic manipulation, whereas the supine thenar is most commonly used for the anterior thoracic and rib manipulative procedures.

Prone

1) From the basic chiropractic arch, the hand and forearm are slowly pronated until the thenar eminence comes into contact with the surface of the table (fig. 5.28). The arch is maintained and the hand is still slightly ulnar deviated. The pronation takes place at the wrist *only*.

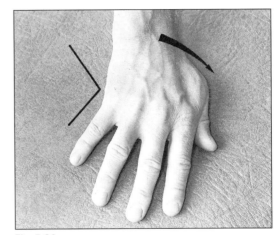

Fig 5.28

2) Tension is produced in the thenar muscles by adducting the thumb towards the index finger and the 4th and 5th digits are slightly elevated (fig. 5.29a). This ensures that the centre of the thenar eminence is in full contact with the table or anatomical landmark (*) (fig. 5.29b). The thumb and first two digits stabilize the hand.

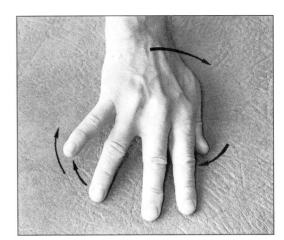

Fig 5.29a

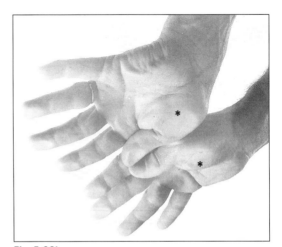

Fig 5.29b

3) There is one minor fault associated with learning this skill, namely over pronating the contact point which places internal torsional stress on the arm and shoulder. This is not a natural posture for the upper extremity and any excessive movement could result in a number of overuse problems in the future.

Supine

1) Begin with the hand flat on the table with the palm side up, fingers together and the thumb adducted close to the palm (fig. 5.30).

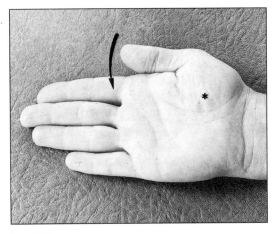

Fig 5.30

2) Adduct the thumb fully bringing it in line with the index finger (fig. 5.31). This maximizes the contraction of the thenar musculature (*) making the contact point firm yet comfortable for the patient.

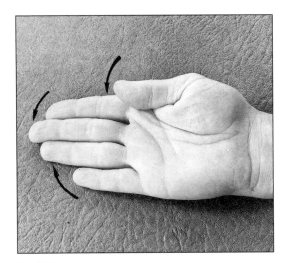

Fig 5.31

3) Flex the distal and proximal interphalangeal joints. This action gives the hand more depth making it a better fulcrum for anatomical contact (fig. 5.32). The hand is relatively relaxed and the thenar eminence is marginally contracted.

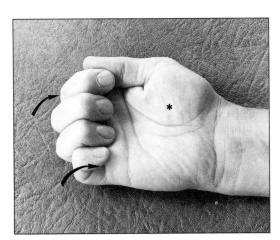

Fig 5.32

Conclusions

This chapter has presented a fairly comprehensive description of the more common hand contact postures associated with chiropractic manipulative therapeutics. The importance of being able to use one's hands skilfully and confidently during the application of spinal manipulative therapy has been emphasized. These are considered first order or basic skills, particularly at the undergraduate level. The significance of maintaining moderately firm hand and arm musculature without excessive joint ranges of motion at the wrist and elbow has also been highlighted to avoid unnecessary injury.

Careful attention and adherence to the sequential steps and fundamental movements adds to the overall process of manipulative skills learning, development and long-term fine tuning. The interface between the practitioner's hands and the patient as an integral aspect of that special clinical communication should not be carelessly overlooked.

References

Bolton, J.E. (1993) Methods of assessing low back pain and related psychological factors. *European Journal of Chiropractic*, **41**, 31–38

Christensen, K.D. (1984) Spinal manual manipulation procedures. In *Clinical Chiropractic Biomechanics*. Foot Levelers, Dubuque, p. 47

Grecco, M.A. (1953) Instruments. In *Chiropractic Technic Illustrated*. Jarl Publishing, New York, p. 51r

Mior, S.A. and Diakow, P.R. (1987) Prevalence of low back pain in chiropractors. *Journal of Manipulative and Physiological Therapeutics*, **10**, 305–309

Molumphy, M., Unger, B., Jensen, G.M. *et al.* (1985) Incidence of work-related low back pain in physical therapists. *Physical Therapy*, **65**, 482–486

Sale, D.G. (1988) Neural adaptation to resistance training. *Medicine Science Sports Exercise*, **20** (Supp), S135–S145

Schafer, R.C. and Faye, L.J. (1989) Introduction to the dynamic chiropractic paradigm. In *Motion Palpation and Chiropractic Technic: Principles of Dynamic Chiropractic*. Motion Palpation Institute, Huntington Beach, p. 35

Scholey, M. and Hair, M. (1989) Back pain in physiotherapists involved in back care education. *Ergonomics*, **32**, 179–190

States, A.Z. (1968) Atlas of Chiropractic Technic: Spinal and Pelvic Technic, 2nd edn. The National College of Chiropractic, Lombard, Illinois

Vernon, H. (1991) Chiropractic: a model of incorporating the illness behavior model in the management of low back pain patients. *Journal of Manipulative and Physiological Therapeutics*, **14**, 379–389

Chapter

6

Thrust skills and other movements

David Byfield

Introduction

Spinal manipulative therapy is heralded as the most commonly used form of treatment for low back pain (Haldeman, 1983) and is growing considerably in popularity and acceptance (Paris, 1983). Of the vast number of manipulative techniques within the field of manual medicine, it has been acknowledged that the high-velocity, low-amplitude, single, impulse-based short lever thrust technique is one of the oldest and most widely practised (Bourdillon and Day, 1987; Greenman, 1989; Bergmann, 1992). Meade *et al.* (1990) have suggested that the high velocity, low amplitude manipulation may be one of the specific components responsible for the effectiveness of chiropractic management in contrast to outpatient hospital care for the treatment of mechanical low back pain.

Definition

The term joint manipulation has always been plagued with an air of misunderstanding (Mennell, 1991). By definition, spinal manipulation is a general term that encompasses different manual techniques to restore and increase joint mobility (Fligg, 1984). It has also been described as any passive physical manoeuvre applied to the spine to increase either regional or segmental range of motion and can be subdivided into joint adjustment and joint mobilization (Byfield, 1991). Joint manipulation has been defined in two ways: a *skilled* passive

movement to a joint or spinal segment either within or beyond its active range of motion (Paris, 1983), or any manual operation or manoeuvre, specifically a *skilled* therapeutic use of a passive movement designed to restore motion (Nyberg, 1993). The terms mobilization, manipulation, and adjustment are regularly used interchangeably, often loosely, without any confusion (Fligg, 1984). However, a clear distinction between the use and application of the terms *adjustment* and *manipulation* continues to be a source of debate within the manipulating professions.

All manipulative procedures employ a high- or low-velocity thrust of variable amplitude applied through a long or short lever. High-velocity techniques may be referred to as adjustments and all low-velocity techniques as mobilizations (Szaraz, 1984). Schafer and Faye (1989) make a very similar classification using the term low-velocity techniques to apply to slow stretching, pulling and compression forces similar to mobilization. High-velocity techniques which incorporate a dynamic thrust are characteristic of a chiropractic adjustment. Mobilizations are low-velocity, repetitive oscillations whereas adjustments comprise a single high-velocity graded amplitude thrust (Fligg, 1984). Spinal manipulation can be classified into two categories (Haldeman, 1983; Shekelle *et al.*, 1992): non-specific, long lever manipulation and specific, high-velocity spinal adjustments closely identified with chiropractic practice. It has been proclaimed that the terms mobilization and manipulation are distinct and require separate definitions (Kirkaldy-Willis and Cassidy, 1985). Mobilization is a slower technique in which the joint remains within its passive range under the control of the patient, whereas manipulation is a faster technique which goes beyond the passive range without patient control (Chapman-Smith, 1991).

The term spinal manipulative therapy has gained popularity to represent all manipulative techniques applied to vertebral and non-vertebral articulations. It includes a very general and broad-based definition which includes all procedures used to mobilize, adjust, massage and stimulate the spine and paraspinal tissues (Grice and Vernon, 1992). Mobilization was defined as a form of non-thrust manipulation within the physiological passive range of joint motion, whereas adjustment is a carefully regulated thrust or force manipulation delivered at the end of the passive range of joint motion (Grice and Vernon, 1992).

A precise and lucid definition of a spinal or joint adjustment was presented by Sandoz (1976). This definition has since been adapted by Cassidy *et al.* (1992): 'manipulation is a *passive* manual manoeuvre during which a synovial joint is *suddenly* carried beyond the normal physiological range of motion without exceeding the boundaries of anatomical integrity'. The dominant characteristic is a *thrust* which is a brief, sudden and carefully delivered 'impulsion' given at the end of the normal passive range of movement and often accompanied by a joint cracking noise or other physiological responses. For the sake of clarity, the terms manipulation and adjustment will be considered the same in terms of manual therapy, and used reciprocally. The common denominator is the high-speed, low-amplitude dynamic impulse thrust.

Thrust Technique

The thrust (or impulse) is the transmission of a controlled force using a combination of muscular power, posture, and body weight. This is delivered at or near the end of the passive range of motion, the limit of the elastic properties of the joint capsule and surrounding soft tissue elements, the 'elastic barrier' or the point of 'tissue tension'. The thrust does not challenge or exceed the anatomical integrity of the joint. This particular skill is an art form of refined balance and accuracy, and a great deal of practice is required in order to acquire the necessary neuromuscular reflexes and competence to control and master it. The thrust has been described as the acceleration phase of the adjustment during which the force required for the correct impact velocity is reached (Haas, 1990a). In addition, quickness and depth control (amplitude) have been identified as the two most important psychomotor skills of joint manipulation (Haas, 1990b).

Quickness is a combination of both the high-velocity and short duration components of the impulse thrust which helps to maximize isolation of a specific joint. The low amplitude functions to protect the joint structures within the boundaries of anatomical integrity. To put this in quantifiable terms, Mennell (1991) has suggested that the extent of any joint play movement in any synovial joint is less than $\frac{1}{5}$ inch (5 mm) in any plane. Although this movement represents the 'give' in the joint's neutral position (Peterson and Bergmann, 1993), it may also give some indication of the depth that may be required during a manipulative thrust.

Manipulative or adjustive procedures are typically applied at the elastic resistance of a joint at the end of the passive range of motion. Movement beyond this point has been recorded in the 3–5 mm range during axial distraction and cavitation of the carpometacarpophalangeal joint (Sandoz, 1976). These are extremely small distances, indicating that the actual depth required for a physical change in joint mobility is probably minute. The results of axial traction of a finger joint should not be extrapolated to portray the complex mechanical behaviour of spinal or pelvic articulations. Nonetheless, the nature of these synovial joints should tolerate some reciprocity.

Furthermore, it could be argued that most of the forces and movement occurring during a manipulative procedure are being dissipated needlessly into the surrounding tissues and joints, whereas most of the skill is in the ability to isolate the manipulable lesion. This highlights the importance of long and short lever control within the physiological limit. Once this has been completed, the amount of force is actually diminutive. Developing the required palpatory and proprioceptive skills regarding tissue and patient tolerance is equally as important as a quick thrust.

Joint Tension Concepts

In addition to accomplishing control of the speed, force and depth components of the thrust, the student must initially learn to appreciate the proprioceptive concept of 'joint prestress' or 'preload' (Grice and Vernon, 1992) or the moment of joint locking (Schafer and Faye, 1989). This concept has also been referred to as 'preadjustive tension' (Haas, 1990b), 'prethrust' (Schafer and Faye, 1989), 'tension-set' (Maigne, 1985) or simply the *joint tension*. It is regarded as a 'feeling' of a gradual development of the point of maximum physiological resistance of the joint holding elements up to and including the elastic barrier of the targetted joint. This tissue feel is equally important during non-thrust mobilization procedures. This feeling or proprioceptive state has been referred to as 'tissue tension sense (TTS)'. It is an appreciation of the amount and quality of stretch or tension during movement of a muscle or joint (Grice *et al.*, 1985). Joint tension has also been associated with a process of *'taking up the slack'* during movement through both active and passive ranges of motion. Practice and experience allows the operator to gauge accurately the amount of force which can be safely applied to any tissue type or condition. TTS also permits the operator to identify the precise moment at which the thrust should be applied. It is analogous to hitting the 'sweet spot' in tennis jargon. This skill

economizes the amount of thrust force and energy required for cavitation and diminishes possible post-treatment injury (Haas, 1990b). A student must learn to appreciate this concept of control physically before thrusting skills are introduced. To do otherwise may contribute to poor skill development and performance. Learning to appreciate the viscoelastic properties of a joint requires a visual working knowledge of joint kinematics, facet angulation and surrounding holding elements. TTS helps the manipulator to coordinate each component of the manipulative procedure into purposeful, slow movements and an overall smooth rhythm. No amount of verbal reassurance can substitute for the patient's awareness of the abilities of the clinician. The contact between the practitioner and the patient is a physical one which is sensitive to the pressure of the doctor's hands. Patient compliance, relaxation and satisfaction are vital components for successful patient management. Developing a refined TTS will at least guarantee that a minimum of force will be applied.

Objective Feedback

The need for objective systems of measuring the performance of chiropractic psychomotor skills during undergraduate training is becoming more apparent. This is of particular importance with respect to the depth and speed of the dynamic thrust. Corlett (1992) investigated the relationship between chiropractic training and the speed and amplitude of a toggle thrust using an adjusting simulator. He found that over the range of 4 years of chiropractic skills training, the speed of the toggle thrust did not change; however the amplitude of a toggle thrust significantly decreased with training and by the fourth year the students had learned to control the amplitude of thrust and maintain a high speed of performance. Byfield *et al.* (1995) have also shown that it is possible to measure quantitatively the forces and displacement occurring during simulated joint play palpation, which may provide valuable feedback during the learning process. The use of such models and possibly high-speed video facilities to record and monitor skill performance may provide more helpful educational feedback.

General Considerations of the Thrust Technique

Characteristics, Localization, Direction, Speed and Modifying Factors

The thrust is only one aspect of the overall manipulative procedure. It is the skill that is applied last and only after a series of doctor and patient preparatory steps have been performed. A combination of patient relaxation, joint isolation, posture and thrust specificity should equate to minimal thrust force. Absolute concentration and attention to the learning task is mandatory. Even though the biomechanical and neurological effects of manipulation are mostly speculative at this point (Cassidy *et al.*, 1992), there is a large body of evidence that documents the deleterious effects of spinal manipulative therapy as a result of inadequate skills and poor technique selection. Applying the same manipulative thrust in terms of depth and speed to each patient with total disregard for their specific needs is not good clinical judgement. It is the *responsibility* of the doctor to apply the appropriate manipulative skill or technique at the most appropriate time. **Not all patients either require or respond favourably to high-velocity thrust manipulation**.

A manipulative or adjustive thrust is a sudden, *non-aggressive* impulse. It has been described as a clean, crisp, sharp, lightning fast, rapid muscular contraction. The speed, direction and force of a thrust are all specific and gaugeable characteristics which are determined by the clinician's skill matched with the patient's needs. The anatomical nature, position and kinematic behaviour of the dysfunctional joint are significant determining factors. The force is adjusted to match the inherent resistance threshold of the patient's tissue, which if exceeded could

cause possible injury. Another characteristic of the thrust is its versatility. The thrust is introduced on a therapeutic basis throughout the entire spine and pelvic girdle and just as effectively treating dysfunction of all the extremities. Above all the most unique characteristics of the thrust are its speed, control and specificity of force application.

Nyberg (1993) suggests that 'a skilled manipulative therapist has *quick acting hands* capable of high speed, low force activity'. The high-velocity decreases the possibility of dissipating the forces and affecting adjacent tissues and joints. A slower thrust velocity requires more force, increasing the chances of local tissue damage. It has been shown that cavitation occurs with greater consistency, at a faster rate and with less force when a manipulative thrust is applied at joint tension when compared to introducing a steady and gradually increasing force (Conway *et al.*, 1992). This rate of change of force was identified as the most significant mechanical factor required for cavitation. The product of time and force ($Ft = M\Delta V$) is called the impulsive force or impulse (LeVeau, 1992). This apparent rate of change of momentum or impulse seems to be a time-dependent variable.

High-velocity procedures are extremely quick and very close to physiological reaction times (Triano, 1992). This may imply that the biomechanical and neurophysiological effects of manipulation may take place before any protective muscle splinting can occur. A patient's muscular response can modify the applied manipulative load, suggesting that a technically slow manipulation will require more force to overcome the patient's muscular reaction. McCarthy (1993, personal communication) suggests that a thrust which is faster than normal reaction time is not compressing the tissues for a long enough period to cause sufficient damage and a nociceptive response. Stretching or compressing sensitive tissue for a very short period is done within the limit of anatomical integrity. If the procedure is performed slowly, the clinician may theoretically have to go much further to sustain the same results, possibly compromising the integrity of the joint. This appears to be directly related to the elastic nature of the tissue. A slow and prolonged procedure could increase tension in the surrounding muscles sufficiently to restrict blood supply, causing local ischaemia. A sustained state of distension or tension along the length of the musculoligamentous system could stretch the collagen/elastin mechanism beyond its elastic limit, resulting in a fatigue state (McCarthy, 1993, personal communication). A skilled manipulative thrust lies within the protective physiological barrier of the joint (elastic barrier) as a direct consequence of the depth.

The duration and quickness of the thrust do not act independently (Haas, 1990b). A relatively large velocity or slow impulse thrust will increase the depth and overdistend local tissue (Haas, 1990b). That brief sharp pain reported by patients during a dynamic thrust may be stimulating the rapidly conducting myelinated A-fibres but not of sufficient enough threshold to trigger the unmyelinated C-fibre system responsible for deep, dull somatic pain. The brisk nature of the thrust may cause a rapid contraction of the local muscles followed by a long slow relaxation recovery period, which could suggest reflex inhibition through activation and modulation by descending fibres. This could be responsible for the immediate and observable changes in local tissue tone, pain appreciation and increase in range of motion. Therefore, the dynamic impulse thrust has many built-in safety features including rapid speed, low amplitude and precise localization which are more effective when a level of competence is attained (Nyberg, 1993).

The ability to localize and focus precisely the thrust force to a single joint is somewhat idealistic. The multisegmental nature and biomechanical effects of the posterior ligamentous system and the thoracolumbar fascia tend to distort this concept. Yet many still regard localization as an important manipulative skill (Maigne, 1972; Bourdillon and Day, 1987). The concept of specificity still remains a source of controversy and great debate. There are simply too many variables to control. The clinical objective is to *minimize* the effects of the mechanical thrust on surrounding healthy joint structures and holding elements. This may become an important factor when segmental instability has been identified. Forces of between 20 and 100 N applied over the L3 spinous during posterior–anterior mobilization have been shown to cause movement in the whole lumbar and lower thoracic spine, indicating that these manual movements do not cause a local response (Lee and Svensson, 1993). Static loading caused less displacement than cyclic application. Therefore methods to moderate this spillover effect would be clinically advantageous. We have to view specificity in a full biomechanical context and not just the effects on the bone. The force of any manipulative procedure must pass through and be absorbed by many layers of muscle and ligaments before the deeper joint structures are affected (Schneider, 1992).

Specificity and force localization implies a high degree of patient control, exactness of hand position for thrust, and postural control. Maigne (1972) states that dexterity and experience are prerequisites for maintaining control and correct patient positioning in order to execute these precise movements. Correctly positioning the patient permits the clinician to stabilize or lock (Bourdillon and Day, 1987; Nyberg, 1993) the joints above and below the targetted lesion. This process requires that the clinician be in absolute control of a relaxed patient at all times during the procedure. The skill also involves a certain amount of palpatory ability. The clinician can monitor the perceived tension in both the joints and the surrounding soft tissues as the patient is being positioned. Any attempt by the patient to assist should be firmly rejected. Patient assistance distracts the clinician and contributes to unwanted tension and poor TTS. Therefore, movements to position the patient should be smooth, slow, methodical and deliberate. The ability to establish patient relaxation and cooperation is one of the most common deterrents encountered during manipulative skills learning. Recognizing and monitoring patient feedback is the total responsibility of the clinician. It is clinically irresponsible to continue to treat an unusually tense and uncooperative patient. The point of joint tension cannot be fully appreciated under these circumstances and applying a dynamic thrust would not be in the patient's best interest.

Precise positioning of both patient and doctor should increase the likelihood that the direction of the thrust will be: (i) parallel to the plane of the intersegmental facets; (ii) in the direction of the loss of joint play, (iii) in the direction of the loss of active movement, (iv) in the direction of pain-free movement and (v) in a direction which stretches the holding elements at the greatest point of resistance. The shape of the articulating facets controls the kinematic behaviour of the motion segment and the effect of the manipulative forces (Grice, 1980). Visual and functional knowledge of these crucial factors should contribute to successful skill acquisition.

Amount of Force Application

Individual Factors

The final stage of the manipulation or adjustment is the introduction of the dynamic thrust. There are several factors which determine the amount of force to apply to the patient. Age, sex, general health, specific condition, stiffness, muscle spasm, chronicity, patient compliance, manipulative position, sizes of the patient and doctor are only a few of the general modulating variables. It has been suggested that 'the skill of a therapist is inversely proportional to the amount of force utilized' (Nyberg, 1993). **The majority of the skill is in the preparation of the patient and the position of the doctor**. Under these circumstances the amount of therapeutic force is minimal.

The amount of tissue between the doctor's hand contact and the anatomical contact on the patient influences the amount of force the patient receives (Plaugher, 1993). The more soft tissue at this interface, the greater the amount of force that is required. Energy is slowly transferred

and the force is dissipated into the surrounding soft tissues, reducing the efficiency of the manipulation. Therefore, contact points that minimize this dampening effect but maintain patient comfort should be selected (Plaugher, 1993). The pisiform traditionally features as a good example of this concept, compared with either the thenar or hypothenar eminences. On the other hand (so to speak), experience has shown that students often hyperextend the wrist and lift the fingers off the patient during a pisiform contact, which may potentially sprain the wrist over a period of time. The force should be transferred from the trunk through the hand to the patient, not the wrist. It is recommended (as discussed in Chapter 5) that a combined pisiform/hypothenar contact be incorporated which still maintains specificity, a stable hand contact and a cushioning effect without significantly compromising the efficiency of the procedure. The finger and thumb pads also represent ideal contact areas. These digital contacts are relatively small, making anatomical location direct and sufficiently padded, providing sufficient comfort to the patient. The fingers provide simultaneous palpatory function during joint tension procedures. The hand and fingers must be strong in order to meet these demands and perform them safely and efficiently. The lateral aspects of the phalanges of the index finger also provide a specific and padded contact point commonly used during cervical manipulation. The thenar and hypothenar eminences are well padded but large in comparison to the finger pads. Learning to contract and isolate these muscle groups ensures reasonable specificity yet maintains some cushioning effect.

Patient Position

The amount of thrust force applied is also significantly influenced by the various patient positions. The ability to control and stabilize patient movement is indirectly proportional to the energy used and applied thrust force. Non-weightbearing postures which naturally reduce muscular tension are optimal for this relationship.

The side posture technique displays less control and consequently more force overall, but the long levers enable the doctor to localize the point of counter-rotation accurately, increasing the specificity of the manipulation. Consequently, more skills are incorporated during this procedure. The prone position affords almost total patient control, but achieving adequate joint tension is more difficult, elevating preload forces and compromising specificity. Using the head as a lever in the prone position for upper thoracic dysfunction improves the situation. Joint tension in the thoracic spine in the supine position is accomplished mainly by trunk flexion; however patient control is marginal and large amounts of the thrust force are dissipated through the rib cage. Supine cervical manipulation with head support has a high degree of control, specificity and low force thrust. Sitting and standing postures are naturally more difficult due to the relative lack of patient control which increases energy used, forces applied and depth of thrust. A good clinician should develop skill to perform competently a variety of manipulative procedures in several postures to meet the demands of the patient. Clinicians should also be realistic with respect to their own abilities, strength and size. It appears that training and experience produce a greater similarity in the recorded thrust forces in the left and right hand in comparison to chiropractic students when using an adjustment simulator (Wood and Adams, 1984). This suggests that an experienced practitioner does develop bilateral dexterity, skill and equality of thrust application with practice. This is an essential characteristic for consistent and controlled thrust application. It has also been shown that stronger subjects were able to deliver more forceful thrusts and that chiropractors were more skilled at using their body weight and height to increase manipulative force when compared to a student group (Adams and Wood, 1984).

Anatomical Lever

The choice of anatomical short lever point at the doctor/patient interface strongly influences the amount of force the patient receives. Short levers encourage specificity but their use requires greater skill acquisition. Long lever manipulation is considerably easier for the doctor, but features a lack of overall patient control and subsequent safety. The spinous and transverse processes, and the PSIS are the most common contact points, yet laminar, mamillary, mastoid and ischial contacts are frequently used. The spinous process is probably the most ideal in terms of specificity compared to the mamillary and transverse contacts partly as a result of the amount of intervening soft tissue. The combination of a pisiform/hypothenar contact on a mamillary process in the lumbar spine equates to a greater amount of manipulative force dissipated compared to a fingertip contact on the spinous process for the same clinical outcome. The ischial tuberosity is a common yet poor contact point due to its size and the amount of overlying muscular tissue, requiring considerable strength and force to achieve mechanical leverage of the sacroiliac joint. The broader hand contact over the patient dissipates force over a larger area, needlessly involving otherwise normal joints and soft tissues. This is not clinically advantageous when specificity is required. A degree of pressure is maintained at the contact point in order to secure accuracy of the thrust. This pressure should be minimal. The size of the patient and the amount of subcutaneous fat also influence the choice of anatomical landmark. In many cases specificity would have to be moderated at the expense of patient comfort and vice versa.

Postural Stance

Posture and balance will be addressed throughout this text as an important modulating parameter when learning manipulative skills. Both patient and doctor considerations will be presented in the individual chapters. The use and position of the doctor's body weight, relative to the patient and the gravity line, should reduce the amount of muscular effort and subsequently decrease the overall forces applied. In the long term this should have beneficial effects in terms of less mechanical stress on the doctor and increased therapeutic compliance by the patient. For example, Kirby *et al.* (1987) verified that foot position is an important determinant of standing balance. They found that postural sway was less with the feet 15 cm apart than with the feet together, but was not affected by a further increase in the base width beyond this point. This suggests that postural balance is significantly improved when the feet are positioned about hip distance apart. This is a recommended stance posture which will be presented in more detail during the skills section of this chapter and relevant subsequent chapters.

The more specific and accurate the contact, all other factors and skills considered, the less manipulative force required. Under these conditions, both doctor and patient benefit. Specific manipulation eliminates many variables, which may improve the likelihood of a positive treatment outcome. Locating anatomical landmarks is not as easy as it seems, but it is an essential prerequisite for specific manipulation. The exact placement of the hand and stabilization of the contact interface throughout the entire procedure are difficult skills to master. However, as palpatory and proprioceptive skills improve, the student will learn to appreciate the physical components of specificity and its overall importance. Slow, methodical movements should be continually reinforced, which promotes an appreciation of the subtle changes taking place in the underlying tissue. Students will begin to learn that safe and effective manipulative procedures are accomplished by applying slow and gentle forces with a strictly controlled amplitude. A common learning error encountered by students is their preoccupation with attempting to contact the periosteum of the pisiform with the periosteum of a transverse process. The student must realize that, in reality, most of our patients are covered by many layers of pain-sensitive soft tissue and are not denuded skeletons as depicted in many technique books published to date.

Summary

The following exercises and movements are designed to help develop efficient dynamic thrusting skills. Con-sideration should also be given to the individual muscles which are primarily involved in each thrust skill. Active visualization of each muscle group and its action will help to facilitate both learning and execution of the particular skill. Of primary importance are the triceps, pectoralis major and minor, biceps, anterior deltoid, serratus anterior and the quadriceps. Understanding the origin, insertion and action of these muscles may assist the learning process. These specific muscle groups are very strong and capable of accelerating body parts at great speed, causing substantial impact velocities. The object of the training exercise is to learn to move these levers as quickly as possible over the shortest distance using the least amount of energy without unnecessary substitution. The following thrust skills should be introduced *immediately* as part of the undergraduate psychomotor motor skills training. Attempting to apply a manipulative thrust without adequate training may result in excessive and forceful movements reinforcing poor professional skills.

Educational Relevance

One may argue that thrusting aimlessly into the air has absolutely no clinical relevance and yields little benefit at the pre-clinical level. This method may reinforce the notion that manipulative thrust has only one speed and one depth. Clearly, this is clinically unrealistic. This approach could also fortify the 'pounding' or 'pile driving' action often observed in undergraduates who typically release the joint preload prior to the thrust (Schafer and Faye, 1989; Grice and Vernon, 1992). This may be the case, but by ranking the importance of these skills as part of a much larger picture and by providing a rationale and clinical perspective, the credibility of these methods may be salvaged. Demonstrating how and when these thrusting skills are actually applied and learning to perform them in their clinical postures may be laudable. Emphasizing the specific thrust skills at the same time as the individual adjustments are being demonstrated may also be of some value in the learning experience. Practising active visualization of the individual tasks may also be of considerable benefit during these simulated exercises. The process should at least introduce the student to the proprioceptive balance and body weight control that will be required.

The primary objective is to learn to contract and isolate specific muscle groups whilst keeping other regions of the body stable. The next objective is to learn to contract them very quickly against resistance, and the last step is to gauge the depth of contraction in a simulated fashion. The muscular power, overall postural control and stability of the body dictate the speed and depth of a manipulative thrust. Speed is attained by practice. The student must realize that the amount of force actually necessary to cavitate or overcome the elastic barrier is extremely small (Cassidy *et al.* 1992).

Each of the following skills is to be practised daily, concentrating on isolating and *contracting the individual muscle first, depth second and speed last.* In order to maximize each practice session, it would be advisable to warmup the major muscle groups using light exercise and slow stretch techniques. Preparing muscle groups for explosive work is advisable to reduce injuries. It is also recommended that students balance their upper body strength and flexibility to develop bilateral dexterity and ensure an equal force is applied with either the left or right hand (Wood and Adams, 1984). A swimming programme complemented with light weights would be of great benefit.

In addition, the practitioner's posture is an important element during the learning and acquisition of these thrust skills. The position of the centre of gravity and the alignment of body weight are major contributions. Even though this is mainly done through simulation, it is important that the exercises re-create the clinical context as closely as possible. Furthermore, understanding that an efficient thrust is a total body commitment is a major hurdle to overcome. Therefore, the doctor must be comfortable, relaxed and flexible. A keen sense of body position and awareness is an additional key factor. The importance of overall good posture not only reduces mechanical overload, but maximizes the efficiency and benefits of the manipulative procedure.

This chapter presents many types of the high-velocity, low-amplitude thrusts. Individual skills should be learned for each set of muscle groups responsible for a particular thrust type. They should be practised in a variety of postures as the required skills are considered specific for a certain movement pattern and non-transferable (Cohen *et al.*, 1993).

Fencer or Lunge Stance

It is recommended that the following postural skill be learned prior to the thrusting skills presented later in the chapter. The optimal position is an angled 45 degrees stance with the majority of the body weight supported by the front leg, which adds symmetry and minimizes torque in the upper back and lumbopelvic regions. This has been referred to as the 'fencer' or 'lunge' stance position (Szaraz, 1984). This position permits the doctor to lean over the patient, providing more efficient use of the arms and upper body weight. The doctor can incorporate valuable visual cues and it also prepares the lower body for an efficient drop thrust.

Ski Stance to Fencer Stance (45 Degree Pivot Shift)

1) Stand with the feet hip distance apart (about 15–18 cm inside foot distance), the knees bent with the centre of the knee joint directly over the transverse metatarsal arch of each foot. The trunk is inclined slightly with the head looking down and focusing on a point just ahead of the feet. This is the *ski stance* (fig. 6.1). The shoulders and arms are relaxed and the majority of the body weight is over the metatarsal joints. There should be a degree of spring in the doctor's legs. The arms are held comfortably in front or behind the back.

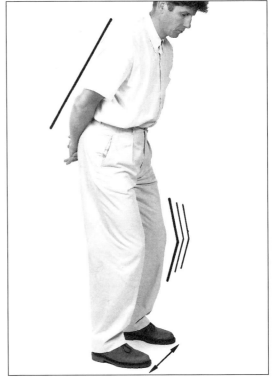

Fig 6.1

2) Push up on the metatarsal pads and slowly shift or twist 45 degrees in either direction maintaining original posture (fig. 6.2). The shoulders, hips, knees and feet are all facing 45 degrees from the coronal plane of the body.

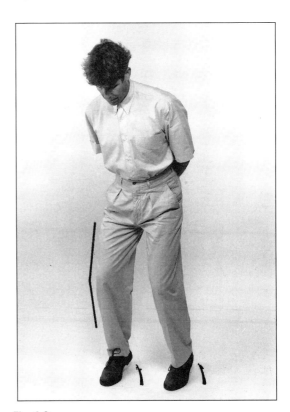

Fig 6.2

3) Pivot complete, plant flex the rear foot of the trailing leg. This effectively pushes the body weight over the front leg (fig. 6.3a). The front leg should be springy, absorbing most of the body weight. The front foot is not completely flat as the weight is borne mainly over the metatarsals. The effect is to transfer the body weight over the front leg to simulate leaning over a patient. Figure 6.3b illustrates a true fencer stance.

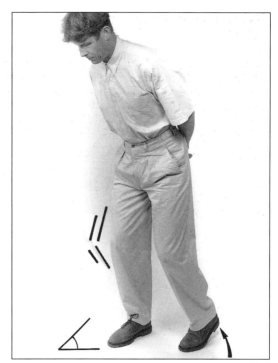

Fig 6.3a

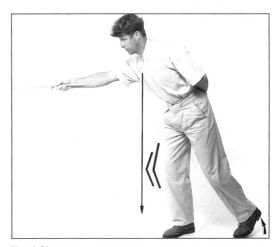

Fig 6.3b

This is a movement pattern that will be repeated thousands of times during the course of a clinical career. It is a very simple yet effective movement for shifting and positioning body weight for many of the side and prone posture manipulative procedures. **Practise in both directions**.

Next repeat the same movement patterns standing next to a chiropractic table.

1) Stand perpendicular to the table with the feet under the edge of the table but still in view from just behind the metatarsal heads and the knees just away from the edge (fig. 6.4). The feet in this approximate position will ensure adequate room to move with a patient. Standing too far away from the table misaligns the centre of gravity. The student must become comfortable and learn to stand very close to the table to stabilize the patient's weight and ensure safe positioning.

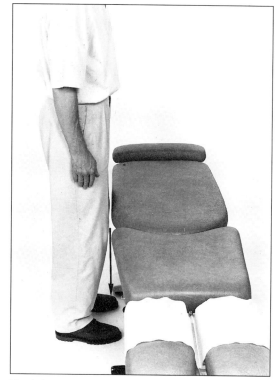

Fig 6.4

2) Pivot shift 45 degrees to the left or right into a fencer stance posture by twisting on the metatarsal pads (fig. 6.5). Keep shoulders, hips, knees, and feet at 45 degrees to the table. Notice how this posture brings the trunk and body weight over the table. The legs are just in contact with the table and the front knee is just slightly away. This doctor/table interface is very close. Practise leaning against the table to learn to feel the table close to the legs.

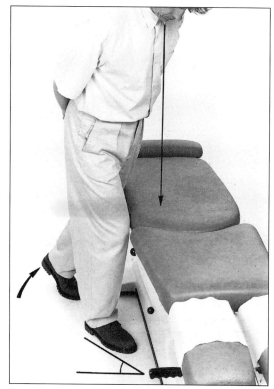

Fig 6.5

3) The most common error encountered is adopting a very wide foot stance and a greater than 45 degrees to the table (fig. 6.6). This position affords little or no spring to the legs and body drop techniques are difficult to perform. The trunk weight is also positioned too far back instead of over the front leg.

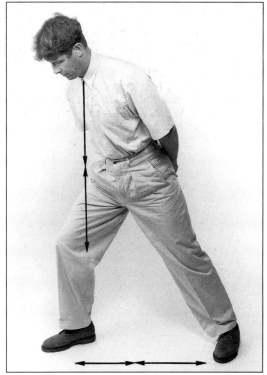

Fig 6.6

Practise this movement skill on a regular basis to become comfortable with the ease of movement and the *small amount of movement actually required*. Perform the movement slowly and deliberately. It does appear easy but it has to be performed automatically when subsequent skills are introduced. Leaning against the side of the table supports some of the body weight but still allows flexibility for doctor movement and body drop thrust. Maintaining the correct distance between the feet ensures that the doctor is dynamic and in control of the patient throughout the entire procedure.

This posture and set of movement skills is an integral and a fundamental part of the following thrust skills. Before introduction to the thrust skills it is advisable that the fencer stance movement sequence is firmly in place. Learning the thrust skills in a common stance provides clinical relevance.

Thrust Skills

Triceps Flick (Unilateral)

This is the most basic of the upper extremity manipulative thrust skills. It is meant to isolate the triceps extensor group which is recruited in many of the common chiropractic manipulative procedures including, most notably, the toggle recoil. The triceps thrust can be used by itself or as part of an overall shoulder/arm thrust through a hand contact. The objective of this introductory exercise is to isolate and contract the triceps equally on left and right sides. Initially, concentrate and visualize isolation of the triceps only and the desired movement. In order to increase the explosive nature of the skill, it may be effective for the student to expel a small amount of air through either the mouth or the nostrils during triceps contraction. This is the essence of the impulse thrust as described by Faye (Schafer and Faye, 1989) as coming from the diaphragm when coughing or spitting. This is only a brief expulsion of air simultaneously with the muscle contraction. The expulsion of air is a skill itself and does assist speed and concentration. No projectile objects please. Naturally, developing skills equally on both sides is recommended (this does not refer to the nose, of course).

1) The doctor stands with feet hip distance apart with slight flexion at both the hip and knee joints (ski stance). The trunk is flexed forward about 20 degrees with the right arm hanging loosely out in front with the natural bend at the elbow. The head is slightly flexed forward. The left arm is held behind the back (fig. 6.7). The entire upper body is relaxed with most of the body weight balanced over the centre of the knees. There is no excess tension in the musculoskeletal system.

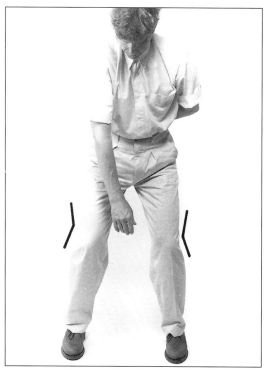

Fig 6.7

2) Contract the triceps slowly to cause extension of the forearm at the elbow only. The forearm should swing like a *pendulum*. The upper arm, shoulder and the entire upper body including the head and trunk remain completely still and relaxed (*) (fig. 6.8). Repeat the contraction with a rest in between. **Do not lift the forearm or hand prior to contracting the triceps or rigidly hyperextend the elbow or push the arm**. After each contraction the forearm should rebound or *recoil* in a bouncing like fashion. The doctor expels a small amount of air through the mouth prior to each contractive thrust. Ensure that there is sufficient time between contractions for adequate recovery. Contraction should be clean and sharp.

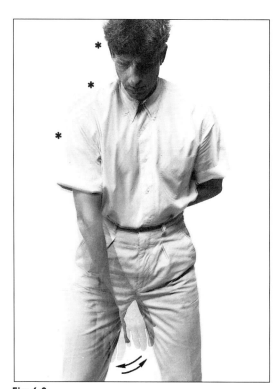

Fig 6.8

3) Repeat with the left arm and then with both arms simultaneously (fig. 6.9). The doctor's posture should be relaxed at all times in the ski stance. There should be no tension in the upper body during this skill.

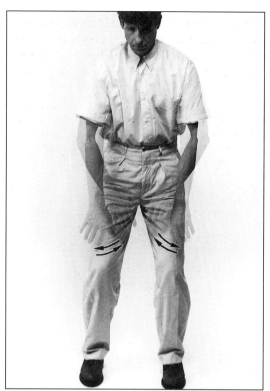

Fig 6.9

The triceps flick represents the basic manipulative reflex thrust. It should be practised for a period of time, on both sides and in various postures until moving on to more advanced movements. The ability to isolate this muscle group is an important step and should not be rushed. Attention should also be given to establishing good and effective posture. This is the time during which postural patterns are reinforced. Initially, there may be an awkward feeling; however with time the patterns will begin to feel more natural.

Double Triceps Flick (Preliminary Toggle Recoil)

1) Begin in the ski stance with both arms hanging freely with the thumbs interlaced. The hands are positioned just below the suprasternal notch (fig. 6.10a). The stance is relaxed at all times with the body weight positioned over the metatarsal pads, upper trunk weight slightly forward and the shoulders relaxed. The knees are bent with a certain amount of natural spring for body flexibility (fig. 6.10b).

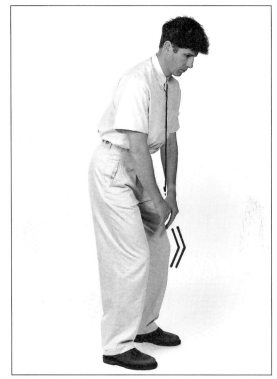

Fig 6.10a

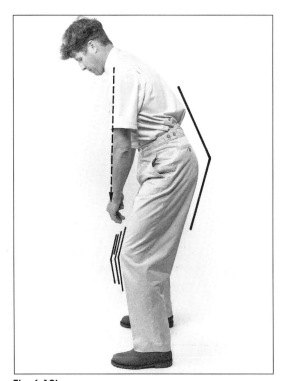

Fig 6.10b

2) Contract both triceps simultaneously in a slow and controlled fashion initially. There will be some contraction of the pectoralis to assist. Expel air during each thrust contraction; *do not lock out* the elbows, and *do not push* the arms. The resultant action is a **rebound or recoiling of the hands** which is due to the natural elastic properties of the tissue. The hands and arms should bounce up and down after each contraction (fig. 6.11). There should be no stress placed upon the elbow joint. The recoil is **not** an active or voluntary action. The head, trunk and upper arms are stable during this exercise (*).

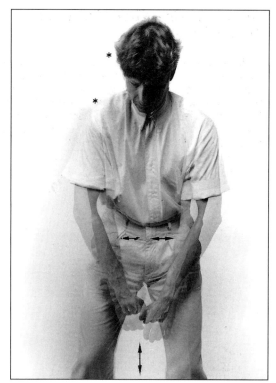

Fig 6.11

This skill should be practised with the same enthusiasm and commitment as the triceps flick. Practise it slowly and try not to see how many contractions you can perform in 60 seconds. The Guinness Book of World Records is not interested. Control each contraction, concentrate, feel what is happening, check your posture, including bent knees, head position over the hands, and expel air through the mouth. The key is to take your time and practise regularly. A few minutes at regular intervals until the skill is performed efficiently is recommended. Intermittently or only during class time is not adequate to reinforce the movement patterns. I know many experienced chiropractors who warm-up in the morning using these skills before they begin treating patients. They perform flexibility exercises as well as thrusting exercises to stimulate the reflex movement patterns they will be using all day. Practise the skills in both the ski and fencer stance to develop symmetry and variety.

Wrist Flick (Unilateral & Bilateral)

1) The arms are held close to the side of the body with the elbows flexed and positioned at 90 degrees. The wrists are held relaxed in a natural ulnar-deviated posture. The doctor is standing in a ski stance posture with the suprasternal notch positioned over the hands (fig. 6.12). There should be spring in both hands and legs but the head and upper body should be completely relaxed and motionless.

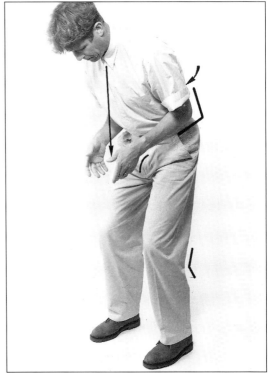

Fig 6.12

2) The wrist **only** is flicked rapidly into ulnar deviation by contraction of the flexor carpi ulnaris alone (fig. 6.13a). The body is totally relaxed especially the head and shoulders. The trunk is also totally immobile′(*). The position of the arms does not change. The doctor expels a small amount of air during each contraction. This particular skill is important during controlled rotary manipulation of the cervical spine. Perform the skill in the sitting posture to increase stability and simulate a clinical situation (fig. 6.13b). Start very slowly and then increase the speed gradually. Try to flick one wrist at a time followed by the two. Keep the head over the hands at all times and the arms tucked in close to the body.

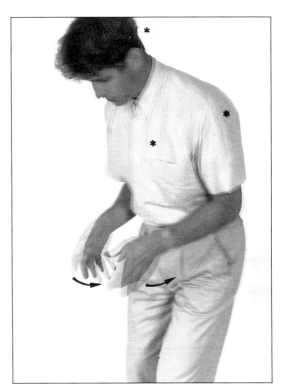

Fig 6.13a

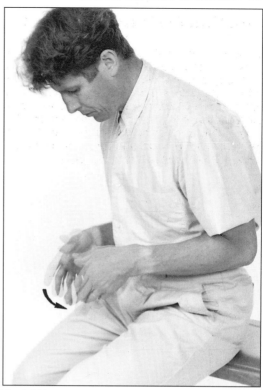

Fig 6.13b

Pectoralis Thrust

A dynamic thrust of pectoralis major muscle is incorporated into many manipulative procedures of the spine and pelvis (Szaraz, 1984). Its anatomical position as an integral part of the shoulder girdle and its function which includes adduction and flexion of the arm provides an excellent lever for a dynamic thrust. Many of the more common manipulative procedures thrust towards or across the body with the arm in a position of flexion. For this reason it is vitally important to learn to isolate and strengthen this muscle group, both sternal and clavicular sections. Start the exercise slowly in order to feel the isolation of the muscle group and then gradually increase the speed and intensity. Do not rush or push this activity. The objective is to learn to contract each pectoralis group individually and then simultaneously. The skills are to be learned in both the ski and fencer stances to simulate clinical postures.

1) The doctor is positioned in the ski stance. The arms are held out and flexed in front of the body and interlaced at the elbows with the web of each hand (fig. 6.14). The contact at the elbow is very light. The arms are in a relaxed state, weight is borne on springy knees and the trunk is totally stable.

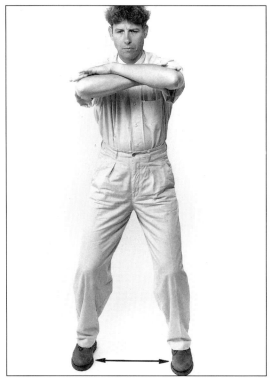

Fig 6.14

2) Rapidly adduct one pectoralis/arm first followed by the second after a small refractory period (clavicular head). The head and trunk are completely motionless and stable (*) (fig. 6.15). The movement will be limited by isometric contraction of the opposite side. Do not pull back and push. As the ability to isolate one muscle group improves, increase the speed and force gradually. **Expel** a small amount of air with each contraction. Rest between each contraction. Use the breath cycle to gauge the next thrust.

Concentrate during the exercise and **visualize** each muscle group contracting.

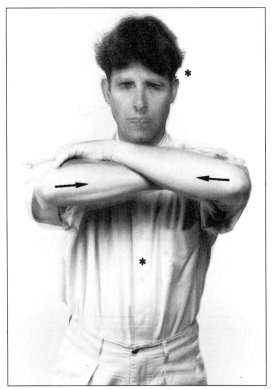

Fig 6.15

3) Adduct each arm individually, contracting the sternal head of the pectoralis major only (fig. 6.16). The head and trunk remain completely motionless (*). **Expel air** and concentrate on the motor action. Start slowly and increase both speed and force of contraction. Do not pull back and push, causing a hitting or slapping effect. The effect is a short, sharp and crisp thrust.

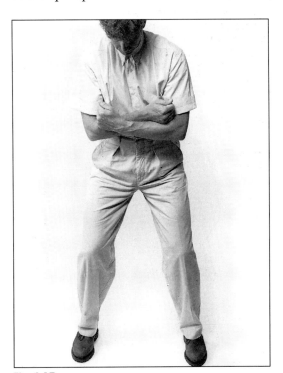

Fig 6.16

Shoulder/Arm Pull Thrust

This is a variation of the pectoralis thrust but performed in the opposite direction. It is incorporated in a variety of manipulative procedures of the extremities and manipulations of both the cervical and lumbar spine, requiring a pulling type action during the thrust. The muscles used are primarily the shoulder extensors and abductors, namely latissimus dorsi, teres major, deltoid, triceps (long head) and supraspinatous.

1) Start in the ski stance. Cross the arms close to the chest wall with the shoulders relaxed. The hands are closed in a loose fist (fig. 6.17) with the body relaxed but spring in the legs and arms. The head and trunk are motionless.

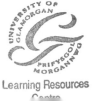

Fig 6.17

2) Rapidly abduct and extend the arms individually and then simultaneously (fig. 6.18). **Expel air** during each contractive thrust to focus the energy (*). The arms are kept tight into the side of the chest wall during the contraction. The distance is very small. A clean, sharp, rapid contraction is the goal.

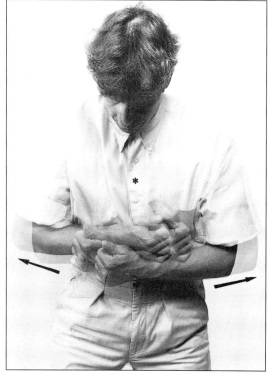

Fig 6.18

3) The straight pull thrust using shoulder extensors is a common variation. The arms are close to the side of the body with the elbows flexed to 90 degrees. The thrust is a rapid extension of the shoulder extensors (fig. 6.19). The head and trunk are motionless (*).

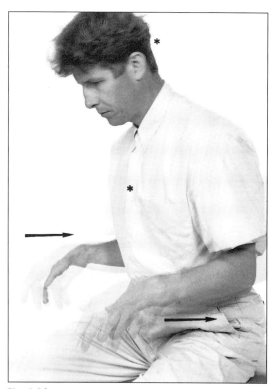

Fig 6.19

Shoulder/Arm Thrust

The shoulder/arm thrust is used in many of the prone and side posture manipulative procedures (Grice, 1980; Fligg, 1984; Szaraz, 1984; Grice and Vernon, 1992). This particular thrusting technique is capable of generating large forces over a longer distance. The force is generated by the shoulder girdle, down the arm across the hand and transferred onto a relatively short anatomical lever (i.e. TP or SP). One of the most common mistakes encountered with students is a pushing or driving effect. They also lift the arm and hand prior to the thrust, resulting in a pile-driving/thumping action. Part of this exercise is to learn to thrust from a neutral position to avoid these common errors.

The ability to isolate and rapidly depress the shoulder girdle musculature cleanly and sharply will be introduced first. The muscles used for this action are primarily the latissimus dorsi, pectoralis major and the serratus anterior. This will be followed later in the chapter using patient simulation and some resistance to practise these newly acquired thrusting skills.

1) The doctor is in the 45 degree fencer stance position with the right arm placed in front of the body. The right hand adopts a firm chiropractic arch and is positioned in line with the jugular notch (note the position of the plumbline *). The upper part of the arm is adducted and held in closely to the chest wall (fig. 6.20). **Do not hyperextend the elbow**; it is comfortably extended. The majority of the doctor's weight is supported by the left leg. The shoulders are relaxed at 45 degrees, the trunk is slightly inclined forward and the head is stable looking down at the right hand.

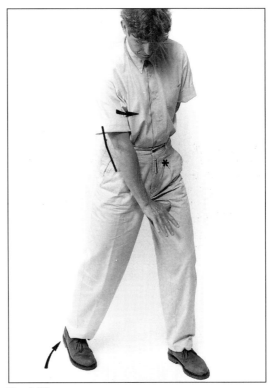

Fig 6.20

2) The shoulder is marginally raised (approximately 0.5–1 inch). Slowly depress the shoulder girdle the same distance to gauge the distance and depth of thrust required (fig. 6.21). The shoulder girdle is the only structure contracting and moving. The head, upper body and lower limbs are motionless (*). Do not assist with a triceps contraction. **Expel air** through the diaphragm with each contraction. Repeat after a brief rest between each contraction. *The contraction should gradually become sharper and crisper in nature during the practice session.* Keep the rest of the body stable and relaxed and keep some spring in the legs. **Practise this skill on both sides of the body to ensure a balanced effect**.

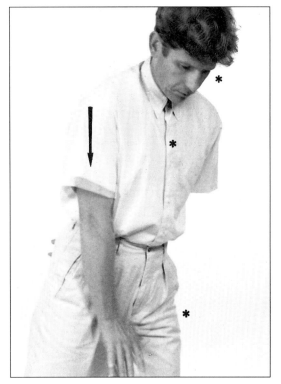

Fig 6.21

3) A variation of this is the *shoulder push thrust*. The arms are held tight against the lateral aspect of the rib cage with the elbows at 90 degrees. The shoulder is elevated marginally and the thrust is a rapid depression of the shoulder girdle produced mainly by the action of the pectoralis minor and the serratus anterior (fig. 6.22). Each arm is contracted individually. The doctor is in both the ski and fencer stance with the head and pelvis stable (*). The key is to expel air and impulse rapidly.

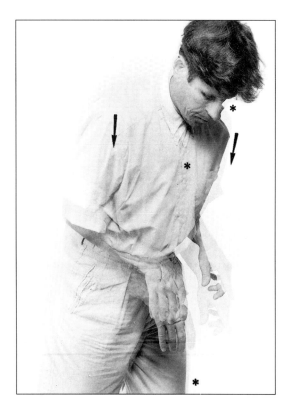

Fig 6.22

Body Drop

The body drop technique is used to increase the force and the efficiency of the manipulative thrust. It is often used during side posture and prone manipulative procedures when there is a greater mass to overcome. The body drop increases the use of the trunk weight in a controlled fashion. The body drop is usually incorporated with the shoulder thrust which is seldom used alone and gives the overall manoeuvre increased acceleration. The body drop constitutes control of the doctor's body weight for a rapid and assisted delivery. The body drop is an important fundamental skill.

Begin the skill in the ski stance and pivot into the fencer stance posture. This helps to prepare the doctor for the initial sequencing required during body weight shift, a basic movement for many of the manipulative procedures described later in this book.

1) Start in the ski stance posture and pivot 45 degrees into the basic fencer or lunge stance position. Slowly push the body weight forward by plantar flexing the back foot. This essentially raises the centre of gravity slightly for the body drop (fig. 6.23). Ensure that there is some spring in the front leg which can be measured by bouncing the weight over the front foot. Notice the position of the plumbline, an indication of body weight alignment over the front knee and the metatarsals of the foot.

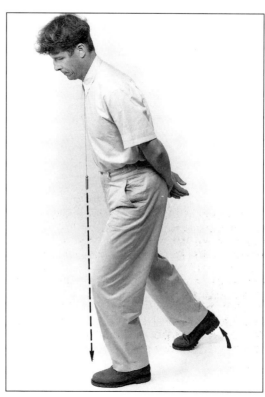

Fig 6.23

2) Let the body drop through the front knee flexion, slowly at first and then increase the speed to the point that the action is similar to a free body fall or impulse drop (fig. 6.24). The body is motionless apart from the vertical drop. The body drop is a controlled movement. Control of the free fall is stopped by the braking action of the quadriceps. **The entire distance dropped is approximately 2–3 inches vertically**. Repeat with a short rest in order to appreciate the movement and appropriate feedback.

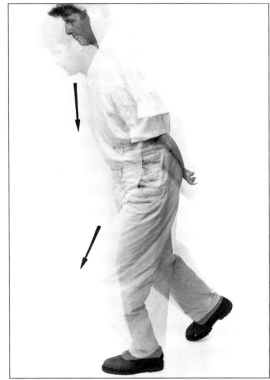

Fig 6.24

Combination Body Drop and Shoulder Thrust

Both skills are combined to produce one action. This should be attempted only after each individual skill is performed with confidence and proficiency. Remember, do not attempt to chew gum at the same time! Many of the manipulative procedures incorporate a variety and combination of thrusting skills depending upon the biomechanical indications and the needs and the size of the patient. The doctor can increase the speed and force of the manipulative thrust by using the whole body as a mechanical lever or compressor. The workload is distributed throughout the system, which places less strain on any one of the individual anatomical structures. The body drop and the shoulder thrust constitute a common method for this purpose.

1) Move from ski to fencer stance. Prepare the shoulder girdle and push the body weight over the metatarsals of the front foot by plantar flexing the back foot as described in Figure 6.20. Simultaneously. and slowly drop and depress the shoulder girdle at the same time, initially to feel the overall movement and then increase the speed gradually (fig. 6.25). **Don't develop a pushing or pounding action with the shoulder**. The body drop is to be a crisp, short movement and not a floating action. The depth of the body drop and shoulder thrust are equal. **Expel air** during each thrust movement.

2) The combination of body drop and shoulder pull and push variations can also be introduced and practised at this stage. Keep the arms in tight against the rib cage and expel air during each thrust, producing a rapid impulse type movement.

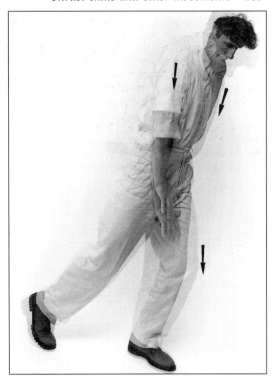

Fig 6.25

Other Movement Skills

Shoulder Flexibility – Protraction/ Retraction

The ability to retract and protract the scapula actively and passively adds to the overall efficiency of the shoulder girdle during the development of thrusting skills. Flexible scapulo-thoracic movement gives a cushioning effect which effectively reduces the potential rigidity of the shoulder/arm thrust when combined with a torso or body drop.

1) Stand in a ski stance with both arms hanging freely in front of the body clasped together by the thumbs. Actively retract both scapulae while keeping the torso and head completely stable (*) (fig. 6.26). Protract the scapulae slowly and eccentrically. The exercise is to isolate actively scapulothoracic movement. Essentially the shoulder girdles move around the torso.

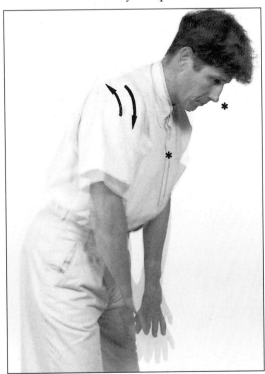

Fig 6.26

Wrist Supination/Pronation

The ability to supinate and pronate both wrists simultaneously is a clinical asset, particularly during skilful manipulation of the cervical spine. The amount of rotation has to be controlled, as well as other potential extreme ranges of motion. The cervical spine is capable of considerable ranges of motion under normal conditions and this feature should not be abused during therapeutic manipulation at the expense of achieving joint cavitation. Control of movement can be accomplished by subjecting the head and neck to the short lever action provided by the **wrists only**. The following is a simulation exercise to develop the motor skills to control any excessive movement of the cervical spine.

1) Stand in a low fencer stance, shoulders relaxed, elbows flexed at 90 degrees and the arms tucked in close to the side of the body. Both wrists are relaxed, naturally ulnar deviated and holding a small ball between the index finger and thumb. The ball represents the patient's head as illustrated in Figure 6.27.

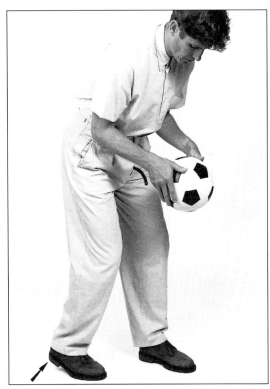

Fig 6.27

2) Simultaneously and slowly pronate and supinate the wrists, balancing the ball between the fingers (fig. 6.28). The pronated hand is the contact and the supinated hand is the support hand usually cupping the occipital rim in a typical clinical combination. The head, shoulders, and arms remain completely stable and motionless during the exercise (*). Repeat the motion in the opposite direction. *Do not allow the arms to drift from the body, as this produces unwanted shoulder motion which effectively increases the size of levers acting on the head.*

Practise this skill with the ball on the head-piece of the table once the pattern is learned. Do not lift the ball; move the ball while the hands are still in contact with the table.

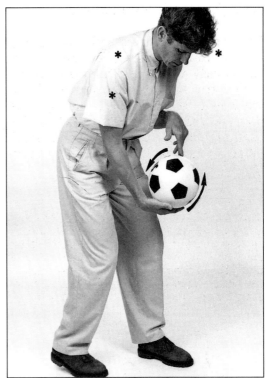

Fig 6.28

Thoracic Compliance Skills

The ability to control and use the compliance of the patient's rib cage is another acquired skill that has to be learned either before or during actual manipulation exercises. This is particularly important when dealing with manipulation of the thoracic spine in any position. The flexibility and expandability of the thoracic cavity and the rib cage permit a great deal of mobility. Therefore, to achieve joint tension without distress or lack of cooperation without any impairment of the patient's respiration, it is important to consider the breathing cycle and thoracic compliance. The premature application of a dynamic manipulative thrust to the thoracic spine may lead to injury and patient dissatisfaction.

It is advisable to introduce and practise these skills during a simulation exercise using a children's beach ball or reasonable facsimile. This is the student's first exposure to the concept of joint preload or prestress ('joint tension') concepts.

1) Stand at the table in a fencer stance posture with a beach ball stabilized by reinforced double hand contact. The suprasternal notch is directly above the hand position (fig. 6.29). Note the position of the plumbline in the middle of the table and ball for more effective use of the doctor's torso weight and body drop through the centre of gravity. The rear foot plantar flexes to push the weight forward. The doctor is in contact with the side of the table to help support body weight.

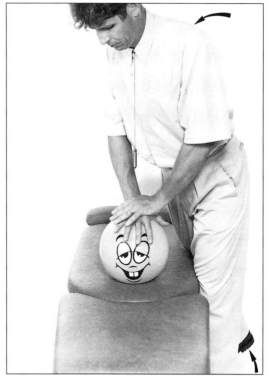

Fig 6.29

2) Push body weight up and forward over the centre of the ball. Keeping the head, shoulders, and arms completely stable, compress the ball very slowly (fig. 6.30). Feel the gradual development of the resistance under the contact and the spring in the ball as the weight and compression are increased. This should be done only during the expiratory stage of respiration in a real clinical setting. Try to visualize the same series of steps on an actual patient and the activity within the rib cage. **Practise on both sides of the table**. Perform this activity very slowly, simulating the speed of patient exhalation.

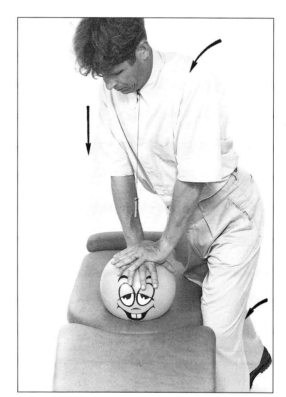

Fig 6.30

Side Posture Squeeze Skills

During the later part of a side posture manipulation, as the patient is breathing out and just prior to the mobilization or dynamic thrust, the doctor localizes and concentrates the forces of the contact levers by slowly squeezing the contact point and the long levers together to increase the available tissue tension around the targetted joint. This squeezing action is in rhythm with the patient's exhalation phase. The student should begin to learn that coordinating breathing cycles with the patient is a very effective clinical tool for stimulating relaxation, increasing tissue tension and focusing the dynamic thrust.

1) Place a beach ball or reasonable equivalent on the table and slowly squeeze the ball together feeling for the resistance that develops in the ball (fig. 6.31). Breathe out as you squeeze. The hands should be positioned in normal bridge postures. Keep the body well over the table to simulate a patient interaction. The squeezing is produced by a slow sustained contraction of the pectoralis group. The body is totally motionless (*) and the doctor is leaning against the table to support body weight.

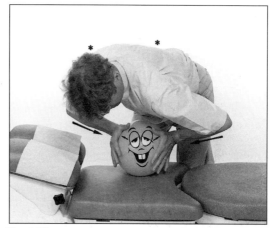

Fig 6.31

Joint Tension Sense Skills

The ability to sense when a specific joint has reached the elastic barrier is a learned skill (tissue tension sense). This is the point at which the dynamic thrust or mobilization force is applied. Tissue tension is the viscoelastic properties of the capsular elements, the surrounding ligaments combined with the flexibility of other articular soft tissue at the end of the passive range of motion. This may include myofascial structures. There are numerous descriptive terms which are used to delineate the condition of the joint and surrounding tissues, such as springy, hard, muscular, bony, etc. However, developing the proprioceptive sense to distinguish between these terms fairly accurately requires some clinical experience. From an educational point of view, simulation provides some realism for the student to begin to build a base of experience for eventual clinical use. The ability to recognize normal joint give or spring provides the student with an early appreciation of this important proprioceptive sense.

Learning to appreciate and isolate the natural joint tension or spring, from either a diagnostic or therapeutic perspective, should be performed slowly and purposefully. This ensures that the natural tensile properties of the soft tissues will gradually create inherent resistance, and time for feedback is accomplished.

1) From the fencer stance slowly pull apart a thick elastic rubber band in order to feel the gradual development of the resistance of the material simulating the natural give in the soft tissues in the body (fig. 6.32). This technique should be practised in a variety of different positions. The key element is to stand always in either the ski or fencer stance and always to exhale as tension is applied. Try to appreciate the elasticity and add more elastic bands if necessary to acquire different amounts of resistance.

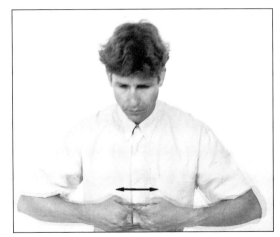

Fig 6.32

Verbal Skills

Patient cooperation depends upon, among other factors, effective communication. This is of utmost importance if the patient is demonstrating signs of distress or apprehension. The patients must know what is going to happen to them and what is expected of them while on the table before spinal manipulative therapy. This requires that the doctor expresses clear, concise and very simple commands to the patient. The doctor has to speak slowly and assertively during a therapeutic encounter. Patient relaxation is a necessary component for successful and efficient manipulation. A lengthy technical explanation just prior to a manipulative thrust to the cervical spine is certainly neither good patient management nor in the patient's best interest.

Read the following aloud slowly and do not mumble or feel embarrassed:

'Lie face (tummy) down on the table, please'

'Lie on your right side (tap the shoulder of the side in question)'

'Take a deep breath in, please'

'Do you feel comfortable in that position?'

'Do you feel any discomfort or pain?'

'Slowly breathe out and let your head and shoulders relax'

'This hurts me more than it hurts you' (usually brings a smile)

'Close your eyes, please' (useful during cervical manipulation)

'Would you hold and interlock your wrists, please' (always demonstrate)

'Place your hands on top of your tummy, please'.

These are just a few examples of some very simple and short commands. Learning to communicate with other students before clinical internship is recommended. The doctor is the director and you simply cannot expect patients to fall into place like your colleagues do in a classroom situation where everyone knows or supposedly knows what they are doing. Providing a patient with an open and relaxed style of effective communication reduces a great deal of frustration and promotes cooperation. This is an ideal situation to apply the KISS principle of, *"keep it simple, stupid"*.

It would be pointless and a total waste of time to develop the complex psychomotor skills of manipulative therapy to be unable to communicate your expertise in a clinical setting for the sake of poor and non-assertive verbal communication.

Thrust Skills – Practice Techniques

Many of the more common types of dynamic thrust skills have now been introduced, learned in principle and practised in terms of muscle groups used and specific motor action required. These have been simulation exercises only with little or no resistance against which to thrust. This has been done for a specific reason. It is more important initially to isolate and develop the reflex motor patterns required. If resistance is introduced at the same time, there may be a tendency to push or thump the targetted object, which may contribute to and reinforce poor motor skills. Learning thrust skills in simulation has its shortcomings, but provided this is kept in perspective with both psychomotor and clinical relevance, the procedure has not been futile. Even though the classroom is unable to supply realism, rudimentary proprioceptive and psychomotor training is provided through these methods. Once the various thrust skills are performed proficiently in a clean, sharp and controlled fashion, it is recommended that some form of resistance be established.

Students of manipulative sciences in a hurry to achieve a joint crack often lose sight of the fact that these procedures are meant to be an integral component and the progressive development of very complex psychomotor skills. There is no easy way. It takes time and practice.

The following thrust skills are somewhat repeated; however this time they are thrusting against some resistance and in various clinical combinations. The same postural and performance rules apply as previously described in this chapter. Perform all skills bilaterally using a chiropractic table. Keep the body weight positioned closely to the table at all times during each exercise. This guarantees optimal weight distribution over the patient and contact point. The legs should be touching the table, but still freely movable. The amplitude of each thrust is very small. Concentrate on the rapidity, explosiveness and quickness of each impulse thrust.

1) *Shoulder Thrust.* High, firm chiropractic arch placed on a cushion positioned just below the suprasternal notch reinforced with the opposite hand. Fencer stance posture. Depress the cushion in a preload simulation by lowering the body towards the table. Apply a relatively straight arm impulse thrust straight down along the line of the arm (fig. 6.33). The torso and pelvis are completely stable (*). The triceps comes into play to add a little elbow extension. The main thrust is from the shoulder girdle. Expel air during each thrust, try not to pound the cushion, and take a rest between each impulse thrust. **This may be performed with single arm thrust.**

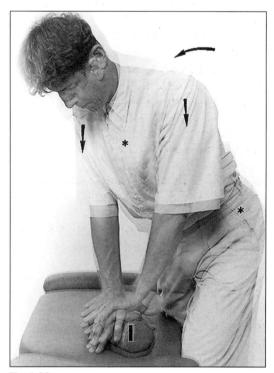

Fig 6.33

2) *Shoulder Thrust and Body Drop.* Same as above but combine the body drop thrust. The body weight is rocked and lifted over the contact point; the contact arm is relatively stable as the force is generated through the shoulder (fig. 6.34). Same additional rules apply as in Figure 6.33. There are degrees of shoulder and body drop depending on the clinical situation.

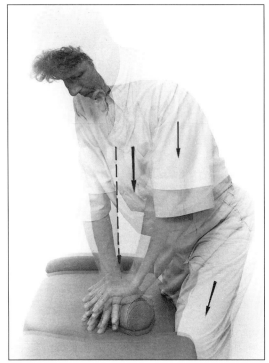

Fig 6.34

3a) *Recoil (Toggle) Thrust.* Stand in a ski stance with a reinforced contact hand and the jugular notch directly over the hands. The arms and shoulders are relaxed and motionless during the whole procedure (*). There is no preload applied. The thrust is a sudden and sharp triceps contraction followed by a biceps recoil (fig. 6.35). The body remains stable during the impulse thrust. Same breathing rules apply. Rest between each contraction.

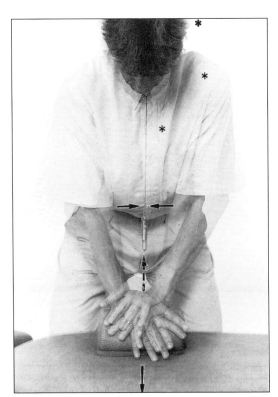

Fig 6.35

3b) *Recoil Thumb Thrust.* This is a variation of 3a (fig. 6.35). Reinforced thumb contact over the cushion replaces the hand/pisiform contact. Perform the same impulse thrust (fig. 6.36).

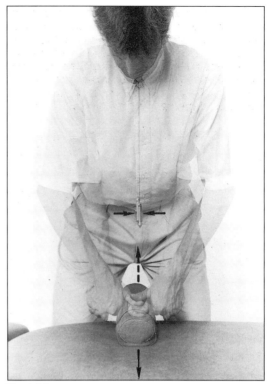

Fig 6.36

4) *Pectoralis Thrust.* Crouch down in a low fencer stance at the head of the table. Contact the table using the web of the contact hand. Arm is at 90 degrees. Sudden short sharp pectoralis/biceps thrust straight across the headpiece (fig. 6.37a). The head and upper body are stable and motionless (*). Practise both ipsilateral and contralateral thrusts (fig. 6.37b). Expel air with each contraction and rest adequately between each contraction.

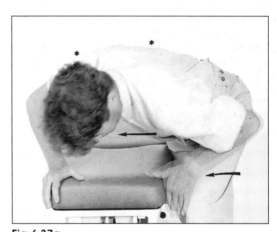

Fig 6.37a

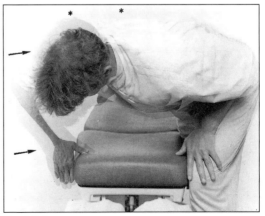

Fig 6.37b

5) *Impulse Wrist Flick Thrust.* Hold a medium sized ball in both hands with the arms tucked in close to the body. The ball represents the head. Pronate/supinate pivot the ball and then apply a sudden, short, sharp contraction causing bilateral ulnar deviation of the wrists **only** (fig. 6.38). The rest of the body remains completely stable (*). As the breath is expelled the forearms are quickly brought towards the side of the body, adding to the impulse nature of this skill.

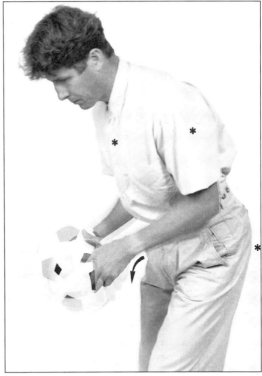

Fig 6.38

6) *Elastic Band Thrust Skills.* There are many different ways to use the bands to practise the impulse thrust. The elastic bands provide an opportunity to feel the preload or joint tension prior to the dynamic impulse thrust. Use your imagination to create more.

i) Double the band and hold it in both hands close to the chest. Distract the bands very slowly apart, feeling the tension developing. As the resistance increases, pause at tension, distract and abduct both shoulders rapidly in an impulse fashion (fig. 6.39a). Expel air with each contraction. The body is motionless (*).

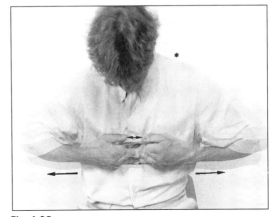

Fig 6.39a

ii) Double the bands over each thumb with the hands close to the chest. Simultaneously push the hands across the body, feeling the tension increase in the bands; pause; apply sudden rapid pectoralis impulse thrust to adduct arms (fig. 6.39b). Expel air with each contraction. The body is motionless (*).

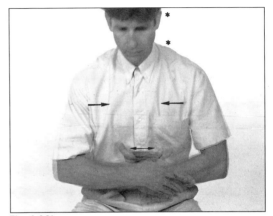

Fig 6.39b

These are just a few of the ways in which the elastic bands can be incorporated into learning joint and tissue tension sense prior to the delivery of an impulse thrust. Practise these skills regularly in association with the other important skills presented in this chapter. For experienced chiropractors, this may help to review and improve existing speed and thrust efficiency.

This chapter has presented a variety of commonly used reflex dynamic thrust techniques associated with many of the manipulative procedures used in the chiropractic profession. It has been the purpose of this chapter to present these skills from very simple movements to more complex ones. The key element of the exercise is to learn to isolate and contract certain muscle groups in a sudden and rapid fashion with controlled amplitude of limb or lever movement. Basic concepts of joint tension or preload and the impulse thrust have also been presented. Pounding and pushing movements have been highlighted and discouraged in an attempt to promote control and muscle isolation. The importance of daily practice to reinforce and develop competent skills has been addressed. The dynamic thrust is only one aspect of the overall manipulative skill learning. Learning to appreciate tissue tension and the proprioceptive sense of joint movement and resistance has also been covered as an important associated skill.

Control of the force of the manipulative or adjustive thrust demands discipline and skill, many hours of practice are needed to attain a competent level of performance. The accuracy and precision of application is the clinical objective. This chapter has presented simulation only. Nonetheless, the importance of introducing these skills to develop an awareness of their existence and potential application may offer a potentially useful teaching strategy. The importance of learning rudimentary movements that can be improved with experience and time has been emphasized.

References

Adams, A.A. and Wood, J. (1984) Changes in force parameters with practice experience for selected low back adjustments. In *Proceedings of the 15th Annual Biomechanics Conference on the Spine* (Boulder, 1984). University of Boulder, Colorado, pp. 143–176

Bergmann, T.F. (1992) Short lever, specific contact articular chiropractic technique. *Journal of Manipulative and Physiological Therapeutics*, **15**, 591–595

Bourdillon, J.F. and Day, E.A. (1987) Manipulation. In *Spinal Manipulation*, 4th edn. William Heinemann Medical Books, London and Appelton and Lange, Los Altos, California, pp. 92–98

Byfield, D. (1991) Lumbar manipulative procedures in relation to segmental specificity and biomechanical properties of the motor unit. *European Journal of Chiropractic*, **39**, 13–19

Byfield, D., Burnett, M., Mealing, D. *et al.* (1995) A method for quantifying the forces and amplitude occurring during simulated joint play palpation: preliminary results using an instrumented device. *European Journal of Chiropractic* (submitted for publication)

Cassidy, J.D., Kirkaldy-Willis, W.H. and Thiel, H.W. (1992) Manipulation. In: *Managing Low Back Pain*, 3rd edn. (eds. W.H. Kirkaldy-Willis and C.V. Burton). Churchill Livingstone, London, pp. 283–296

Chapman-Smith, D. (1991) The RAND study – manipulation for low-back pain. *Chiropractic Report*, **5**, 2

Cohen, E., Triano, J., Papakyriakow, M. *et al.* (1993) Experienced vs. novice manipulator performance measures. In *Proceedings of the 1993 International Conference on Spinal Manipulation* (Montreal, 1993). Foundation for Chiropractic Education and Research, Arlington, p. 91

Conway, P., Herzog, W., Zhang, Y. *et al.* (1992) Identification of the mechanical factors required to cause cavitation during spinal manipulation in the thoracic spine. In *Proceedings of the 1992 International Conference on Spinal Manipulation* (Chicago, 1992). FCER, Arlington, p. 18

Corlett, D. (1992) Relationship between chiropractic training and speed and amplitude of a toggle thrust. BSc (Chiro) Thesis, Anglo-European College of Chiropractic, Bournemouth, UK

Fligg, B. (1984) The art of manipulation. *Journal of the Canadian Chiropractic Association*, **28**, 384–386

Greenman, P.E. (1989) Principles of high-velocity, low-amplitude thrust technique (mobilization with impulse). In: *Principles of Manual Medicine*, Williams and Wilkins, Baltimore, Maryland, pp. 94–100

Grice, A.S. (1980) A biomechanical approach to cervical and dorsal adjusting. In: *Modern Developments in the Principles and Practice of Chiropractic*, 1st edn. (ed. S. Haldeman). Appleton-Century-Crofts, New York, pp. 331–358

Grice, A., Fligg, B. and Szaraz, Z. (1985) *Biomechanics Course Notes*. Canadian Memorial Chiropractic College, Toronto

Grice, A. and Vernon, H. (1992) Basic principles on the performance of chiropractic adjusting: historical review, classification, and objectives. In: *Principles and Practice of Chiropractic*, 2nd edn. (ed. S. Haldeman). Appleton and Lange, San Mateo, California, pp. 443–458

Haas, M. (1990a) The physics of spinal manipulation. Part I. The myth of F = ma. *Journal of Manipulative and Physiological Therapeutics*, **13**, 204–206

Haas, M. (1990b) The physics of spinal manipulation. Part III. Some characteristics of adjusting that facilitate joint distraction. *Journal of Manipulative and Physiological Therapeutics*, **13**, 305–308

Haldeman, S. (1983) Spinal manipulative therapy: a status report. *Clinical Orthopaedic*, **179**, 62–70

Kirby, R.L., Price, N.A. and MacLeod, D.A. (1987) The influence of foot position on standing balance. *Journal of Biomechanics*, **20**, 423–427

Kirkaldy-Willis, W.H. and Cassidy, J.D. (1985) Spinal manipulation in the treatment of low back pain. *Canadian Family Physician*, **31**, 535–540

Lee, M. and Svensson, N.L. (1993) Effect of loading frequency on response of the spine to lumbar posteroanterior forces. *Journal of Manipulative and Physiological Therapeutics*, **16**, 439–446

LeVeau, B.F. (1992) Dynamics. In *Biomechanics of Human Motion*, 3rd edn. W.B. Saunders, London, pp. 196–197

Maigne, R. (1972) Localization of manipulation of the spine. In *Orthopaedic Medicine: A New Approach to Vertebral Manipulations* (ed. W.T. Liberson). Charles C. Thomas, Springfield, Illinois, pp. 131–136

Maigne, R. (1985) Manipulation of the spine. In *Manipulation, Traction and Massage*, 3rd edn. (ed. J.V. Basmajian). Williams and Wilkins, London, p. 73

Meade, T.W., Dyer, S., Browne, W. *et al.* (1990) Low back pain of mechanical origin: randomised comparison of chiropractic and hospital outpatient treatment. *British Medical Journal*, **300**, 1431–1437

Mennell, J. (1991) The manipulatable lesion: joint play, joint dysfunction, and joint manipulation. In *Functional Soft Tissue Examination and Treatment by Manual Methods. The Extremities*. Aspen Publishers, Gaithersburg, pp. 191–196

Nyberg, R. (1993) Manipulation: definition, types, application. In *Rational Manual Therapies*, 1st edn. (eds. J.V. Basmajian and R. Nyberg). Williams and Wilkins, London, pp. 21–47

Paris, S.V. (1983) Spinal manipulative therapy. *Clinical Orthopaedics and Related Research*, **179**, 55–61

Peterson, D.H. and Bergmann, T.F. (1993) Joint assessment principles and procedures. In *Chiropractic Technique* (eds. T.F. Bergmann, D.H. Peterson and D.J. Lawrence). Churchill Livingstone, London, pp. 81–96

Plaugher, G. (1993) Clinical anatomy and biomechanics of the spine. In *Textbook of Clinical Chiropractic: A Specific Biomechanical Approach* (ed. G. Plaugher & assoc. ed. M.A. Lopes). Williams and Wilkins, London, pp. 12–51

Sandoz, R. (1976) Some physical mechanisms and effects of spinal adjustments. *Annals Swiss Chiropractic Association* **VI**, 91–142

Schafer, R.C. and Faye, L.J. (1989) The thoracic spine. In *Motion Palpation and Chiropractic Technic: Principles of Dynamic Chiropractic*, 1st edn. The Motion Palpation Institute, Huntington Beach, California, p. 187

Schneider, M.J. (1992) Soft tissue effects of sacroiliac and lumbosacral joint manipulation. *Chiropractic Technique*, **4**, 136–142

Shekelle, P.G., Adams, A.H., Chassin, M.R. *et al.* (1992) Spinal manipulation for low-back pain. *Annals of Internal Medicine*, **117**, 590–598

Szaraz, Z.T. (1984) *Compendium of Chiropractic Technique*, Canadian Memorial Chiropractic College, Toronto, Canada

Triano, J.J. (1992) Studies on the biomechanical effect of a spinal manipulation. *Journal of Manipulative and Physiological Therapeutics*, **15**, 71–75

Wood, J. and Adams, A.A. (1984) Comparison of forces used in selected adjustments of the low back by experienced chiropractors and chiropractic students with no clinical experience: a preliminary study. *The Research Forum, The Palmer College of Chiropractic*, **1**, 16–23

Further Reading

Cassidy, J.D., Thiel, H.W. and Kirkaldy-Willis, W.H. (1993) Side posture manipulation for lumbar intervertebral disc herniation. *Journal of Manipulative and Physiological Therapeutics*, **16**, 96–103

Curtis, P. (1988) Spinal manipulation: does it work? *Occupational Medicine*, **3**, 31–44

Nyberg, R. (1985) Role of physical therapists in spinal manipulation. In *Manipulation, Traction and Massage*, 3rd edn. (ed. J.V. Basmajian). Williams and Wilkins, London, pp. 22–46

7

Patient positioning skills

David Byfield

Introduction

Patient compliance and comfort during spinal manipulation is paramount. There are many different postures that are used to perform manipulative therapy which are governed by clinical indications, patient's needs and individual tolerances. Some positions are more advantageous in terms of maximizing patient relaxation and clinical efficiency. Other positions furnish the most mechanical advantage for joint isolation, specificity and accuracy of force application. These represent a group of skills which are usually difficult to learn, but once mastered combine to yield efficient manipulative procedures. The side posture supplies all the ingredients necessary for mechanical leverage and advantage, but may subject both the patient and the clinician to twisting actions and mechanical deformation of pain-sensitive tissues. The supine and prone positions are less demanding of both the practitioner and patient due to the inherent patient control. As a result of this fact alone, all the other factors which determine the success of manipulative procedures are substantially improved. The sitting and standing positions are useful clinically, but limited due to the additional effects of weight-bearing and gravity on patient relaxation and cooperation.

Positioning the patient is a learned skill and forms an integral part of the overall therapeutic encounter. This following chapter will present the skills associated with the most common patient positions.

Emphasis is placed once again upon employing slow and methodical movements in order to appreciate the complexity of the movements involved. Frequent practice is encouraged as part of the learning and conditioning process.

Side Posture

The side posture is one of the more traditional and seemingly one of the most effective positions used by the chiropractic profession in the treatment of the lumbar spine and pelvic girdle. This manipulative method is incorporated into the management of dysfunction syndromes of the lumbar spine and pelvis with great success (Kirkaldy-Willis and Cassidy, 1985). Manipulation of the lumbar spine and sacroiliac joints is most often performed with the patient in the side posture (Cassidy et al. 1985; Cassidy et al. 1993). The side posture is by far the most difficult to learn. It is difficult to gain clinical proficiency in the use of the side posture and manipulation performed using this posture is infinitely more complex than manipulation performed in the prone, supine or even sitting positions. This is partly due to the fact that the clinician has to learn to balance both the patient's and his or her weight simultaneously. Subsequently, the number of psychomotor skills in this procedure are numerous. This requires a great deal of time and effort on behalf of the student to learn and develop repeatability. The side posture provides optimal mechanical counter-rotation of the lumbar intervertebral segments, which improves segmental isolation and the likelihood of safer thrust localization of the intended segmental level. The side posture is unique in that it incorporates both long and short levers to introduce a biomechanical effect. The lumbar motion segments are well suited and biologically designed to withstand very large compressive and torsional loads, possibly induced during side posture manipulation (Pearcy, 1989).

The essence of side posture skill is the ability to control the patient in order to isolate and restore very small joint movements characteristic of the lumbar intervertebral and sacroiliac joints (Sturesson *et al.* 1989). This is accomplished by manoeuvring long levers of the shoulder and pelvic girdles and the short levers characteristic of the targetted joint complexes. The palpatory skills and the ability to process proprioceptive information regarding joint movement and resistance are integral parts of the overall skill. Developing joint preload or 'joint tension' at the precise physiological barrier guarantees minimal force and patient movement. This type of skilful positioning of the patient requires considerable balance and control on the part of the practitioner before an adjustive thrust is considered. Both patient and practitioner should be comfortable and balanced throughout the entire manipula-

tive procedure. Ultimately, there is a connection between the balance of the practitioner against the balance of the patient and it is this balance which provides the minimum use of force and the maximum use of finesse. It is this important symbiotic relationship that will build effective clinical procedures, improve patient compliance, enhance therapeutic outcome, and reduce possible injury.

The following description will provide the basis for a sequential learning process for side posture skills. Each of the steps represents an important building block for the acquisition and patterning of these specific movements. These movements or steps are to be performed each and every time a patient is placed in side posture. These skills will allow the doctor to establish clinical *consistency*, as well as clinical *flexibility* when dealing with a wide range of patient types and presenting complaints. Learning the ability to repeatedly and efficiently apply positioning skills should be the goal of the student of spinal manipulative sciences. Effective and structured daily practice is one method of attaining this goal. Naturally, the student should endeavour to attain the skill, coordination and dexterity required for handling patients in both left and right side postures.

Side Posture Skills – Patient Positioning

1) The patient is instructed to lie on his or her right side from a sitting position facing the doctor with the head comfortably placed on the raised headpiece. The patient folds his/her arms across the chest so that he/she is lying on the posterior aspect of the shoulder and scapula on the down side. The patient then flexes both hips and knees to finish in the semifetal position approximately in the middle of the table (fig. 7.1). This maintains patient relaxation and spinal flexion. If the patient is in pain and needs assistance then the doctor will help to lower his or her body weight down onto the table and assist in bringing the knees up.

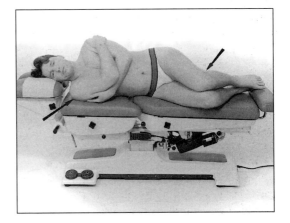

Fig 7.1

2) *Position the upper torso first.* Grasp the arm closest to the table by the wrist just above the radial and ulnar styli (*) and by the elbow just above the medial and lateral condyles (*) with your thumb and index finger. **Gently** pull the arm towards you and cephalad to take out the soft tissue slack in the upper back and shoulder girdle (fig. 7.2). This will essentially increase the tension in the upper back. Try not to pull any hairs or skin. The arm is slowly pulled forward and down.

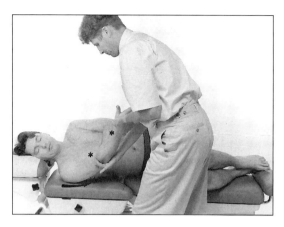

Fig 7.2

3) Place the hand of the bottom arm on the anterior deltoid region of the opposite arm (*) and ask the patient to grasp the side of the table with the other hand for a sense of security (+) (fig. 7.3). Make sure the patient's elbows are not too high. NB: There are many ways to position the patient's hands and arms according to the preference of the practitioner. This arrangement represents a very basic approach from which the student can build during the acquisition of more advanced manipulative skills.

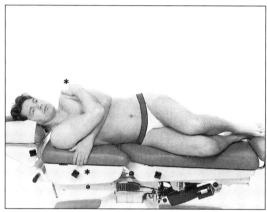

Fig 7.3

4) Finally, the patient should be lying on the posterior aspect of the shoulder girdle with no excessive torque in the full length of the spine (fig. 7.4). It is good practice to ask the patient if he/she is comfortable during these procedures.

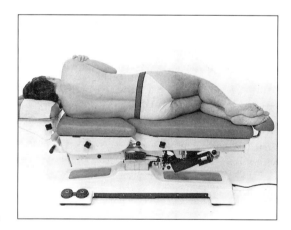

Fig 7.4

5) Position the lower legs next by flexing the upper leg at the hip and placing the dorsum of the foot into the popliteal fossa of the bottom leg (*). This places the upper hip at about 90 degrees of flexion. The bottom leg is flexed at about 20–25 degrees to reduce any tension on the hamstrings (fig. 7.5). The other option is to place the medial malleolus in the popliteal space, essentially reducing the amount of stress in the ankle mortice joint (*) (fig. 7.7).

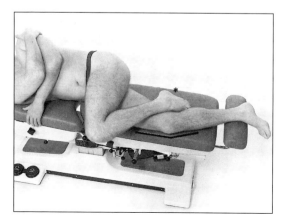

Fig 7.5

6) Bring the patient closer to the edge of the table from the initial central position. This will permit better use of doctor's body weight and also increase the leverage of the lower leg. This should always be done **facing** the patient. *Never* turn your backside toward the patient under any circumstances while performing any manipulative skill!

Push the top knee down slightly with the left hand and place the right hand under the iliac crest (fig. 7.6). From this point scoop the pelvic girdle forward towards the edge of the table. The amount of movement is minimal. Ask for the patient's assistance with a clear and concise command: 'Please, bring your body towards me'.

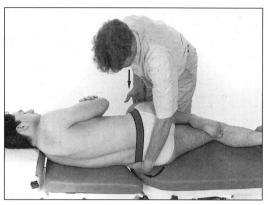

Fig 7.6

7) How far forward should the patient be positioned? This is important relative to patient balance and comfort, and as a starting point it is suggested that the practitioner should use the anterior edge of the lower leg thigh as a marker. The patient should be brought forward so that the lower thigh is just behind the edge of the table and the pelvis is slightly supinated with the superior ASIS just behind the centre line (fig. 7.7).

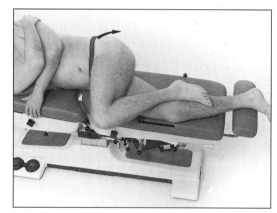

Fig 7.7

8) This completes patient side posture positioning so that when complete the patient should be relaxed, comfortable and stable on the table so that if pushed on either the upper or lower part of the body, he or she will not fall forward (fig. 7.8). The shoulders and pelvis should be lined up in a longitudinal fashion so that the shoulders are not too far back or the pelvis is not too far forward. The patient should lie motionless and unassisted on the table without feeling unsteady, establishing confidence. Clinically, if you are suddenly called away to the telephone the patient would be in a position to rest quietly and motionless with only a minimum amount of readjustment of body position. **This control is essential before other skills are introduced**.

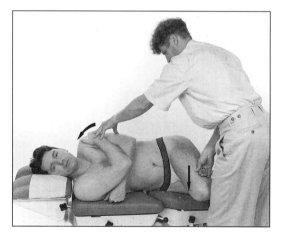

Fig 7.8

9) There are three commonly encountered errors to recognize during the learning of this part of the skill.

i) Pulling the patient's arm by the wrist only (*) causes excessive skin pulling at both the wrist and shoulder, and neck discomfort (fig. 7.9). This may contribute to patient resistance during the next steps of the manipulative procedure. Forcing the arm out shows very little concern for the wellbeing of the patient, compromising patient confidence.

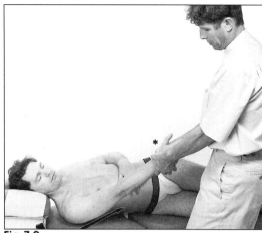

Fig 7.9

ii) Not pulling the arm through enough and leaving the patient lying on the tip of the deltoid region, cramping both the shoulder girdle and the cervical spine (fig. 7.10). This places the patient's weight forward instead of slightly posterior, reducing the balance that you want to achieve before the next step can be effectively performed.

iii) Don't lift the patient to the edge of the table unassisted. It is difficult and awkward. The patient under most circumstances (**except during extremely acute situations**) is quite capable of assisting the doctor in shifting body weight.

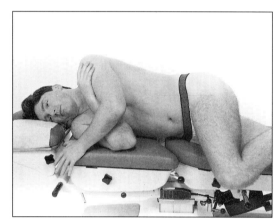

Fig 7.10

Side Posture Skills – Doctor Position

Once the patient is comfortable and secure on the table the next step is to correctly position the practitioner's body weight over the patient. The next series of steps is very important in terms of balancing the weight of both the practitioner and the patient on the table. One of the most commonly observed mistakes by students is to rush this series of skills and maul the patient into submission. The movements should be slow and methodical. Repeat them in sequence as often as required until the pattern becomes smoother.

1) The practitioner directly faces the patient at 90 degrees to the table and places the cephalad hand over the patient's hand on the shoulder, keeping the arm relatively straight while applying **minimal** pressure down and slightly cephalad. This maintains patient position and controls patient upper body weight. Simultaneously, the doctor pushes the patient's top leg down very slowly **only a few inches** with the fingertips to be gently placed between the doctor's thighs just above the knees (fig. 7.11). This is the *thigh sandwich* or *thigh squeeze*. This controls patient leg weight and position. The feet should be about hip distance apart. The patient's top leg should be flexed 90 degrees at the hip, flattening the lumbar lordosis which is a key factor in side posture manipulation.

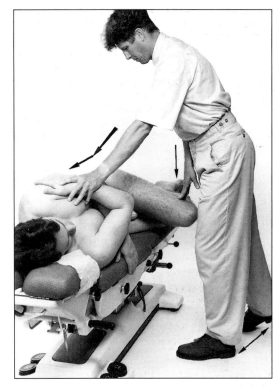

Fig 7.11

2) There are four commonly encountered errors to note during this part of the skill.

i) The doctor should not lie on the patient with the forearm when stabilizing the upper body. This shifts the doctor's centre of gravity cephalad and has a tendency to drag the patient forward, compromising the efficiency and success of the procedure (fig. 7.12). Compare this to the upright stance depicted in Figure 7.11.

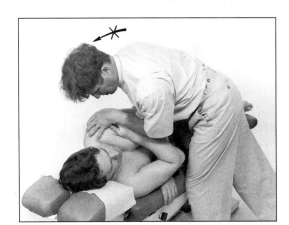

Fig 7.12

ii) DON'T push the patient's upper body back with the support hand to counter the force being applied to the pelvis. This creates unwanted torque in the spine and increases patient resistance (fig. 7.13). The support hand should be used to maintain the patient on the table for a sense of security with the pressure directed down towards the table.

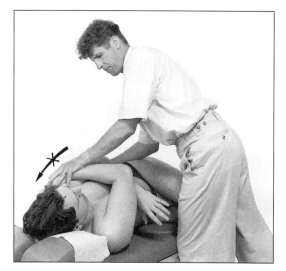

Fig 7.13

iii) DON'T climb aboard or mount the patient and ram his or her knee into your groin when attempting to secure and position the patient's upper leg, while precariously balanced on the tips of the toes (fig. 7.14). This is very clumsy and may simply require a table height change.

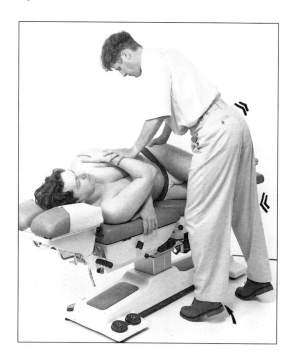

Fig 7.14

iv) DON'T squeeze the patient's knee and leg too tightly with your own legs during the thigh sandwich manoeuvre. This compresses the knee, causing excessive flexion which may cause discomfort and pain (fig. 7.15). This may disrupt comfort and compliance. *Provide* feedback for each other on this point. The sandwich or squeeze should be very light for the best results and control.

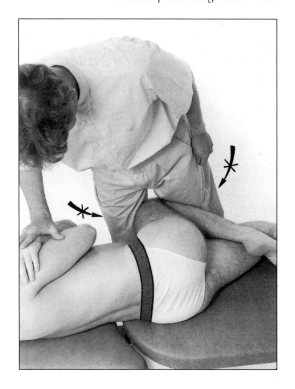

Fig 7.15

3) *The next step is critical transition* for overall doctor positioning and control. The doctor begins to shift and position body weight over the patient. The most advantageous position is with the doctor placed at a 45 degree angle to the table in a LOW FENCER or LUNGE STANCE POSITION described in Chapter 6. The actual movement sequence will be called the 45–45 pivot shift. This starts with the feet hip distance apart as described in Figure 7.11. With the feet maintained in this position, the doctor swivels on the metatarsal pads to face the table at a 45 degree angle (fig. 7.16). This has to be done very slowly to maintain control of both the doctor and the patient. Maintain a light **thigh sandwich** throughout the pivot shift. The patient **should not** move during this procedure. The doctor's head, shoulders, pelvis, knees, and feet should all finish at 45 degrees to the table. Patient's position is stable (S). The fencer posture reduces any torsional stress to the doctor and patient.

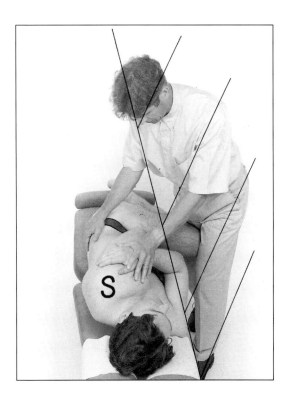

Fig 7.16

4) i) Transfer the doctor's body weight forward towards the patient and over the front foot by **plantar flexing the rear foot**. Consciously maintain a light thigh squeeze during the weight transfer to control leg weight and position. This action is extremely important for all side posture manipulative procedures. Transferring the weight over the metatarsal heads gives the doctor more spring and control of body weight and position. This shifts the weight towards and down over the patient to position the doctor's centre of gravity as close to the target joint as possible (fig. 7.17a). Additional support and spring come from flexion of the front knee (*). The back foot is maintained in a plantar flexed posture. The patient's flexed leg is stabilized in the same position during the pivot shift to the fencer stance. There should be no muscular tension or excess weight on the patient.

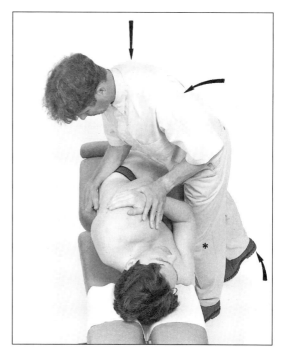

Fig 7.17a

ii) Learn to feel the play in the lumbar spine and pelvis without creating too much tension from the position established in Figure 7.17a. Pull the pelvis towards the doctor in succession several times to appreciate the give and play in the spine while stabilizing the upper body (fig. 7.17b). Don't push down on the pelvis.

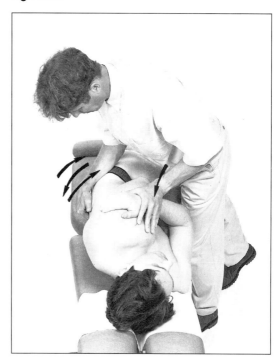

Fig 7.17b

iii) Now pull the pelvis towards the doctor as described in (ii) above and simultaneously drop the body weight through the front knee in time with the arm pull on the pelvis (fig. 17.7c). This will give appreciation of body weight dropping and tension in the lumbar spine. The upper body is stable and there should be no excess compression over the pelvis. Feel the spring in both the legs and the spine/pelvis.

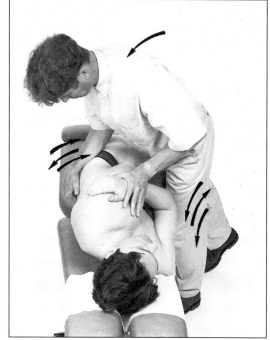

Fig 7.17c

5) There are four commonly encountered errors to be aware of during the performance of this procedure.

i) DON'T separate the feet more than hip distance. This effectively eliminates thigh sandwich control. Loss of control of the patient's leg subsequently jeopardizes control of the entire lower body of the patient (fig. 7.18).

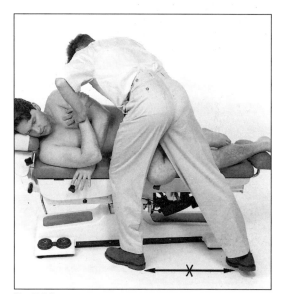

Fig 7.18

ii) The angulation of the feet (optimally 45 degrees) has a tendency to drift into an exaggerated fencer stance position with the front foot parallel to the table and the hind foot perpendicular and flat on the floor (fig. 7.19). A thigh sandwich is impossible to perform in this position. This reduces the spring on the feet, keeps the doctor's body weight back from the table, compromising the overall efficiency of the manipulative procedure. The back leg should not be straight (*).

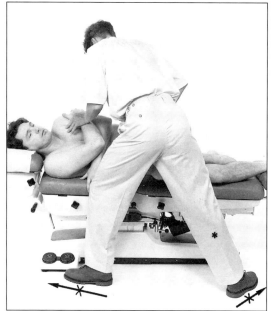

Fig 7.19

iii) DON'T over-rotate one part of the body during the pivot shift, producing unwanted torsion in the spine (fig. 7.20). This usually occurs due to the sequence being performed too quickly. The lower leg often compensates by kicking out to balance the trunk torsion (*). This could result in repetitive torsional injuries to both the lumbar and thoracic spines and shoulder. **The body moves as a single unit**.

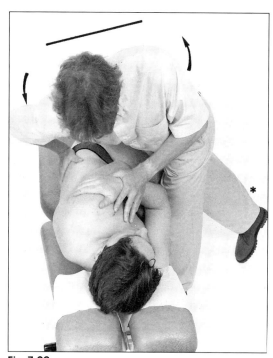

Fig 7.20

iv) The doctor's body weight can be too far from the table and the patient. This will undermine patient stability, increase the lever arms acting on the patient and affect the quality of the body drop (fig. 7.21). Compare this posture to the more acceptable situation in Figure 7.17. Note the distance between the doctor and the targetted joint (*).

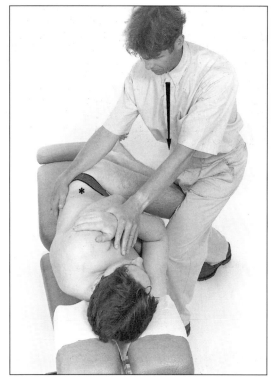

Fig 7.21

Supine Posture Skills – Patient

1) The patient lies with knees and hips flexed to relax the abdominals and the hamstrings. Flexion of the hips also flattens the lumbar lordosis and relaxes the paraspinal musculature. The hands are comfortably interlaced and placed across the lower part of the chest. This ensures relaxed shoulders. The head is supported on a flexed and upright headpiece according to the clinical needs of the patient (fig. 7.22). There are many alternatives of this basic theme which are tailored to the needs of the patient. All of the above cater to patient comfort and relaxation.

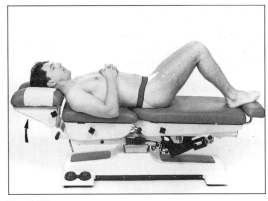

Fig 7.22

Prone Posture Skills – Patient

The patient lies face down with the headpiece dropped slightly to flex the upper thoracic lower cervical region. The feet are slightly elevated, which takes the tension off the posterior leg musculature (fig. 7.23). The arms are placed over the table supports (*) to maintain shoulder relaxation and prevent the doctor from stepping on the patient's hands. Support is introduced for the lumbar region on a case by case situation. Some patients require more lordosis than others.

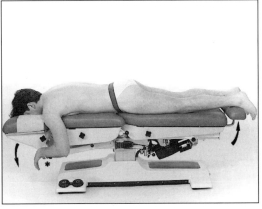

Fig 7.23

Recommended Table Height

This is a personal preference in most instances. For the uninitiated, the ideal height is the top of the table lined up just at or above the level of the knee joint line in the fencer stance (fig. 7.24). This height will change according to the size of the patient. If the table height is wrong for the practitioner the efficiency of the manipulation will be affected due to inappropriate weight distribution and patient control. A vertically adjustable table is a clinical necessity to maintain this ideal height relative to the patient.

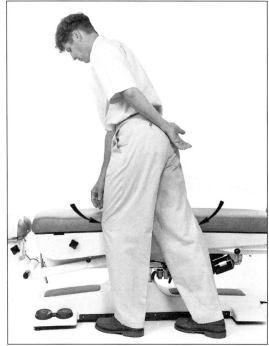

Fig 7.24

The overall effect of this step-by-step procedure is to produce an effortless process for patient comfort and relaxation with a minimum amount of effort by the practitioner. Both patient and practitioner weight distribution are considered fundamental factors in maintaining overall management and control. The above skills should be learned **slowly**, and practised until they become a smooth series of movements in preparation for more advanced skills learning.

This chapter has presented a fairly comprehensive description of side posture positioning skills and, to a lesser extent, both supine and prone positions associated with chiropractic manipulative therapeutics. These skills will form the foundation for the introduction of specific manipulative techniques covering the spine and pelvis to be presented in subsequent chapters. Balance, control and mutual comfort considerations have been emphasized.

References

Cassidy, J.D., Kirkaldy-Willis, W.H. and McGregor, M. (1985) Spinal manipulation for the treatment of chronic low-back and leg pain: an observational study. In: *Empirical Approaches to the Validation of Spinal Manipulation* (eds. A.A. Buerger and P.E. Greenman). Charles, C. Thomas, Springfield, IL, pp. 123–128

Cassidy, J.D., Thiel, H.W. and Kirkaldy-Willis, W.H. (1993) Side posture manipulation for lumbar intervertebral disk herniation. *Journal of Manipulative and Physiological Therapeutics*, **16**, 96–103

Kirkaldy-Willis, W.H. and Cassidy, J.D. (1985) Spinal manipulation in the treatment of low-back pain. *Canadian Family Physician*, **31**, 535–540

Pearcy, M. (1989) Biomechanics of the spine. *Current Orthopaedics*, **3**, 96–100

Sturesson, B., Selvik, G. and Uden, A. (1989) Movements of the sacroiliac joints: a roentgen stereophotogrammetric analysis. *Spine*, **14**, 162–165

8

Pelvic/sacroiliac manipulative skills

David Byfield

Introduction

The role of the sacroiliac joint as a source of low back pain is still the subject of great debate and controversy among health care professionals (Bernard and Cassidy, 1991; Cassidy, 1992). There is still a poor understanding of the actual pathogenesis of mechanical pain syndromes and a lack of objective diagnostic evidence to support this view. Nonetheless, the chiropractic profession has always contested the fundamental role of the sacroiliac joint in the production of low back and leg pain. This supposition is strengthened by a vast amount of foundation knowledge concerning the functional anatomy, histology and pathomechanics of the sacroiliac joint which has provided a rational basis for manipulative intervention (Bowen and Cassidy, 1981; Vleeming et al., 1990; Bernard and Cassidy, 1991). Even though attempts have been made to describe and measure sacroiliac motion, discussions regarding joint biomechanics are still largely speculative and its biomechanical function is still regarded as uncertain (McGregor and Cassidy, 1983; Cassidy, 1992; Cassidy and Mierau, 1992).

Biomechanical Considerations

Recent evidence suggests that sacroiliac joint mobility is minimal and variable, particularly influenced by increasing age and sex. Movement has been found to be greatest around the transverse axis in the order of 2.5 degrees with a mean translation of 0.7 mm (Sturesson et al., 1989). A more recent investigation found the sacroiliac joints in the elderly were mobile, allowing up to 4 degrees of rotation (Vleeming et al., 1992), whereas other workers have established that rotation of the sacrum was much less in the sacroiliac joints of males (0.6–1.2 degrees) than females (1.9–2.8 degrees) (Brunner et al., 1991).

The mechanical influence of a musculo-ligamentous interplay has been closely associated with various kinematic chains influencing sacroiliac joint mobility (Vleeming et al., 1989). It is their contention that contraction of the gluteus maximus, for example, could strongly affect the nature of sacroiliac joint motion via its attachment to the sacrotuberous ligament. This could shed some light on the aetiology of mechanical irritation of the sacroiliac joint by way of asymmetrical contraction of these large stabilizing muscles. It has been stated that very little attention has been given to the role of these influential soft tissue structures during spinal manipulation therapy (Schneider, 1992). Schneider feels that the forces applied during pelvic manipulation are gradually dissipated through several layers of soft tissue before actually affecting the joint surfaces. It is difficult to visualize absolute joint isolation during manipulation of the lumbopelvic articulations, especially considering the complex arrangements of supporting soft tissue that are common to both regions. Therefore, an adjustive thrust directed towards the sacroiliac joint may influence the lumbosacral articulation and vice versa. This may be one explanation why poorly applied manipulative skills often achieve some clinical success (Grice, 1980). Since the sacroiliac joint displays extremely small movements, it is unlikely that the response to manual therapy is simply a reduction of a subluxation or dislocation (Bernard and Cassidy, 1991). These workers imply that the role of high-velocity, low-amplitude manipulation lies in restoring the balance between joint kinematics and associated muscle function, which subsequently normalizes the arthrokinetic reflex and breaks the pain cycle; it is active stimulation and stretch of these large pelvic muscles which causes reflex myofascial relaxation and pain inhibition. These concepts would certainly support the notion that skilled manipulation is mandatory to discriminate the complex interaction of so many influential and pain-sensitive structures.

Clinical Considerations

Despite the lack of objective evidence to define the role of the sacroiliac joint in mechanical low back pain, its pathogenesis, some diagnostic criteria, and the treatment of the sacroiliac syndrome have been described in detail (McGregor and Cassidy, 1983; Kirkaldy-Willis, 1988; Cassidy and Mierau, 1992).

Sacroiliac joint dysfunction is prevalent in the population. Sacroiliac disorders have been implicated in 50–70% of adults presenting with low back pain (Chapman-Smith, 1990), whereas 26% and 33.5% of a sample of school-aged children had low back pain and some form of sacroiliac joint dysfunction, respectively (Mierau *et al.*, 1984). The older age group of students (12–17 years) had a 41.5% prevalence of sacroiliac dysfunction, which is lower than that reported for adults but represents a very high incidence for a young age-group population. The role of the sacroiliac joint as a mechanical source of pain during pregnancy has also been established (Berg *et al.*, 1988). They found a complete resolution of presenting symptoms in 70% of those manipulated. Furthermore, 93% improvement overall was achieved in a group of patients with sacroiliac syndrome treated by manipulative therapy (Cassidy *et al.*, 1985; Kirkaldy-Willis, 1988). Even though the true pathophysiology of the sacroiliac joint and the aetiology of the pain remain unclear, there is a growing body of evidence that suggests a positive response to manipulative intervention. Even though there is no compelling data supporting any specific treatment approach as of yet, there still appears to be more support for manipulative management (Chapman-Smith, 1993). Therefore, chiropractors have a professional responsibility to learn and execute manipulation of the sacroiliac joint in a highly skilful manner.

Force of Manipulation

The magnitude of the thrust force recorded during prone manipulation of the sacroiliac joints was in the range of 220–550 N (50 lb (23 kg) and 120 lb (56 kg)) which equates to roughly 1/3 to 3/4 the body weight of an average 150 lb man (Hessel *et al.*, 1990). Height, weight and grip strength have been identified as physical characteristics that appear to play an important role in a clinician's ability to generate efficient manipulative forces (Adams and Wood, 1984). Since height and weight do not fluctuate greatly, improving strength generally may improve the ability of the practitioner, and especially the student, to deliver a range of manipulative thrust forces required for each clinical situation and patient type.

There is a multitude of different methods reported in the literature to treat clinical manifestations of sacroiliac dysfunction, including a variety of manipulative techniques.

Sacroiliac Manipulative Skills

There are many different techniques available to manipulate the sacroiliac joints in a variety of postures including the supine, prone and side positions. Several different techniques have been described by various professions, including physiotherapy, osteopathy and chiropractic (States, 1968; Nwuga, 1976; Gitelman, 1980; Grice, 1983; McGregor and Cassidy, 1983; Szaraz, 1984; Bourdillon and Day, 1987; Blackman and Prip, 1988; Greenman, 1989; Schafer and Faye, 1989; Bernard and Cassidy, 1991; Cassidy *et al.*, 1992; Cassidy and Mierau, 1992; Gitelman and Fligg, 1992; Cassidy *et al.*, 1993).

It appears that any number of techniques are equally as effective in eliminating the symptoms of mechanical low back pain due to sacroiliac dysfunction. A clinician should become proficient in a number of different mobilization and manipulative styles, depending upon the clinical presentation of the patient. Many of these techniques are only variations of a common theme which is based upon a biomechanical model of reciprocal movement of the innominates and nutation/counter-nutation of the sacrum (Grice and Fligg, 1980; McGregor and Cassidy, 1983; Bernard and Cassidy, 1991). This model includes the mechanical influence of the stabilizing ligaments and the contractile elements of the pelvis which form a kinematic chain.

The student should begin at a point that will provide the basis for the introduction of other manipulative methods used for treatment of the sacroiliac joint. This hinges on a fundamental understanding of the anatomy, biomechanics, pathogenesis and diagnosis of sacroiliac dysfunction. It has been reported that the side posture method is the most effective method for treating sacroiliac dysfunction (Kirkaldy-Willis and Cassidy, 1985; Cassidy *et al.* 1985; Bernard and Kirkaldy-Willis, 1987; Bourdillon and

Day, 1987; Cassidy and Mierau, 1992). It is for this reason that a description of side posture skills for the sacroiliac joint will be presented. Reference will be made to the anatomical landmark and not the therapeutic indications for pelvic correction. Three anatomical contact points will be presented:

Posterior superior iliac spine (PSIS)

Ischial tuberosity (IT)

Sacral base (SB).

The following skills are based upon a standardized and fairly reliable palpatory diagnostic method (Gillet and Liekens, 1981) and a chiropractic model of the functional aspects of the sacroiliac joint (McGregor and Cassidy, 1983; Cassidy and Mierau, 1992). Specific clinical criteria necessary to accommodate both patient tolerance and other sensitive structures, such as the lumbosacral spine and hip joints, will be included. It may be noted that modifications of the following skills may be adapted to any analysis system.

Posterior Superior Iliac Spine (PSIS) Contact

This contact point is used for adjustments commonly referred to as PI (Walters, 1993), upper joint flexion fixation of the sacroiliac joint (Gitelman, 1980), upper sacroiliac joint fixation (Schafer and Faye, 1989), flexion of the sacrum, flexed innominate, flexion malposition of the innominate (Szaraz, 1984).

1) Follow and complete the basic side posture procedural skills as described in Chapter 7 to the point where the doctor is directly facing the patient and supporting the upper leg (*thigh sandwich*) with minimum of 90 degrees of hip flexion. With the index and middle finger of the contact (left) hand, the doctor palpates the space just medial to the PSIS to appreciate the tissue tension around the sacroiliac joint during increased hip flexion (fig. 8.1). Increased hip flexion is achieved by moving the doctor's hips and thigh sandwich in a cephalad direction. At the point of perceived tissue tension further hip flexion is unnecessary. The patient's hip should be stabilized to prevent loss of flexion and tension by the doctor's firm foot placement and stance. The lumbar spine will be flattened and there should be no excess tension placed on the patient's hip. The doctor is supported by the table and the patient. The patient's pelvis is perpendicular or slightly supinated relative to the table as indicated by the superior ASIS (*).

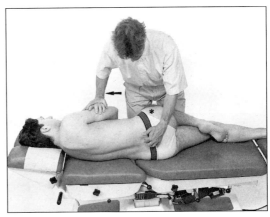

Fig 8.1

2) Once appropriate hip flexion and medial joint tissue tension has been accomplished, the hip is stabilized. Additional or excess tissue slack is drawn cephalad directly towards the doctor using the index and middle fingers of the indifferent hand (right) prior to the application of the contact hand (fig. 8.2).

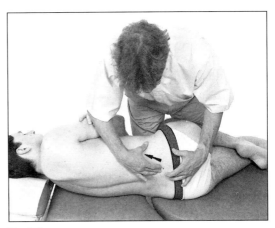

Fig 8.2

3) A bridge arch formed by the contact hand and the hypothenar/pisiform contact point is placed **lightly** over the most medial aspect of the PSIS and drawn up in the same direction as the tissue slack hand to tighten and increase the specificity of the contact hand. The contact arm is relaxed and positioned parallel to the patient's body (*) (fig. 8.3). The shoulders should be in a relaxed position with no muscular tension in either the contact or indifferent hands. There is minimal wrist extension (*). The doctor is still directly facing the table.

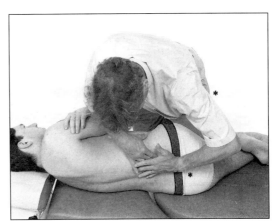

Fig 8.3

4) The contact arm is brought in line with the joint by pivoting the arm **around the wrist**, bringing the arm almost perpendicular to the contact point until the angle at the wrist is comfortably placed, with no muscular tension in the arm or shoulder girdle (fig. 8.4). The contact is **firm but light** and not **stiff**. The wrist is kept straight with no radial or ulnar deviation. The doctor must not pivot from the shoulder, disturbing the symmetry and balance already established (*). The doctor is still positioned perpendicular to the patient and the table, standing firmly in place. *Note that the shoulder posture does not change before or after the pivot shift.* Note the lack of upper back torsion during this procedure.

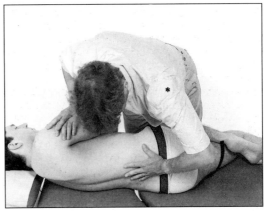

Fig 8.4

5) The doctor begins the 45 pivot shift into a fencer stance while at the same time maintaining tissue tension, hip flexion and patient comfort. The pivot procedure is described in Chapter 4; a full body 45 degree turn. This brings the contact hand and arm into position without excess shoulder torsion (fig. 8.5). The fencer stance position places the body weight slightly forward on the front leg and the heel of the back leg is slightly raised with both legs flexed. The suprasternal notch should be slightly ahead of the PSIS (*). There should be **absolutely no force** on the PSIS or muscular tension in the upper body of the doctor. Minimal tension and effort should be expended to support the patient on the table. *Note the shoulder posture does not change.* The patient is relaxed with no twist or tension in the body. Compare position in Figure 8.4. The patient's pelvis remains perpendicular to the table.

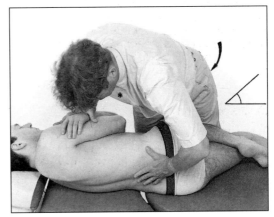

Fig 8.5

6) The next step is to shift doctor's body weight forward and onto the patient to further stabilize the patient on the table and position the body weight over the joint prior to the dynamic thrust. The doctor *very slowly* pushes his/her weight forward by plantar flexing the foot of the back leg, which will project the body forward towards the patient so that the front leg assumes a majority of the doctor's body weight (fig. 8.6). This is done while all other previous skills remain intact to maintain patient control. A gentle thigh squeeze is essential at this point. The doctor slides the rear leg over the patient's tibia to control the amount of leg drop (*). As the doctor moves forward, the rear foot will elevate off the floor as the front leg supports the majority of the body weight.

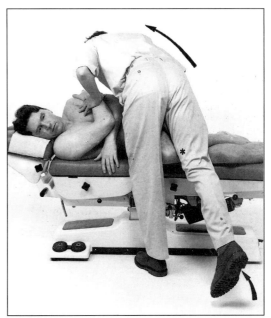

Fig 8.6

7) The doctor continues to move up and forward until the patient's tibia falls into the suprapatellar fossa (*) (fig. 8.7). The patient's leg is not forced towards the table. This controls leg drop and excess twist in the hip and lumbosacral region. The hip is maintained at a minimum of 90 degrees during this entire procedure. The contact arm and shoulder should not change. Nor should there be any tension felt by the patient. He or she should be relaxed and cooperative. Don't squeeze the patient's leg and **don't let it drop**. The amount of leg drop and hip flexion assists sacroiliac joint isolation and tension.

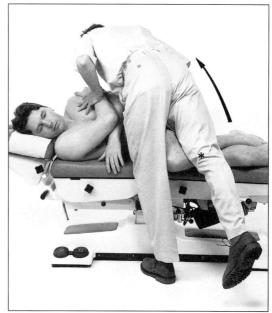

Fig 8.7

8) Once body weight is over the patient, the doctor brings the rear foot down to the floor in a plantar flexed posture, which permits flexibility in the doctor's stance. This action will bring the patient's leg down towards the table to increase the tension in the sacroiliac joint (fig. 8.8). Note the position of the patient's knee in Figure 8.8 as compared to 8.7 to get an appreciation of the amount of drop involved. Notice that the doctor has dropped his weight down over the patient and the rear leg is slightly flexed supporting under the patient's leg with a thigh sandwich. The doctor gently squeezes his legs together to hold the leg in place without compressing the patient's knee. The doctor's feet are still only hip distance apart and 45 degrees to the table. **There are many other methods of stabilizing the patient's leg**.

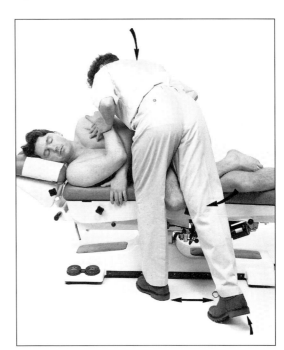

Fig 8.8

9) There are many errors to be aware of during this sequence of skills.

i) The contact arm pivot at the shoulder instead of the wrist will produce unwanted torque and tissue stress at the shoulder (fig. 8.9). This can also be produced by over-pivoting the lower body. Note the amount of internal rotation of the contact (right) shoulder. A dynamic thrust applied through this joint may cause injury.

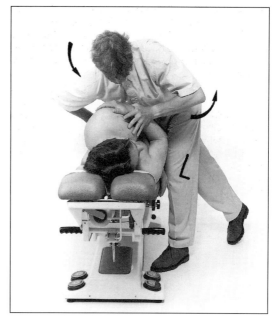

Fig 8.9

ii) The feet and legs can drift apart during the pivot to a low fencer stance. This will contribute to loss of control of the patient's leg and body weight. (fig. 8.10). Some find this stance clinically useful, but they have developed other patient control skills to compensate.

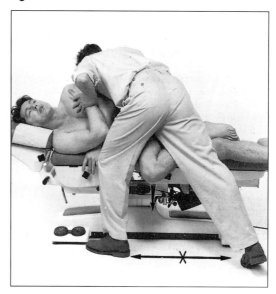

Fig 8.10

iii) Losing soft tissue tension at the sacroiliac joint during the pivot shift to a 45 degree fencer stance, by letting the patient's hip drop below the minimal 90 degrees of hip flexion increasing paraspinal muscular laxity and the lumbar lordosis (*), decreasing joint stability. It is essential to maintain tension prior to the thrust (fig. 8.11).

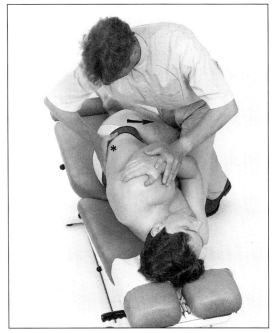

Fig 8.11

iv) The doctor may tend to lean on the patient's upper body instead of elevating the torso and centre of gravity above the joint to maximize the use of body weight to develop joint tension prior to the dynamic thrust (fig. 8.12).

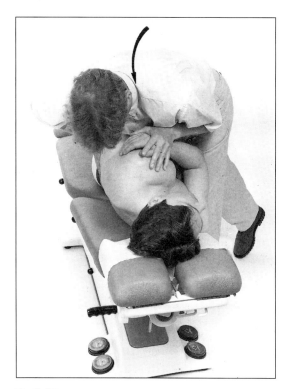

Fig 8.12

v) Positioning the torso too high, whereby the angle of the contact arm could create a pile-driver or pushing effect over the contact point, is another error. This increases the length of the lever arm which amplifies the amount of force applied (fig. 8.13). The balance of torso weight is somewhere between (iv) and (v).

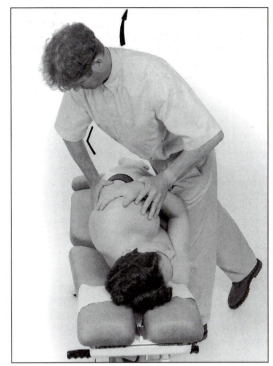

Fig 8.13

One of the most common errors at this stage is the excessive use of muscular force while developing tension on the PSIS contact. It is a natural tendency to work harder than is necessary. The awkward movements trying to control patient motion often result in an increase in pressure over the patient. Another assumption that the firmer the contact the better the manipulative technique is not valid. The procedure revolves around positioning, slowly isolating small joint motion, and patient comfort. Keep things light at all times with no excessive movements.

Up to this point there should be no excessive tension across the lumbosacral joint complex. The skills have been introduced in order to position the patient and isolate the joint movement effectively using the longer levers of the skill. The next series of steps will bring the sequence to the point of maximum joint tension appreciation just before joint preload or prestress is applied, concentrating on incorporating the short levers. Move *slowly and methodically*. The movement sequence should not be hurried. It is a natural tendency to rush the process and

attempt an adjustive thrust. This may reinforce unwanted habits which are sometimes difficult to alter in the long term.

At this point the patient should be relaxed and comfortable in the side posture, the doctor positioned with body weight forward, centre of gravity close vertically to the sacroiliac joint (suprasternal notch), contact shoulder, arm and hand relaxed with **no** compressive force placed over the PSIS and **no** muscular tension in any part of the doctor's body apart from the front leg. It is recommended that students must not proceed past this point until the skills and sequence thus far are efficiently performed. The movements of both the doctor and the patient are very small in relation to the whole manipulative skill. This is the essence of control – limit the amount of movement.

The following steps of this manipulative skill will function to introduce the short levers to develop joint tension and apply preload prior to the adjustive thrust. During this final step, it is recommended that the patient's breathing pattern be incorporated as part of the overall skill sequence. The patient will be requested to breathe in and then slowly out as tension and joint preload are applied across the sacroiliac joint and surrounding soft tissues. This action may help to focus the patient's attention and assist overall relaxation. It is recommended that the doctor also coordinate his/her breathing pattern with that of the patient, which may help to focus the effort required for the eventual dynamic thrust. This breathing pattern may quite simply distract the patient's attention from the impending manipulation by reducing muscular tension, maintaining trunk flexibility and patient control.

10) From the sequence of movements described in Figures 8.1 to 8.8, the doctor's body weight moves forward and down by slightly flexing the legs at the knees. At the same time the patient's pelvis is **slowly** rolled forward from a perpendicular position (*) (fig. 8.14a) to a position that is slightly angled towards the table (fig. 8.14b). This is controlled by the doctor's leg position and body weight. The indifferent hand maintains upper body position and stability by **pressing down** and **not backwards**, but allowing the upper torso to roll very slightly forward to eliminate excess upper body torque.

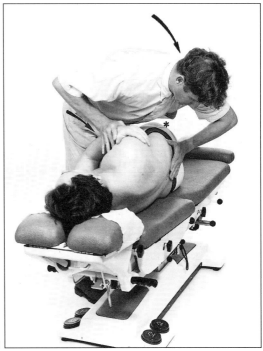

Fig 8.14a

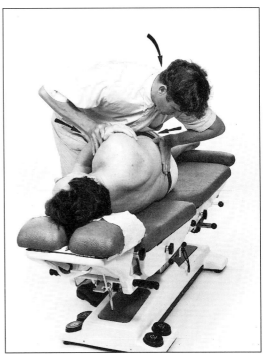

Fig 8.14b

11) The suprasternal notch and the body weight should be located just ahead of the PSIS as a result of the forward movement of the doctor's weight and after the pelvis has been moved forward. This should still align the doctor's centre of gravity and weight distribution optimally for the dynamic thrust (fig. 8.15a). The indifferent arm (right) is brought in to the side of the doctor's body to make a more compact thrust application. The patient is aligned in a straight longitudinal fashion along the table, reducing overall torque and spinal stress (fig. 8.15b)

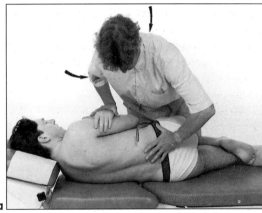

Fig 8.15a

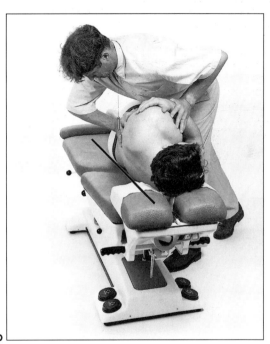

Fig 8.15b

12) The contact arm begins to apply force gradually to the contact point using, primarily, the shoulder adductors (fig. 8.16). This is likened to a *squeezing action* between the contact hand and the doctor's body to isolate and localize preload or tension to one primary target joint (*refer back to Chapter 6, Figures 6.30 and 6.31*). The pelvis is virtually stationary at this point as the doctor's body weight is placed to block further movement. This is the point at which the short levers are introduced and controlled by very slow application until a resistance is appreciated at the point of contact. The student should consider this a mock thrust, a repetitive oscillation at joint tension to feel the point of maximum joint give. **This is the only time that any significant muscular tension is produced by either the contact or indifferent hand and arm over the contact point.**

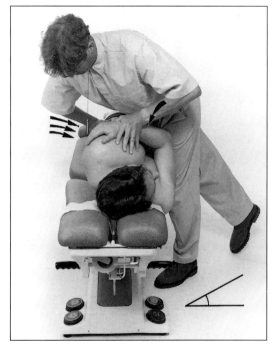

Fig 8.16

A dynamic thrust should not be applied at this stage; only mock preloads to learn to appreciate joint resistance and the tightening of the targetted joint and surrounding tissue. Care must be taken not to stress the tissue over a period of time, which may cause unwanted reactions during practice sessions.

13) There are a few errors to be aware of during this last section.

i) Over-rotating the pelvis forward and too quickly causes excessive twist in the thoracic spine and thoracocolumbar region and loss of control of the patient before the dynamic thrust. The upper back is pushed too far back and the pelvis too far forward (fig. 8.17). Compare the pelvic rotation to Figure 8.16. Also note the tension in the shoulder girdle (*). It is difficult for the patient to relax under this excessive tension.

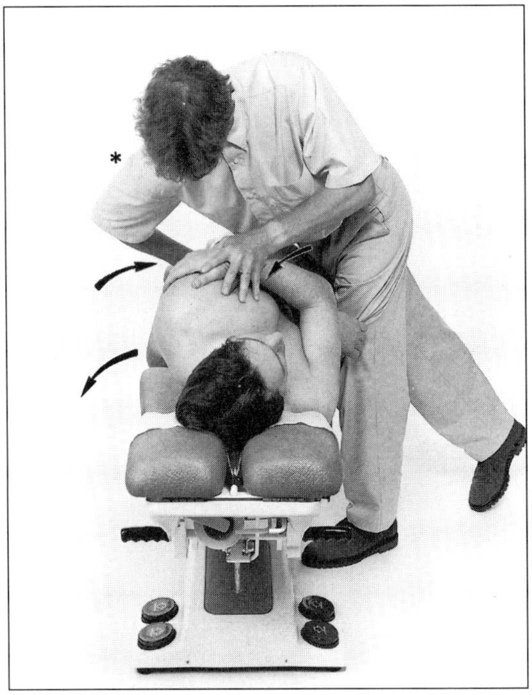

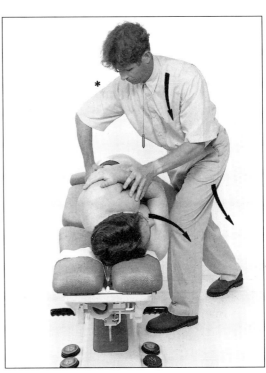

Fig 8.17

ii) The most common mistake encountered occurs during transferring of body weight. The tendency is to push up and then straight down instead of forward and over the patient to centre the body weight. In this instance the body weight is over the front of the table (fig. 8.18). This movement brings the patient too far forward on the table and the doctor's jugular notch and weight are not centred over the sacroiliac joint. Further movement will compromise the patient's stability on the table and the patient may automatically roll uncontrollably forward, resulting in emergency evasive action by the doctor to keep the patient on the table. Note the stress on the contact arm (*).

iii) Students have a tendency to focus all of their energy on the PSIS contact point. Unnecessary muscular forces may cause fatigue and possible patient distress if the contact is also painful. Patients will react by displaying protective resistance, which decreases the efficiency and smooth performance of the skill.

Fig 8.18

Tension in the contact arm should take place only during the final stages of the manipulative skill. This tension should be applied gradually. All aspects of the sequence are equally important.

Ischial Tuberosity (IT) Contact

This contact point is commonly used for adjustments referred to as AS (Walters, 1993), lower joint extension fixation of the sacroiliac joint (Gitelman, 1980), lower sacroiliac joint fixation (Schafer and Faye, 1989), extension of the sacrum, extension of the innominate and extension malposition of the innominate (Szaraz, 1984).

This manipulative procedure involves *the same sequential steps* previously described for the PSIS contact above and side posture skills in Chapter 7 up to where the contact hand is applied to the IT. It should also be pointed out that the IT represents a very large and broad contact which has a tendency to distribute the manipulative forces over a wider area. With this in mind, the muscular power required for this set of skills may seem to exceed the student's capabilities. Keep this in perspective and concentrate on the slow movement and gradually develop the necessary strength to perform an efficient overall manipulative procedure. The majority of the muscular power is used only at the end of the sequence, just as the preload is applied, and during the manipulative thrust itself. On a clinical note, this particular manipulation is not recommended during the treatment of suspected lumbar intervertebral disc herniation (Cassidy *et al.*, 1993).

1) The doctor is perpendicular to the patient prior to the pivot shift and in a fairly low fencer stance posture. The indifferent hand (right) is in place, with the patient in a comfortable and relaxed position. The heel of the bridged contact hand is placed on the buttock next to the sacrum well above the ischial contact. The contact is **light but firm** and not **stiff**. The wrist is kept straight with no radial or ulnar deviation (*). The contact arm is subsequently positioned almost parallel to the patient and the patient's hip is flexed to 90 degrees and secured by the doctor's legs with a thigh sandwich. The doctor's torso is positioned directly in line with the hand contact and elevated above the pelvis (fig. 8.19). There is no tension or torque in the shoulder girdle.

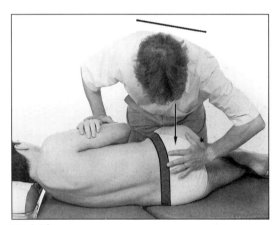

Fig 8.19

2) In order to develop tension in the surrounding soft tissues, three simultaneous actions are required.

i) The contact hand is pulled caudad and around the IT drawing tissue and at the same time the contact arm is brought in toward the body in a slow controlled **scooping** movement (arm is extended and adducted across the chest wall) (fig. 8.20). This causes dorsiflexion (extension) of the wrist during this movement (*).

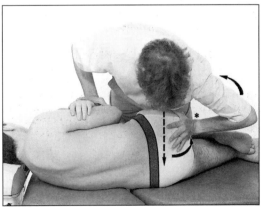

Fig 8.20

ii) The doctor assists the innominate flexion by pivoting and moving the hips cephalad with the knees bent and feet planted hip distance apart at the same time, thereby keeping the torso in the same position, which is now positioned behind the contact point. There is only a minimal pivot shift into a semi-fencer stance (fig. 8.21). If additional tension is required, the patient's leg is allowed to drop towards the floor.

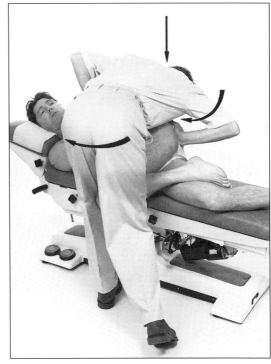

Fig 8.21

iii) As the hips pivot forward, the doctor's torso becomes positioned closer and behind the contact hand and arm for additional support (fig. 8.22). The contact arm is positioned close to the body in order to reduce any torsional effects. This is a very large and stable structure that cannot be moved by the arm only. Effective use of the shoulder girdle and the body weight will minimize any mechanical effects. The torsion in the lumbar region is minimal (*). Appreciation of both joint and soft tissue tension and the muscular force required for joint preload should be introduced gradually.

3) The indifferent hand (right) adds slight traction and downward pressure in a cephalad direction. The indifferent arm is kept close to the doctor's body (fig. 8.22).

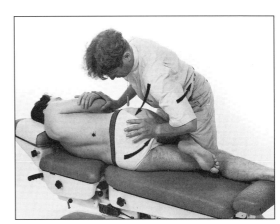

Fig 8.22

4) An alternative forearm contact may be used and is just as effective. The flexor region of the contact forearm contacts the IT in the same way as the pisiform/hypothenar contact (fig. 8.23). The arm is pulled toward the body in a similar scooping action to cause flexion of the innominate. The use of this contact does not subject the shoulder girdle to the same physical demands. Note the lack of torsion in the lumbar spine (*).

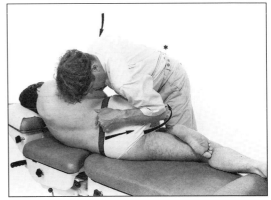

Fig 8.23

5) *There is one major error to be aware of while learning this particular set of manipulative skills combined with those already presented in the section on PSIS contact (above).*

The doctor's torso drifts ahead of the contact point, increasing the mechanical stress on the arm and shoulder (fig. 8.24). This places the centre of gravity at a disadvantage. The whole body moves forward during the hip pivot action in the cephalad direction, causing unnecessary torque of the doctor's shoulder. Due to the lack of an efficient scooping action of the contact arm and hand to assist flexion of the innominate, the student attempts to push the IT cephalad against considerable resistance (fig. 8.24).

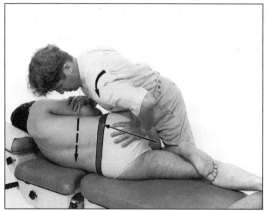

Fig 8.24

Sacral Base (SB) Contact

This anatomical contact point is often used for adjustments referred to as upper sacroiliac joint and posterior superior subluxation of the sacrum. Gitelman (1980), Grice (1983) and Gitelman and Fligg (1992) describe alternate contacts for manipulation of the various sacroiliac fixations. Grice (1983) describes in detail a sacral contact to correct sacroiliac dysfunction, called the sacroiliac cross fix adjustment, which is based upon specific motion palpation patterns. **The sacrum represents a smaller anatomical landmark and lever compared to the larger PSIS and IT, which may provide additional biomechanical advantage to both** the patient and the manipulator. Nonetheless, a substantial amount of control is necessary to manoeuvre the small levers prior to the dynamic thrust. The biomechanical effects upon the joint should be almost identical.

This particular manipulative skill is almost self-explanatory. The anatomical contact point is on the sacral base just superior and lateral to the second sacral tubercle. The sequence of skills is exactly the same as that described and practised for the PSIS contact, except for some minor modifications related to the contact hand and arm and the position of the doctor. The side posture positional skills have previously been described. Position the patient accordingly.

1) The hypothenar/pisiform or thenar contact points can be used. The hypothenar is the easiest adaptation already described above for the PSIS. Virtually everything is the same except that after the tissue has been drawn, the contact hand is placed just lateral to the first sacral segment on the base of the sacrum (fig. 8.25). Then proceed with the other steps as described above. Remember, the bridged hand posture is essential. Note the symmetry in the shoulder girdle, the position of the body weight over the contact point and the lack of torque in the shoulder (*).

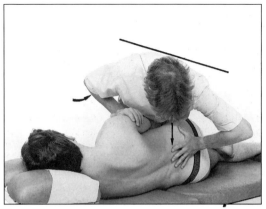

Fig 8.25

2) The thenar eminence is slightly more difficult to perform as the wrist is pronated which may cause some torque at the shoulder joint (*) (fig. 8.26). Note the symmetry of the shoulders. The doctor slowly rotates the pelvis forward as the body weight drops to develop preload prior to the dynamic body drop thrust.

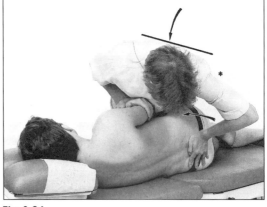

Fig 8.26

3) As a result of the movement of the arm to position the thenar contact the shoulder has to rotate forward. To reduce this effect upon the shoulder the doctor's torso has to move the centre of gravity cephalad, (fig. 8.27). This is not the most advantageous posture for the optimal use of the doctor's body weight and the efficiency of the overall manipulative skill. The thenar eminence offers advantages in terms of comfort and ease of localization.

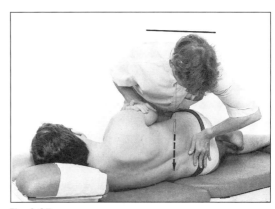

Fig 8.27

4) There are similar errors to be aware of while learning this set of manipulative skills.
    The most common one encountered for both the hypothenar/pisiform and thenar contacts is the excess torque of the shoulder when the hand contact is made (fig. 8.28). The shift of the body weight forward reduces the efficiency of the manipulative response.

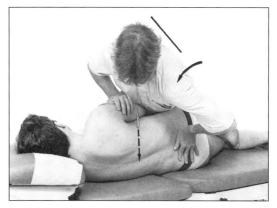

Fig 8.28

This chapter has presented three of the most common anatomical landmarks used for manipulative procedures associated with dysfunction of the sacroiliac joint. The presentation has been careful *not* to over-emphasize the dynamic thrust, but has more importantly, emphasized the sequence of skills for both patient and doctor up to the point of joint/tissue tension and the application of joint pre-load.

The dynamic thrust is a highly skilled manoeuvre that should be introduced only after proficiency in all other aspects has been demonstrated. Finesse, control and balance have been highlighted.

References

Adams, A.A. and Wood, J. (1984) Forces used in selected chiropractic adjustments of the low back: a preliminary study. *The Research Forum, Palmer College of Chiropractic*, **1**, 5–9

Bernard, T.N. and Kirkaldy-Willis, W.H. (1987) Recognising specific characteristics of non-specific low back pain. *Clinical Orthopaedics*, **217**, 266–280

Bernard, T.N. and Cassidy, J.D. (1991) The sacroiliac syndrome: pathophysiology, diagnosis, and management. In *The Adult Spine: Principles and Practice* (ed. J.W. Frymoyer). Raven Press, New York, pp. 2107–2130

Berg, G., Hammer, M., Moller-Nielsen, J. *et al.* (1988) Low back pain during pregnancy. *Obstetrics and Gynecology*, **71**, 71–75

Blackman, J. and Prip, K. (1988) Sacroiliac joint. In *Mobilisation Techniques*, 2nd edn. Churchill Livingstone, London

Bourdillon, J.F. and Day, E.A. (1987) Treatment of the joints of the pelvis. In *Spinal Manipulation*, 4th edn. William Heinemann Medical Books, London, Appleton and Lange, Los Altos, California, pp. 99–117

Bowen, V. and Cassidy, J.D. (1981) Macroscopic and microscopic anatomy of the sacroiliac joint from embryonic life until the eighth decade. *Spine*, **6**, 620–628

Brunner, C., Kissling, R. and Jacob, H.A.C. (1991) The effects of morphology and histopathologic findings on the mobility of the sacroiliac joint. *Spine*, **16**, 1111–1117

Cassidy, J.D., Kirkaldy-Willis, W.H. and McGregor, M. (1985) Spinal manipulation for the treatment of chronic low-back and leg pain: an observational study. In *Empirical Approaches to the Validation of Spinal Manipulation* (eds. A.A. Buerger and P.E. Greenman). Charles C. Thomas, Springfield IL, pp. 123–128

Cassidy, J.D. (1992) The pathoanatomy and clinical significance of the sacroiliac joints. *Journal of Manipulative and Physiological Therapeutics*, **15**, 41–42

Cassidy, J.D. and Mierau, D.R. (1992) Pathophysiology of the sacroiliac joint. In *Principles and Practice of Chiropractic*, 2nd edn. Appleton and Lange, California, pp. 211–224

Cassidy, J.D., Kirkaldy-Willis, W.H. and Thiel, H.W. (1992) Manipulation. In *Managing Low Back Pain*, 3rd edn. (ed. W.H. Kirkaldy-Willis and C.V. Burton). Churchill Livingstone, London, pp. 283–296

Cassidy, J.D., Thiel, H.W. and Kirkaldy-Willis, W.H. (1993) Side posture manipulation for lumbar intervertebral disc herniation. *Journal of Manipulative and Physiological Therapeutics*, **16**, 96–103

Chapman-Smith, D. (1990) Sacroiliac dysfunction. *The Chiropractic Report*, **5**, 1–6

Chapman-Smith, D. (1993) The sacroiliac joints revisited. *The Chiropractic Report*, **7**, 1–6

Gillet, H. and Liekens, M. (1981) *Belgium Chiropractic Research Notes*, 11th edn. Motion Palpation Institute, Huntington Beach, California

Gitelman, R. (1980) A chiropractic approach to biomechanical disorders of the lumbar spine and pelvis. In *Modern Developments in the Principles and Practice of Chiropractic* (ed. S. Haldeman). Appleton-Century-Crofts, New York, pp. 297–330

Gitelman, R. and Fligg, B. (1992) Diversified technique. In *Principles and Practice of Chiropractic*, 2nd edn. (ed. S. Haldeman). Appleton and Lange, San Mateo, California, pp. 483–501

Greenman, P.E. (1989) Principles of diagnosis and treatment of pelvic girdle dysfunction. In *Principles of Manual Medicine*, 1st edn. Williams and Wilkins, London, pp. 225–270

Grice, A.S. (1980) A biomechanical approach to cervical and dorsal adjusting. In *Modern Developments in the Principles and Practice of Chiropractic* (ed. S. Haldeman). Appleton-Century-Crofts, New York, p. 340

Grice, A. and Fligg, B. (1980) Biomechanics of the pelvis. In *Biomechanics of the Pelvis* (ed. P. Laufenberg). Denver Conference Monographs, Council on Technique ACA, Iowa

Grice, A. (1983) Sacroiliac cross fix adjustment. *Journal of the Canadian Chiropractic Association*, **27**, 162–163

Hessell, B.W., Herzog, W., Conway, P.J.W. *et al.* (1990) Experimental measurement of the force exerted during spinal manipulation using the Thompson Technique. *Journal of Manipulative and Physiological Therapeutics*, **13**, 448–453

Kirkaldy-Willis, W.H., and Cassidy, J.D. (1985) Spinal manipulation in the treatment of low back pain. *Canadian Family Physician*, **31**, 535–540

Kirkaldy-Willis, W.H. (1988) The site and nature of the lesion. In *Managing Low Back Pain*, 2nd edn. (ed. W.H. Kirkaldy-Willis). Churchill Livingstone, London, pp. 133–154

McGregor, M. and Cassidy, J.D. (1983) Post-surgical sacroiliac syndrome. *Journal of*

Manipulative and Physiological Therapeutics, **6**, 1–11

Mierau, D.R., Cassidy, J.D., Hamin, T. *et al.* (1984) Sacroiliac joint dysfunction and low back pain in school aged children. *Journal of Manipulative and Physiological Therapeutics*, **7**, 81–84

Nwuga, V.C. (1976) Techniques of spinal manipulation. In *Manipulation of the Spine*. Waverly Press, Baltimore, pp. 47–66

Schafer, R.C. and Faye, L.J. (1989) The pelvis. In *Motion Palpation and Chiropractic Technic – Principles of Dynamic Chiropractic*. Motion Palpation Institute, Huntington Beach, California, pp. 241–292

Schneider, M.J. (1992) Soft tissue effects of sacroiliac and lumbosacral joint manipulation. *Chiropractic Technique*, **4**, 136–142

States, A.Z. (1968) *Atlas of Chiropractic Technic: Spinal and Pelvic Technics*, 2nd edn. National College of Chiropractic, Lombard Il., USA

Sturesson, B., Selvik, G. and Uden, A. (1989) Movements of the sacroiliac joints: a roentgen stereophotogrammetric analysis. *Spine*, **14**, 162–165

Szaraz, Z.T. (1984) *Compendium of Chiropractic Technique*. Canadian Memorial Chiropractic College, Toronto, Canada

Vleeming, A., Stoeckart, R. and Snijders, C.J. (1989) The sacrotuberous ligament: a conceptual approach to its dynamic role in stabilizing the sacroiliac joint. *Clinical Biomechanics*, **4**, 201–203

Vleeming, A., Stoeckart, R., Volkers, A.C.W. *et al.* (1990) Relation between form and function in the sacroiliac joint, Part 1: Clinical anatomical aspects. *Spine*, **15**, 130–132

Vleeming, A., Van Wingerden, J.P., Dijkstra, P.F. *et al.* (1992) Mobility in the sacroiliac joints in the elderly: a kinematic and radiological study. *Clinical Biomechanics*, **7**, 170–176

Walters, P.J. (1993) Pelvis. In *Textbook of Clinical Chiropractic. A Specific Biomechanical Approach* (eds. G. Plaugher and M.A. Lopes). Williams and Wilkins, London, p. 161

Further Reading

Bogduk, N. and Twomey, L.T. (1991) The lumbar muscles and their fascia. In *Clinical Anatomy of the Lumbar Spine*, 2nd edn. (eds. N. Bogduk and L.T. Twomey). Churchill Livingstone, Edinburgh, pp. 83–105

Pearcy, M. (1989) Biomechanics of the spine. *Current Orthopaedics*, **3**, 96–100

Vleeming, A., Volkers, A.C.W., Snijders, C.J. *et al.* (1990) Relation between form and function in the sacro-iliac joint, Part 2: Biomechanical aspects. *Spine*, **15**, 133–136

9

Lumbar spine manipulative skills

David Byfield

Introduction

The magnitude of the social and economic effects of low back pain is a well known fact of life. The impact of low back pain has been described as enormous and extremely costly in terms of treatment and lost productivity (Burton and Cassidy, 1992). There is little doubt that low back pain affects the quality of life for a substantial number of people in contemporary western society (Kelsey, 1982; Kirkaldy-Willis and Cassidy, 1985). When estimates of 6.8% of the US population are suffering from at least a 2-week spell of low back pain at any given time with a lifetime prevalence of 13.8% (Deyo and Tsui-Wu, 1987), it is not unrealistic to suggest that modern societies may be facing an epidemic of lower back disability (Waddell, 1993). The magnitude of this problem is clearly indicated when 60–80% of the general population will suffer low back pain at some time during their lives and between 20% and 30% are suffering at any given time (Kelsey and White, 1980). Consequently, it should not be unexpected that due to a cumulative lifetime incidence as high as 65% (Deyo and Tsui-Wu, 1987), more than one half of the working population will suffer low back pain during the working life (Cassidy and Wedge, 1988).

Chronic back pain represents the most rapidly growing cause of any other form of disability (Waddell, 1993) and has been identified as the leading cause of disability and most expensive health care problem in the 30–50 year old age group

(Spengler *et al.*, 1986). More alarming is the fact that there appears to be no evidence of any change in the nature, severity or biological basis of back pain (Waddell, 1993). To date, the medical contribution to this expanding problem has been ineffective and minimal. This state of affairs has been attributed, in part, to a lack of understanding of the pathophysiological and pathoanatomical principles associated with low back pain (Waddell, 1987). It is reasonable to assume that therapeutic intervention is going to have limited measurable value when the aetiological factors are unknown. Musculoskeletal pain has been described as both multidimensional and multifactorial in nature, which represents a much wider view of the potential aetiological parameters associated with low back pain (Troup and Videman, 1989). These authors have attempted to redirect and focus the attitude of the health care community into viewing the problem as more of a social dilemma rather than a single identifiable lesion. This is equally as relevant and of considerable importance to the chiropractic profession, which traditionally has proclaimed that a patient is treated as a whole person, encompassing many contributory aspects of the individual's lifestyle. Furthermore, the treatment of pain and dis-ability can be altered by appropriate conservative care (Wiltse, 1987).

The aetiology of most spinal pain remains obscure and in most cases unknown (Waddell, 1987). This has been attributed, in part, to the complex innervation of the intrinsic spinal structures which could provide valuable information as to potential pain sources, but presently only confounds the issue (Bogduk, 1983). Therefore, it is not surprising that between 20% and 80% of medical diagnoses of low back pain are still considered idiopathic in nature (White, 1982). As a result of the complexity of its pathogenesis, which still remains a poorly understood chain of events (Acker *et al.*, 1990). Even though there is little agreement upon the nature of the aetiology of low back pain, clinical models and management strategies have been developed based upon available information regarding its natural history, biochemical and biomechanical characteristics (Kirkaldy-Willis, *et al.*, 1978). There is no doubt that our sedentary lifestyle and escalating socioeconomic tensions have contributed to the problem. In an attempt to address this issue, medical treatment and management of back pain has failed because of a seemingly passive role and a sustained focus on structural disorders rather than more relevant functional, psychosocial and environmental factors (Waddell, 1987; Vernon, 1991; Liebenson, 1992).

Conventional Treatment

The more traditional and acceptable forms of medical treatment for low back pain have largely gone untested and remain questionable. Deyo *et al.* (1986) have shown that bed rest is of little therapeutic value after 2 days and prolonged use is potentially harmful. In another study, patients receiving no bed rest returned to work significantly faster than those receiving 4 days' rest (Gilbert *et al.*, 1985). The Quebec Task Force on Spinal Disorders (1987) concluded that bed rest should be reserved for acute cases only and in most cases limited to a few days. Notwithstanding, a large proportion of UK general practitioners still prescribe bed rest for low back pain (Waddell, 1993). Other more popular forms of treatment, most notably corticosteroid injections into the facet joints of the lumbar spine, have been shown to be ineffective

and of little benefit in the treatment of low back pain (Carette *et al.*, 1991; Frank, 1993). Widely used methods of pain control such as transcutaneous electrical nerve stimulation (TENS) and epidural anaesthetic injections can support minimal proof of efficacy and evidence is mounting to suggest that they can actually contribute to the development of long-term chronic pain patterns (Bennett, 1990; Frank, 1993). Therefore, it can be concluded that inactive forms of treatment provide no advantage in the management of low back pain and should be used with caution. These conclusions are supported by recent evidence demonstrating the pathological effects of long periods of immobilization (Videman, 1987). This is of significant clinical importance to the chiropractic profession, because it supports a more active treatment intervention strategy including skilled manipulative management.

Therefore, it appears that restoring function could be the most significant factor in preventing chronic disability (Mayer *et al.*, 1987). The emphasis should focus equally on symptomatic relief and the early return to functional capacity of both joints and muscles, providing a rapid resumption of daily activities (Waddell, 1993). The patient willingly participates and assumes a responsibility for his/her continuing rehabilitation throughout the entire integrated process (Hazard *et al.*, 1989). This constitutes the basis of the chiropractic functional approach and with effective use of spinal manipulative therapy, may play a key role in the future management of low back pain disability (Vernon, 1991). Ebrall (1992) suggested that the cost-effectiveness of chiropractic management of mechanical low back pain compared to medical treatment was due to a prompt restoration of function. He concluded that the success of chiropractic management was attributed to a complex interaction of clinical activities which emphasize diagnostic classification and clinical management protocols, including patient responsibilities, attention to optimal spinal function and rehabilitative aftercare. It has been observed that work-related disability could be lessened by prompt manipulative intervention by chiropractors (Ebrall, 1993). A recent report commissioned by the government of Ontario, Canada concludes unequivocally that chiropractic management is superior to medical management for low back pain in terms of scientific effectiveness, cost-effectiveness, safety and overall patient satisfaction (Chapman-Smith, 1993a and b; Manga *et al.*, 1993)

Role of Manipulation

The role of skilled manipulation in this dynamic and functional approach can no longer be reasonably questioned, especially in light of more recent evidence illustrating its clinical efficacy. Manipulation has been shown to be highly instrumental in the treatment and management of both acute and chronic forms of low back pain. A contemporary review recently published by Shekelle *et al.* (1992) concluded that manipulation was appropriate for acute and uncomplicated forms of low back pain, but was undecided on its role in chronic pain management. However, Meade *et al.* (1990) concluded that chiropractic manipulative management was highly successful in the long-term management of chronic and severe forms of low back pain compared with outpatient hospital care. These conclusions were echoed in a recent study by Koes *et al.* (1992b) who demonstrated the long-term benefits of manipulative therapy compared to medical treatment and physiotherapy for chronic non-specific neck and back pain over a 12-month period. Manual therapy has also been shown to improve performance levels of active spinal movements faster and greater compared to medical and physiotherapy (Koes *et al.*, 1992a). The role of chiropractic manipulation as part of a multidisciplinary approach is becoming increasingly more clear and will hopefully be more effectively defined over the next few years.

What makes chiropractic management superior to other forms of treatment for mechanical low back pain? Skilled manipulation and the dynamic thrust, among others, have been identified as a common denominator (Kirkaldy-Willis and Cassidy, 1985; Lewit, 1986; Meade *et al.*, 1990). Even though injuries to lumbar spine following manipulation are rare (Curtis, 1988), a clinical awareness of the absolute and relative contraindications of manual therapy should reduce the frequency of post-treatment reactions. This is particularly relevant since a larger number of elderly patients with osteoporosis are now seeking chiropractic care (Haldeman and Rubinstein, 1992). Manipulative complications of the lumbar spine are substantially fewer than the cervical spine and are attributed to long lever rotational manipulation methods (Dvorak *et al.*, 1992). There is an unwritten belief and fear within the chiropractic profession that rotational manipulation will cause or aggravate a pre-existing disc herniation. Fortunately, these cases are infrequent (Quon *et al.*, 1989).

Several factors have been identified as partially responsible for the complications of manipulation of the lumbar spine, including inadequate history, insufficient patient assessment, lack of knowledge, diagnostic errors, incompetent technical skills and inappropriate technique selection (Kleynhans, 1980; Terrett and Kleynhans, 1992). Finesse, positioning the patient, technique used and the area of the spine manipulated have been proposed as factors which may reduce the number of complications (Kleynhans, 1980). Standardizing patient assessment procedures has been targetted as a means of reducing these complications (Kleynhans and Terrett, 1985). It becomes increasingly clear that the clinical efficiency and consistency of spinal manipulative therapy depends upon not only the use of clever skills, but on the interaction of these skills with an in-depth knowledge base upon which meaningful decisions can be made concerning patient care.

Biomechanical Considerations (Disc and Facet)

It has been shown that forced rotation of the intervertebral joints *in vitro* will produce a torsional injury (Farfan *et al.*,

1970; Farfan, 1973). Cassidy *et al*. (1993) indicate that the direct relationship between torsion and disc failure is an erroneous notion. They contend that the intervertebral disc is well suited to withstand rotation based upon, among other factors, the orientation of the annular fibres. This has created a long-standing attitude in both medical and chiropractic communities. It only stands to reason that if you twist something hard enough, it will eventually break. However, evidence is now emerging which states that about 25% of the population have asymptomatic lumbar disc hernias which would be considered for surgical intervention if they were symptomatic (Dickson and Butt, 1992). They go on to say that 'the notion that one single injurious event, such as spinal manipulation, can induce a disc hernia is not tenable'. From a clinical perspective, Quon *et al*. (1989) have demonstrated that, even though a massive central herniation was demonstrable on CT scan, rotational manipulation for 2 weeks reduced the signs and symptoms. A follow-up scan at 4 months showed no change in the size or position of the disc herniation, yet the patient was pain free. They implied that the posterior joints played an important role in limiting the torsional strain on the disc and concluded that injury to the disc from manipulation is negligible. More recently, Cassidy *et al*. (1993) observed 14 patients undergoing treatment for disc herniation using side posture manipulation for a 2–3-week period improve their overall spinal mobility. The results showed that all but one patient benefited from the treatment and in most cases the disc herniation did not alter in size. They concluded that the pain associated with disc herniation was due to an inflammatory response and not due to the size of the herniation. Observations such as these begin to confirm the efficacy of side posture manipulation for the treatment of what has been considered in the past a condition that required specialist surgical intervention and bed rest. In light of this present study, side posture manipulation as a direct cause of disc rupture has to be reconsidered seriously. Careful appreciation of the underlying

pathological process combined with the **confidence** to perform these manipulative procedures takes considerable skill.

Yamamoto *et al*. (1989) established kinematic magnitudes of 1.5–2.6 degrees of axial rotation in each lumbar motion segment with the least motion occurring at the L5–S1 level. This evidence may indicate that the facet joints are more susceptible to torsional stress during side posture rotational manipulation than the disc (Byfield, 1991). Torsional loads that normally damage the facet joints have been shown to have no effect on the integrity of the disc (Adams and Hutton, 1981). This is not to imply that the intervertebral disc and related soft tissues are totally immune from the torsional effects of manipulation. Under normal conditions within the physiological range, there is minimal strain on the disc. Excessive torsional strain will be resisted by the intact facet joint (Stokes, 1988), which if applied repetitively may disrupt the axis of motion, increasing the lateral shear across the plane of the disc, causing torsional failure and peripheral tears in the annulus (Bogduk and Twomey, 1991). Lumbar facet asymmetry, once considered an aetiological factor associated with disc herniation, has recently been unsupported (Cassidy *et al*., 1992b). It is, therefore, difficult to imagine that daily practice methods could produce such a catastrophic event.

Nonetheless, the intervertebral disc is not totally exempt from injury. It has been reported that the disc will prolapse as a result of a sudden hyperflexion action, sometimes associated with industrial lifting accidents (Adams and Hutton, 1982). The disc has also been demonstrated to prolapse gradually over a period of time due to microtrauma under repetitive compression and flexion loads (Adams and Hutton, 1985). These two mechanisms are common aetiological processes seen clinically with patients presenting with both acute and chronic insidious back pain. The lumbar spine in a flexed position can sustain very large forces as a result of the tension developed in the posterior ligamentous system (PLS), which includes the joint capsules, interspinous and supraspinous ligaments (Adams and Hutton, 1986). In terms of side posture rotational manipulation, the lumbar spine is normally flexed, which increases the tension in the PLS. One of the more important manipulative skills is the ability to isolate one specific motion segment and concentrate the thrust force by selectively using the posterior elements to stabilize the segments above and below the targeted facet, minimizing force dissipation and injury to neighbouring tissues.

Maintaining a lordotic spine may impair the protective effects of the PLS, leaving the posterior elements and other contractile tissue susceptible to injury during rotational manipulation. These mechanical properties may provide a rationale for safe and controlled manipulative procedures. The fact that the patient is in the non-weight bearing posture could minimize the mechanical effects of the PLS.

Manipulative Considerations

The lumbar spine is subjected to the effects of both long and short levers during therapeutic manipulation. This is unavoidable as the upper torso and lower limbs are involved in the procedure. Therefore, methods to control long lever and emphasize short lever action would no doubt be clinically advantageous. Sandoz (1976) describes the mechanism of side posture adjustment in a series of steps which results in a mechanical helicoidal type of traction effect on the disc. The point of counter-rotation or maximum torque is achieved by flexing the lower leg towards the chest, thereby flattening the lumbar lordosis, creating tension in the PLS and protecting the segments below (Cassidy *et al.*, 1992a). Gently pushing the patient's torso slightly posterior and down towards the table produces tension in the PLS above the point of counter-rotation which essentially focuses the manipulative forces to one intervertebral level. Directing the patient to breathe in and then out just prior to the manipulative thrust introduces a small, but stabilizing effect of increasing the intra-abdominal pressure (Byfield, 1991). The mechanical

effects of this may be negligible, but could simply help to relax the patient. Any increase in the intrathoracic tension would provide a more solid base of support for the doctor's indifferent hand and body weight. Therefore, the concept that the disc is susceptible to excessive rotational strain is no longer justified in view of the biomechanical and clinical evidence.

Summary

Chiropractic is poised to play a key role in the future management and rehabilitation of musculoskeletal dysfunction, particularly acute and chronic back pain. The chiropractic profession possesses all the elements to accept this responsibility fully.

Manipulative Skills

The following manipulative skills represent the basic and fundamental movements required to perform safe and efficient side posture manipulation, the most common position for manipulation of the lumbar spine (Barrale *et al.*, 1989; Cassidy *et al.*, 1992a). The skills section will concentrate on the introduction and use of both long and short levers, plus a sample of the more common errors encountered during the acquisition of these complex psychomotor skills. The skills are a series of building blocks which form the basis of diversified side posture manipulation. There are other postures, most commonly the sitting (DeCamillis, 1977) and prone positions (Barrale *et al.*, 1989) which, although frequently used, are generally considered more advanced clinical skills that should be introduced later in the student's undergraduate technique development. This would provide the basis for a second volume.

The skills presented should be learned as a sequence and executed slowly and methodically up to the point of joint tension. Each manipulative procedure will incorporate several planes of movement in order to illustrate the concept of joint specificity and segmental isolation for localizing thrust forces. The key element is to maintain patient control and relaxation at all times. This will enhance palpatory skills and provide essential proprioceptive feedback information. Deliberate movements and courteous positioning of the patient will be stressed.

The manipulative skills will concentrate on the spinous and mamillary process of the L34 intervertebral motion segment as the anatomical contact points. Specific reference to the posterior facet on the up side during the description of the skills will be described. The following three specific anatomical landmarks will represent the specific contact points for the manipulative skills discussed in this chapter:

Double spinous process (DSP)

Single spinous process (SSP)

Mamillary process (MP).

1) Place the patient in the side posture as described previously in Chapter 7 with no torso rotation. The doctor is positioned at 90 degrees to the patient with the patient's top leg flexed to 90 degrees and secured between the doctor's legs (thigh sandwich) (*) (fig. 9.1). The doctor's body weight is forward over the patient and the upper body is stabilized. The patient should be positioned in line with the table. The patient's upper leg should be parallel to the table.

2) With the doctor in this position (fig. 9.1) the patient is requested to interlock the hands around the midforearm region (fig. 9.2). This is the average position of the hands. If the patient has particularly long or short arms then adjust the position accordingly. Make sure the patient is secure on the table before attempting this procedure.

Double Spinous Process

The manipulative procedure using this anatomical contact combination is often referred to as: (i) a zygapophyseal rotatory adjustment (Paris, 1983; Schafer and Faye, 1989); (ii) modified Bonyun; (iii) Bonyun's discal techniques (Bonyun and Brunner, 1976); (iv) the double spinous rotary adjustment; and (v) the double spinous hook technique (Gitelman, 1980; Gitelman and Fligg, 1992) otherwise classified as a combined short–long lever specific contact procedure (Grice and Vernon, 1992). It has also been described as THE technique of side posture manipulation (Cassidy *et al.*, 1985; Kirkaldy-Willis and Cassidy, 1995; Cassidy *et al.*, 1992a; Cassidy *et al.*, 1993). The double spinous procedure is presented initially as it provides *the basic hand, arm and body skills that will be required for the next three lumbar side posture manipulative procedures.*

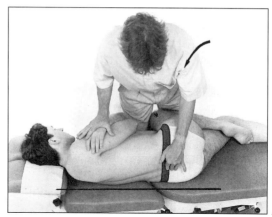

Fig 9.1

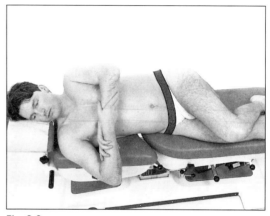

Fig 9.2

3) The doctor then brings the cephalad arm under and through the patient's interlocked arms up to the cubital fossa. The forearm of the caudad arm is placed with the flexor side down over the fleshy part of the buttock just below the pelvic crest (*). **Care is taken not to place the caudad arm over the sciatic nerve at the postero-medial third of the pelvis.** Both hands adopt a reinforced fingertip contact posture (fig. 9.3). Notice the position of the plumbline.

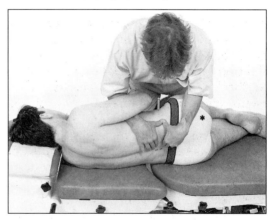

Fig 9.3

4) Specific segmental localization and intersegmental tension are accomplished by flexing the patient's hip **beyond** 90 degrees until the point at which the contact fingers begin to feel slight tension or stretching in the L34 interspinous space (*). This is the point at which counter-rotation is reached and no further hip flexion is required (fig. 9.4). This is a difficult skill, but an absolute requirement for segmental specificity and isolation. Locating anatomical landmarks is the first step to accomplish this goal. There should be no pressure over the patient.

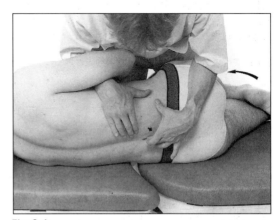

Fig 9.4

5) Once interspinous tension has been determined, double finger/spinous contact is made. Try to stabilize hip flexion with a gentle thigh squeeze. L3 ipsilateral lateral spinous contact is made first with the cephalad hand. The thumb of the caudad hand draws tissue slack down towards the table followed by the reinforced finger pad contact of the cephalad contact hand. The DIP joints are firm and extended (fig. 9.5).

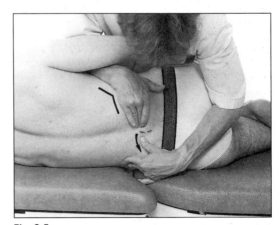

Fig 9.5

6) The caudad hand hooks the contralateral lateral border of the L4 spinous by pulling excess skin slack towards the doctor. The finger pad contact follows by flexing the DIP joint of the middle finger in the hooking process (fig. 9.6). The contact points should be light and the hand postures should be relaxed at all times with no tension or pressure over the spinous processes. Body weight should be directly over the contact hands and the doctor is still facing the patient. Note the flat lumbar curve and the relaxed upper back (*). Both contact hands are in the same goose-neck posture angled at 90 degrees to each other with a firm yet light contact on the osseous landmark. The thumbs are extended and out of the way so as to not interfere with the overall hand position.

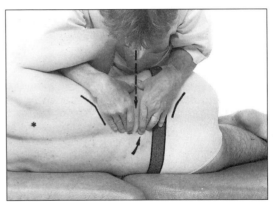

Fig 9.6

7) Shift 45 degrees to the low fencer stance bringing body weight slightly forward. Maintain patient hip flexion with the thigh sandwich to secure segmental isolation and finger contact on each spinous process (fig. 9.7). **Absolutely no force or pressure** is to be applied to the contact hand or the patient's arms at this point. Patient comfort and cooperation is essential.

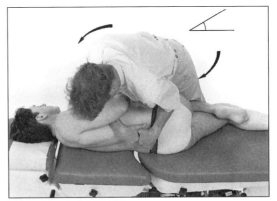

Fig 9.7

8) Control patient leg drop to regulate the amount of tension in both the hip joint and lumbar spine using the legs (*) (fig. 9.8). The rear foot is plantar flexed ready to shift weight forward and maintain foot/hip distance ratio. Note the relaxed and symmetrical posture of the doctor.

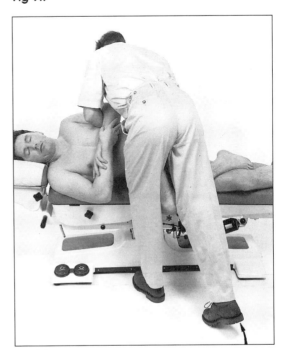

Fig 9.8

9) Prior to the weight transfer, politely ask the patient to **gently squeeze** the cephalad arm against their own rib cage in order to stabilize the upper body (*). Transfer the weight up and forward by plantar flexing the rear foot. Note the position of the plumbline (fig. 9.9a). This brings the body weight over the targetted joint. The doctor's trail leg slides up and over the patient's tibia until it reaches the supra-patellar fossa while maintaining a thigh squeeze (*) (fig. 9.9b). (*Refer to Figures 8.6 & 8.7 for more detail of this procedure.*) The rear foot re-plants with the leg flexed at the knee and the foot plantar flexed and the weight forward over the front leg (fig. 9.9c). (*Refer to Figure 8.8 for more detail.*)

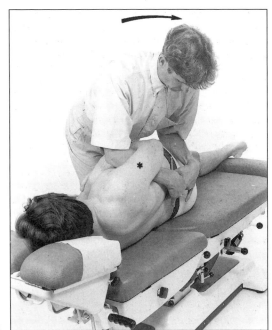

Fig 9.9a

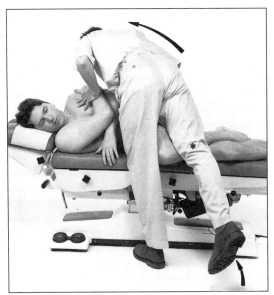

Fig 9.9b

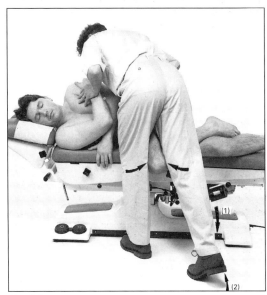

Fig 9.9c

10) As the weight drops slowly towards the table, the doctor **simultaneously and slowly** pulls the pelvis with the caudad arm towards the edge of the table and the cephalad arm resists patient forward movement by pressing down and slightly cephalad (fig. 9.10). This maintains upper body in a neutral position with very little torque (*). *Be careful not to push down on the patient's rib cage and push back too far creating a torquing action in the lumbar spine.* **Remember** to ask the patient to take a breath in as the doctor's weight is transferred and breathe out slowly as the weight is brought down over the spine in time with the various lever movements. The hand postures remain firm over the spinous contact points to detect spinous and soft tissue movement. As the weight comes down and the arms separate, tension should be developing at the L34 segment. Remember to breathe and don't thrust. Feel the joint tension developing.

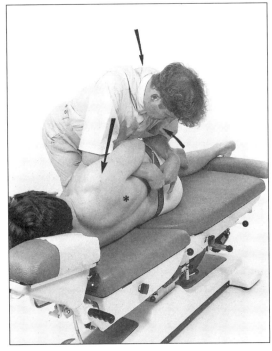

Fig 9.10

11) There are several errors to be aware of during the development of this manipulative procedure:

i) the standard over-rotating during weight shift causing torque in the doctor's upper and lower back; improper hand posture and contact affects force localization and specificity (*); pushing patient's upper body back too far producing torque in the patient's spine; lifting the caudad arm off the pelvic contact completely changes the lever system (*) (fig. 9.11);

ii) applying a compressive or pushing force to both the upper body and the pelvic crest.

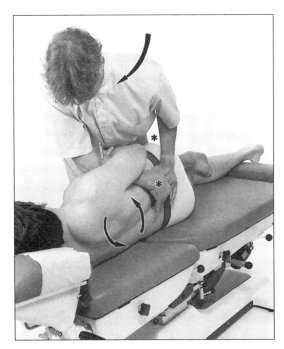

Fig 9.11

The soft tissues of the pelvic crest region are very sensitive to pressure, especially when dealing with painful mechanical syndromes of the lumbopelvic spine. The doctor may risk compressing the sciatic nerve if the arm placement is too low over the buttock which could elicit a painful response and a protective reaction by the patient. Additionally, compressing and leaning too heavily on the rib cage will have a similar effect and may compromise patient breathing. Both will potentially distress the patient and compromise the performance of the manipulative procedure. Other faults to consider have been presented in Chapter 8 covering the sacroiliac joint. Foot spread, hip flexion and lumbar lordosis are all factors to consider in the area of potential errors.

The aim is to begin to feel the concept of joint resistance or tension without applying a dynamic thrust. This should be seen as a gradual process.

Single Spinous Process

There are several manipulative procedures which use an SPP as an anatomical lever point. These manipulations use the upper body, lower limb and pelvic structures as long levers to produce a counter-rotation at a specific segmental level. These manipulative procedures are commonly referred to as the spinous hook or pull (States, 1968; Gitelman, 1980; Szaraz, 1984; Gitelman and Fligg, 1992; Cassidy *et al.*, 1993) and the spinous push adjustments (Gitelman, 1980; Grice, 1983; Fligg, 1984; Szaraz, 1984; Gitelman and Fligg, 1992) and are classified as a combined short–long lever specific contact procedure (Grice and Vernon, 1992). These manipulations are performed in the side posture and present skills which are both common and unique, such as those presented above. The skills presented in this section of the chapter are a continuation of the common building skills already presented. These manipulative procedures utilize all the planes of motion of a typical lumbar motor unit. A sensible approach to segmental isolation and specificity is considered.

Spinous Hook/Pull

1) Place the patient in the side posture as described previously (Chapter 7, fig. 7.1) with the patient's arms folded and the hand placed on the anterior deltoid area and no torso rotation. The doctor is in the starting posture perpendicular to the patient with hip flexed to 90 degrees and parallel to the table (fig. 9.12). The doctor's cephalad hand supports the patient's upper body and the caudad arm is resting on the lateral pelvic crest region just above the greater trochanter. The patient's pelvis should be at right angles to the table or just slightly supinated.

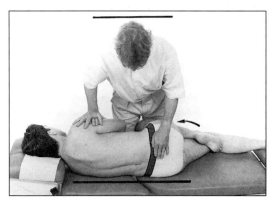

Fig 9.12

2) L34 intersegmental location and isolation is secured as described above except that the interspinous space is palpated with the fingers of the caudad hand only (fig. 9.13). Hip flexion is stopped once tension and separation in the interspinous soft tissue of L34 is perceived (*).

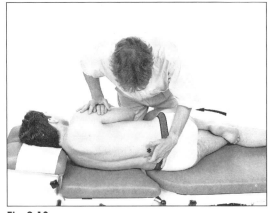

Fig 9.13

3) A reinforced fingertip hand posture is formed with the caudad hand. The middle finger is flexed at the PIP and DIP joints in a cup-like fashion and is placed on the contralateral, lateral edge (down side) of the spinous of L4 providing a **hooking** action of the fingers. The middle finger of the cephalad hand can be used to pull any excess tissue towards the doctor in order to make a more secure contact for the reinforced finger. The flexor aspect of the forearm (fleshy part) is simultaneously and gently placed over the gluteus medius portion of the pelvis just below the region of the pelvic crest and just above the greater trochanter, forming a 90 degree angle (fig. 9.14). There should be no downward pressure of the arm on the pelvic musculature or sciatic nerve. The arm and hand are basically placed in position with little or no tension. Monitor patient relaxation and reactions at all times.

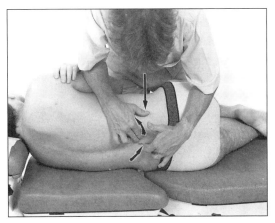

Fig 9.14

4) Prior to the pivot shift and weight transfer, the doctor should be in a relaxed position with both cephalad and caudad arms and hands in position with the patient's weight balanced on the table. Note the placement of the cephalad arm close to the body (*) to shorten that lever and ensure control of the counter-rotation of the upper body (fig. 9.15). The patient is in line on the table. **There is no downward pressure over the iliac crest or spinous.**

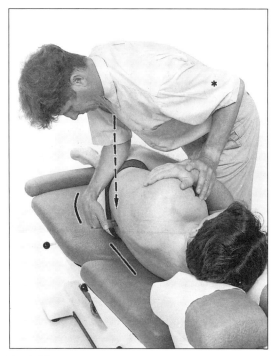

Fig 9.15

5) Pivot 45 degrees maintaining patient control and hand contact position. Transfer weight by lifting and flexing the plantar flexors of the back leg (*this has been described in Chapter 8, Figures 8.6, 8.7 & 8.8 and above, fig. 9.9a-c*). During this action the contact arm is rolled slightly forward on the pelvic position, increasing the angle at the wrist in order to increase the leverage (fig. 9.16).

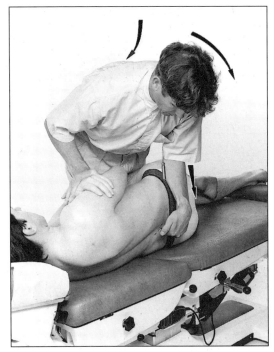

Fig 9.16

6) With the weight positioned over the contact and hand posture, the doctor slowly lowers body weight towards the patient and simultaneously slowly **pulls** the contact arm back towards the body pulling the pelvis anterior at the same time (fig. 9.17a). The support arm/hand maintains the upper body in place on the table being careful not to push posterior. This provides the mechanism for some of the counter-rotation. The main component of counter-rotation and tissue slack elimination is a direct result of the anterior movement or pronating of the patient's pelvis towards the table (fig. 9.17b). The cephalad hand holds the upper torso down on the table with **minimal superior and posterior traction**. The purpose of the support hand is to secure the patient on the table and help to stabilize the doctor's weight. The support arm blocks forward movement of the patient. The hand posture is maintained throughout the entire procedure.

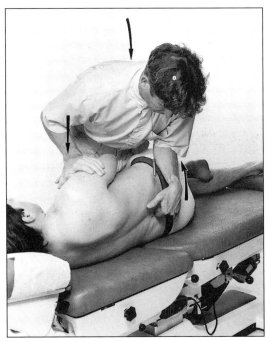

Fig 9.17a

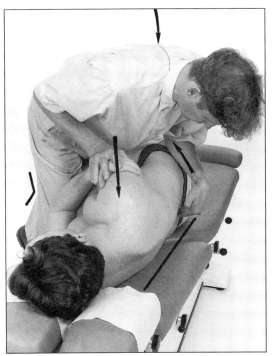

Fig 9.17b

7) With doctor's weight forward over the front leg and coming down through the patient's leg, the contact arm **very slowly** continues to pull the pelvis forward by keeping the arm close and tucked into the body. This ensures that all the slack is taken out (end of the passive range of motion near the elastic barrier) and the segments below the L34 are stabilized (fig. 9.18a). The pelvis continues to roll anterior to increase counter-rotation (fig. 9.18b). The cephalad arm is also kept in close to the body in order to make the doctor more compact prior to the delivery of a 'mock' thrust at the end of the passive range of motion. At this point only appreciate the tension. As the weight is coming down on the patient instruct him to breathe out to assist the weight transfer. Note the position of the plumbline, indicating the position of the body mass. Compare the subtle movements between Figures 9.17 and 9.18. The hand posture is maintained throughout the entire procedure. There should be no pressure down on the pelvis. The action is a pulling one.

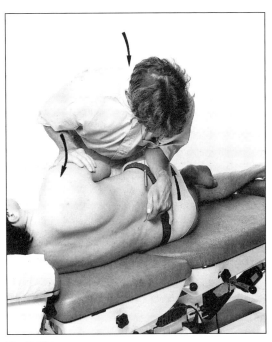

Fig 9.18a

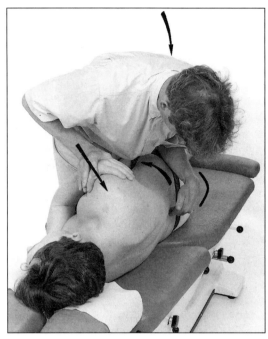

Fig 9.18b

8) There are several common errors to be aware of during the learning of this manipulative procedure.

The errors associated with this manipulative skill are the same as those encountered with the double spinous skills. Over-rotating and torquing the spinal elements at the wrong level, poor hand skills and goose-neck hand posture, excessive leaning and compression over the sensitive tissue of the buttock region and permitting the patient's leg to drop below the 90 degree threshold of hip flexion which may compromise segmental specificity are similar skills to note during the development of these manipulative skills.

Figure 9.19 illustrates several errors including over-rotating the doctor's upper back, pushing the patient's upper back too far posteriorly torquing the spine, applying downward pressure on the sensitive iliac crest instead of pulling, and loss of hand posture on the spinal segment (*).

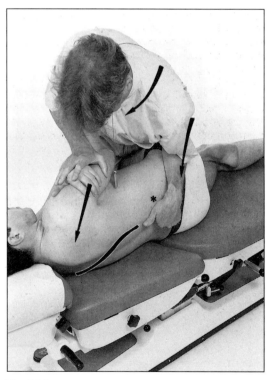

Fig 9.19

Spinous Push

This manipulative procedure is far more complex than the spinous pull in terms of performance and overall psychomotor skills. This manipulative procedure is essentially the same as the single spinous–spinous pull except for the following subtle differences: (i) segmental localization and specific facet contact stabilization takes place from above the contact on the spinous instead of from below (i.e. finger pad contact is on L3); (ii) reinforced fingertip contact is placed on the ipsilateral side of the spinous process of the upper segment of the motion segment being isolated; and (iii) the short levers are controlled by a pull–push action on the pelvis rather than just a pulling action.

Therefore, the patient is placed in the side posture as described above in Figures 9.15 and 9.16 including the pivot shift into a fencer stance with the appropriate amount of body weight transfer up and towards the patient. To this point the only significant difference is the placement of the contact hand and finger pad which is described below and in Figure 9.5 above.

1) A reinforced middle finger in a goose-neck hand posture is placed on the ipsilateral lateral edge of the spinous process of the L3. The skin slack is initially removed by pulling the skin with the support hand thumb towards the table. The interphalangeal joints are positioned at 90 degrees with slight ulnar deviation of the wrist. The flexor portion of the forearm is gently placed upon the lateral aspect of the buttock just below the pelvic crest with both arms held relaxed and close into the body (fig. 9.20). Note the position of the plumbline relative to the hand. There should be no downward pressure over the iliac crest and no excess cephalad push with the indifferent arm.

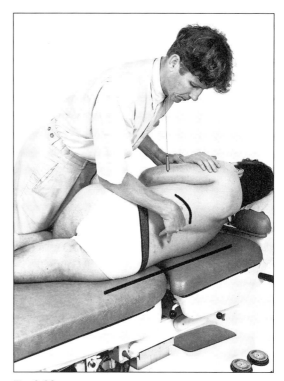

Fig 9.20

2) The doctor transfers body weight forward by plantar flexing the rear foot (fig. 9.21a). Note the 45 degree position of the doctor and the bend in the legs to add spring and control the patient's leg drop (thigh sandwich) (*). At the same time the contact arm is also brought slightly forward on the pelvic contact, exaggerating the hand posture (fig. 9.21b). This will provide the doctor with more leverage across the pelvis to reach joint tension and apply preload. *(Refer to Figures 8.6–8.8 for more details or above for a similar explanation.)*

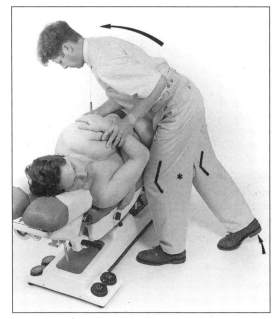

Fig 9.21a

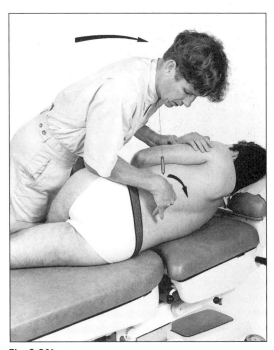

Fig 9.21b

3) Very slowly

i) pull the pelvic contact towards the body, tucking the contact arm into the body to the point when movement of the L3 spinous is perceived and tissue resistance between the contact finger pads and the pelvic contact is increasing. This should occur at a point when the contact arm is in a 90 degree angle at the elbow (fig. 9.22a). At this point the pulling action is stopped (as opposed to the spinous pull described above) and the doctor

ii) simultaneously pushes gently down on both the contact point on the spinous and the pelvic contact with the arm (fig. 9.22a). This is assisted by the natural movement of the doctor's weight down through the long levers of the patient's leg (fig. 9.22b). Compare the relative amount of body drop between Figures 9.21a and 9.22b. The pull/push action needs to be equally balanced. This overall movement increases the tissue tension below the L3 contact point.

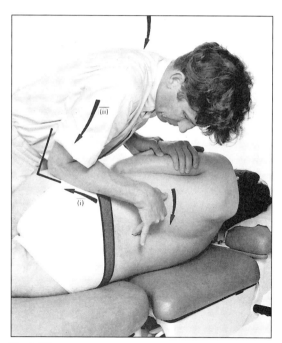

Fig 9.22a

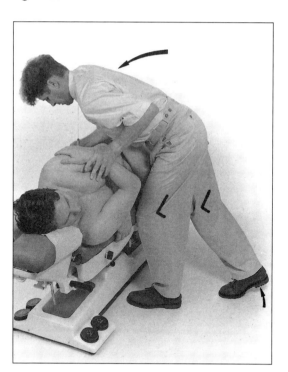

Fig 9.22b

4) *There are several potential learning errors to be aware of during this set of manipulative skills.*

These are very similar to those associated with any of the side posture skills learned thus far. This is particularly applicable to the double spinous and the single spinous described above. The spinous push provides a very safe and efficient procedure for side posture lumbar spine manipulation but there are some very specific and subtle skills that must be adhered to for successful performance of these procedures. The following are of particular note.

There is a tendency to over pull the pelvis and push down with too much force on the sensitive pelvic musculature (*). The pulling/pushing action has to be balanced. This occurs if the doctor is too far back and the weight is not over the appropriate spinal level (fig. 9.23). Often these actions are performed too quickly. There is also a tendency to just pull the pelvis similar to the spinous pull skills and not incorporate a push component.

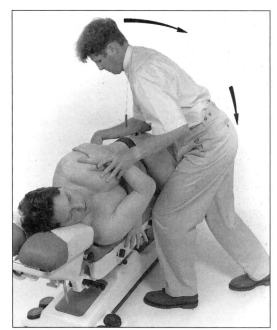

Fig 9.23

Mamillary Process

The manipulative procedures which use this anatomical landmark are often referred to as the lumbar roll adjustment (States, 1968; Szaraz, 1984), mamillary process rotary adjustment (Gitelman, 1980; Gitelman and Fligg, 1992) or the extension move (Cassidy *et al.*, 1993). It represents one of the more traditional and most widely used manipulative procedures in the chiropractic profession to correct inter-segmental rotation restrictions (Barrale *et al.*, 1989) and is one of the more difficult to learn and perform. Breen (1988) describes a specific derivative of this manipulative procedure using a mamillary contact for the treatment of lateral recess encroachment. Although reported to be an effective alternative, it is a very difficult and strenuous manipulation to perform due to the lack of effective levers to isolate and preload the specific segmental level. The forces and energy consumed are substantial, which places additional strain on the doctor's own back and shoulder girdle.

The manipulative skills are different from those presented previously in this chapter mainly due to the fact the contact arm is positioned much further away from the body. This essentially makes the contact arm a longer lever. This could compromise the stability of the patient and the overall proficiency of the skill. The longer lever of the contact arm could place the upper back and shoulders under greater mechanical load and result in potential overuse injuries. The point of contact is the mamillary process of the superior articulating process. This contact point is much more difficult to control because it is not a superficial one such as the spinous process. Therefore, this could also compromise segmental specificity and increase the forces applied which are subsequently dissipated in the surrounding tissues. This reduces its clinical efficiency and increases the amount of work required.

To begin this manipulative skill execute the same sequential steps and skills as described above and in Chapter 7 covering side posture and positioning skills. This procedure is also similar to the PSIS pelvic manoeuvre described in Chapter 8. Therefore, the basic skills and rationale have already been presented.

To review: the patient is placed in the right side posture recumbent position, hip flexed to 90 degrees and leg placed gently between the doctor's thighs (thigh sandwich) in order to stabilize the position of the lower body. The upper torso is supported by the cephalad hand with no excessive torque to strain the spine. The doctor is perpendicular to the patient and the table. The patient's hip is flexed and the L3–L4 interspinous movement is monitored by the index and middle finger of the caudad contact hand. Once tension in the L34 interspinous space is perceived,

further hip flexion is unnecessary and the segment is stabilized by dropping the patient's leg down slightly towards the table, but still controlled by the doctor's thigh squeeze. This step is necessary for patient comfort and stability. The patient will begin to roll off the table if the leg is allowed to drop too close to the table. The cephalad arm is kept in close to the body to reduce fatigue.

1) Interspinous movement and tension is monitored by the caudad hand during hip flexion (*) and excess tissue slack is drawn laterally towards the doctor by the index and middle finger pads of the cephalad hand (fig. 9.24). Note the relative flatness of the patient's spine and its relaxed nature.

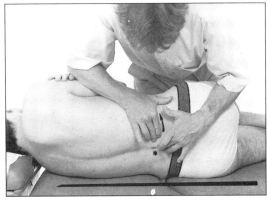
Fig 9.24

2) Replace the palpating fingers with the pisi-form/hypothenar eminence contact point of the caudad hand at the same time assisting tissue tension by rolling off the spinous processes of L3 and L4 on to the mamillary process of the superior articulating process of L4 (fig. 9.25). The contact hand should be arched and the fingers should be pointing cephalad with the hypothenar eminence and the 5th digit parallel to the spinal column.

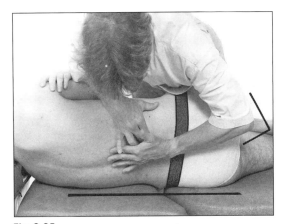
Fig 9.25

3) The cephalad or indifferent hand is placed on the shoulder in order to support the upper torso with gentle downward pressure and no backward rotation. The caudad contact arm is held parallel to the spine and the doctor is still positioned 90 degrees to the patient (fig. 9.26).

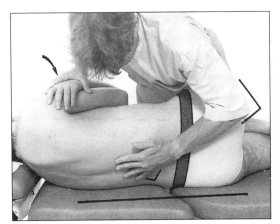
Fig 9.26

4) Pivot shift 45 degrees into fencer stance maintaining hip flexion (thigh sandwich), upper torso and hand contact control. This is performed very slowly to maintain position and control. **The contact arm pivots with the rest of the body at the wrist and not the shoulder** (fig. 9.27). This protects the shoulder from excess torsion (*) and strain on the soft tissues. The caudad arm is positioned comfortably at about 45 degrees to the patient's spine.

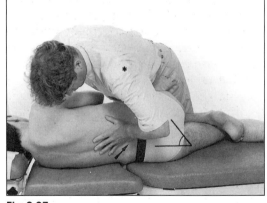

Fig 9.27

5) With the arm angled away from the body the doctor has to lean forward and over the patient to a much greater degree when compared to the spinous contacts described above (fig. 9.28). The doctor is just not as upright or in control of body weight to the same degree. This places potentially greater loads over the whole spine and shoulder even before tension and 'mock' thrust are applied (*). The patient's leg is controlled very effectively by the clamping action of the thigh sandwich (*).

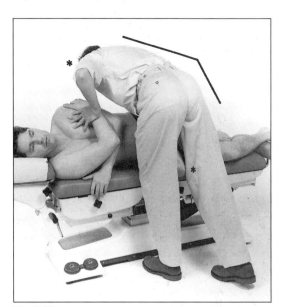

Fig 9.28

6) Transfer the body weight forward and over the patient by plantar flexing the rear foot in the same way as described previously (fig. 9.29). Care has to be taken to watch the torsion in the shoulders and the flexion strain on the lower back. Keep the legs flexed and springy to absorb some of the load (*). Patient leg control is described in Chapter 8, Figures 8.6–8.8 or above for optimal leg drop control. There are other methods to secure the leg and transfer weight, for example by pinning the patient's leg to the table.

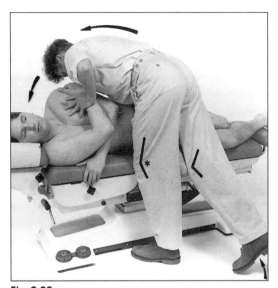

Fig 9.29

7) The final sequence is the weight distribution and the patient 'roll'. The sequence starts with Figure 9.30a where the weight is positioned over the contact, comfortable arms and no pressure over a relaxed patient. As the weight comes down slowly over the L34 segment and contact point, the doctor allows the patient to begin to 'roll' slightly forward towards the edge of the table from a 90 degree position (fig. 9.30b). The patient is instructed to breathe in and out slowly at this point and the doctor moves in unison with the breathing cycle. This roll continues to about 45 degrees to the table applying pressure to the contact point at the same rate as the weight is being dropped (fig. 9.30c). There should be no excessive tension on the contact point, no torque in the spine (both the upper body and pelvis roll forward). The roll is performed slowly so that the patient does not react, feel unsteady and tense up. When the roll is complete the doctor can begin to preload the long levers initially and then the short lever of specific segment (L34). The cephalad hand pushes down, cephalad and only slightly posterior to avoid torquing the spine. The doctor 'locks' in against the patient's leg and stops any further forward pelvic movement (fig. 9.30c).

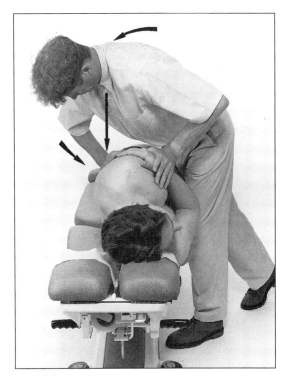

Fig 9.30a

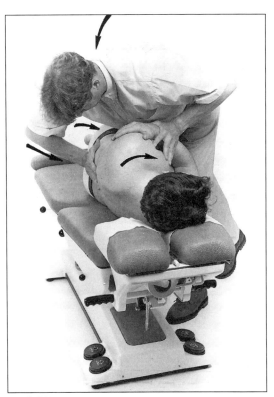

Fig 9.30b

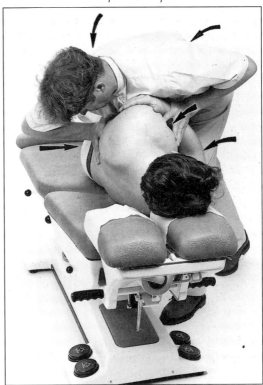

Fig 9.30c

8) As the long levers are engaged with a comfortable stretch (*long elastic tension*) in the surrounding tissue, the doctor can start to engage the short lever by compressing (*squeezing*) the tissue over the mamillary contact. The contact arm should be almost parallel to the table but not 90 degrees to the patient placing excessive stress on the soft tissues of the shoulder (fig. 9.31). The patient is once again asked to breathe in and then out as the short lever is engaged to assist overall control and focus the patient's attention.

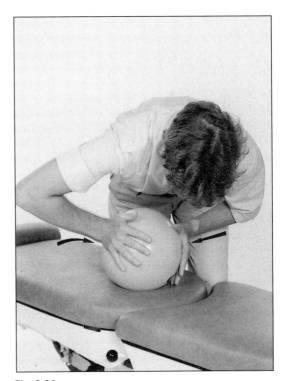

Fig 9.31

9) **There are several potential errors associated with learning these side posture skills**.

i) The most common is 'rolling' the patient too fast and too far, thus losing complete control.

ii) Torquing the contact arm placing it 90 degrees to the spine to get more push on the short lever contact, producing a pile-driver effect. This can introduce mechanical compression to already irritated soft tissues and compromise patient cooperation.

iii) Pushing the upper body backwards instead of cephalad subjecting the thoraco-lumbar spine to potentially hazardous torsional stress.

This chapter has presented the basic skills necessary for a variety of side posture manipulative procedures that are used within the chiropractic profession. Supine or prone procedures have been avoided as they represent procedures that are specifically selected under special clinical circumstances. Students would be exposed to these skills in more advanced years and during problem solving exercises requiring specific clinical decisions. The side posture is more difficult to learn in terms of skill acquisition because the doctor has to learn to control both himself or herself and the patient simultaneously. Supine and prone skills are simply easier to learn, not used as often and do not generate the same amount of tension and leverage characteristic of side posture manipulative procedures. A typical example would be the use of an articulated or motorized adjusting table: though requiring specific skills, the overall procedure is dictated by the quality of the instrument being used. This is not to detract from the use of such tables and the skills necessary, but once the mechanics of the table are conquered it could be reasoned that most patients will fit the manipulative therapy. There are advantages for the use of these tools for both patient and practitioner alike.

Certain biomechanical properties of the tissues of the lumbar spine act harmoniously to protect the structure during specific tasks and movements. During side posture rotational manipulation the spinal elements are subjected to unknown, as yet, compressive and torsional loads. These forces could be similar to those generated during the performance of a lift, for instance. I feel that even though side posture is a non-weight bearing position, mechanical advantage can be maintained. This will promote integrity of the soft tissues of the motion segment, as long as specific technique skills and biomechanical principles are used to accomplish segmental isolation, patient comfort and motion segment stability.

This chapter has presented the most common manipulative skills and procedures associated with dysfunction of a lumbar motion segment. It illustrates how a group of common psychomotor skills can be repeatedly incorporated to develop specific manipulative procedures for a distinctive region of the spine. The objective has been to develop and organize these skills slowly in context with the designated joint. The presentation has been careful not to overemphasize the dynamic thrust component of the overall manipulation, but has more importantly defined the sequence of events for both the practitioner and patient leading up to joint tension. The dynamic thrust is only one aspect of the overall skill that is learned after the basic skills are perfected.

References

Acker, P.D., Thiel, H.W. and Kirkaldy-Willis, W.H. (1990) Low back pain: pathogenesis, diagnosis and management. *American Journal of Chiropractic Medicine*, **3**, 19–24

Adams, M.A. and Hutton, W.C. (1981) The relevance of torsion to the mechanical derangement of the lumbar spine. *Spine*, **6**, 241–248

Adams, M.A. and Hutton, W.C. (1982) Prolapsed intervertebral disc – a hyperflexion injury. *Spine*, **7**, 184–191

Adams, M.A. and Hutton, W.C. (1985) Gradual disc prolapse. *Spine*, **10**, 524–531

Adams, M.A. and Hutton, W.C. (1986) Has the lumbar spine a margin of safety in forward bending? *Clinical Biomechanics*, **1**, 3–6

Barrale, R., Diamond, R., Filson, R. *et al.* (1989) Manipulative management of lumbar disc bulge. *Chiropractic Technique*, **1**, 79–87

Bennett, W.I. (1990) Low back pain: the scoreboard. *Harvard Medical School Health Letter*, **15**, (Sept)

Bogduk, N. (1983) The innervation of the lumbar spine. *Spine*, **8**, 286–293

Bogduk, N. and Twomey, L.T. (1991) Nerves of the lumbar spine. In *Clinical Anatomy of the Lumbar Spine*, 2nd edn. Churchill Livingstone, London, pp. 107–120

Bonyun, J. and Brunner, D. (1976) *The Bonyun Technique for Lumbar Intradiscal Instability.* Sturgeon Lake Publishing, Fenelon Falls, Ontario

Breen, A. (1988) Dynamic lateral recess encroachment in minimal degenerative states: diagnosis and management. *European Journal of Chiropractic*, **36**, 3–9

Burton, C.V. and Cassidy, J.D. (1992) Economics, epidemiology, and risk factors. In *Managing Low Back Pain*, 3rd edn. (eds. W.H. Kirkaldy-Willis and C.V. Burton). Churchill Livingstone, London, pp. 1–6

Byfield, D. (1991) Lumbar manipulative procedures in relation to segmental specificity and biomechanical properties of the motor unit. *European Journal of Chiropractic*, **39**, 13–19

Carette, S., Marcoux, S., Truchon, R. *et al.* (1991) A controlled trial of corticosteroid injections into facet joints for chronic low back pain. *New England Journal of Medicine*, **325**, 1002–1007

Cassidy, J.D., Kirkaldy-Willis, W.H. and McGregor, M. (1985) Spinal manipulation for the treatment of chronic low-back and leg pain: an observational study. In *Empirical Approaches to the Validation of Spinal Manipulation* (eds. A.A. Buerger and P.E. Greenman). Charles C. Thomas, Springfield, Illinois, pp. 119–148

Cassidy, J.D. and Wedge, J.H. (1988) The epidemiology and natural history of low back pain and spinal degeneration. In *Managing Low Back Pain*, 2nd edn. (ed. W.H. Kirkaldy-Willis). Churchill Livingstone, London

Cassidy, J.D., Kirkaldy-Willis, W.H. and Thiel, H.W. (1992a) Manipulation. In *Managing Low Back Pain*, 3rd edn (eds. W.H. Kirkaldy-Willis and C.V. Burton). Churchill Livingstone, London, pp. 283–296

Cassidy, J.D., Loback, D., Yong-Hing, K. *et al.* (1992b) Lumbar facet joint asymmetry intervertebral disc herniation. *Spine*, **17**, 570–573

Cassidy, J.D., Thiel, H.W. and Kirkaldy-Willis, W.H. (1993) Side posture manipulation for lumbar intervertebral disc herniation. *Journal of Manipulative and Physiological Therapeutics*, **16**, 96–103

Chapman-Smith, D. (1993a) The chiropractic profession. *The Chiropractic Report*, **7**, 3

Chapman-Smith, D. (1993b) Cost-effectiveness – the Manga report. *The Chiropractic Report*, **7**, 1

Curtis, P. (1988) Spinal manipulation: does it work? *Occupational Medicine*, **3**, 31–44

DeCamillis, D. (1977) Chiropractic adjustive technique using pelvic and spinal stabilization. *Journal of the Canadian Chiropractic Association*, **21**, 74–77

Deyo, R.A., Diehl, A.K. and Rosenthal, M. (1986) How many days bed rest for acute low back pain? *New England Journal of Medicine*, **315**, 1064–1070

Deyo, R.A. and Tsui-Wu, Y-J. (1987) Description epidemiology of low-back pain and its related medical care in the United States. *Spine*, **12**, 264–268

Dickson, R.A. and Butt, W.P. (1992) Mini-symposium: surgery for back pain. (i) Clinical/radiological evaluation. *Current Orthopaedics*, **6**, 3–11

Dvorak, J., Kranzlin, P., Muhlemann, D. *et al.* (1992) Musculoskeletal complications. In *Principles and Practice of Chiropractic*, 2nd edn. (ed. S. Haldeman). Appleton and Lange, San Mateo, California, pp. 549–577

Ebrall, P.S. (1992) Mechanical low-back pain: a comparison of medical and chiropractic management within the Victorian work care scheme. *Chiropractic Journal of Australia*, **22**, 47–53

Ebrall, P.S. (1993) Residual disability from delayed manipulative treatment for mechanical low back pain: a case review. *Chiropractic Journal of Australia*, **23**, 54–58

Farfan, H.F. (1973) Torsion and compression. In *Mechanical Disorders of the Lumbar Spine*. Lea and Febiger, Philadelphia, pp. 74–92

Farfan, H.F., Cossette, J.W., Robertson, G.H. *et al.* (1970) The effects of torsion in the lumbar intervertebral joints: the role of torsion in the production of disc degeneration. *Journal of Bone and Joint Surgery*, **52**, 468–497

Fligg, B. (1984) The art of manipulation. *Journal of the Canadian Chiropractic Association*, **28**, 384–386

Frank, A. (1993) Low back pain. *British Medical Journal*, **306**, 901–909

Gilbert, J.R., Taylor, D.W. and Hildebrandt, A. (1985) Clinical trial of common treatments for low back pain in family practice. *British Medical Journal*, **291**, 791–794

Gitelman, R. (1980) A chiropractic approach to biomechanical disorders of the lumbar spine and pelvis. In *Modern Developments in the Principles and Practice of Chiropractic*, 1st edn. (ed. S. Haldeman). Appleton-Century-Crofts, New York, pp. 297–330

Gitelman, R. and Fligg, B. (1992) Diversified technique. In *Principles and Practice of Chiropractic*, 2nd edn. (ed. S. Haldeman). Appleton and Lange, San Mateo, California, pp. 483–501

Grice, A. (1983) Lumbar closure adjustment. *Journal of the Canadian Chiropractic Association*, **27**, 75–77

Grice, A. and Vernon, H. (1992) Basic principles in the performance of chiropractic adjusting: historical review, classification, and objectives. In *Principles and Practice of Chiropractic*, 2nd edn. (ed. S. Haldeman). Appleton and Lange, San Mateo, California, pp. 443–458

Haldeman, S. and Rubinstein, S.M. (1992) Compression fractures in patients undergoing spinal manipulative therapy. *Journal of Manipulative and Physiological Therapeutics*, **15**, 450–454

Hazard, R.G., Fenwick, J.W., Kalisch, S.M. *et al.* (1989) Functional restoration with behavioural support. A one-year prospective study of patients with chronic low-back pain. *Spine*, **14**, 157–161

Kelsey, J.L. and White, A.A. (1980) Epidemiology and impact of low-back pain. *Spine*, **5**, 133–142

Kelsey, J.L. (1982) Idiopathic low back pain: magnitude of the problem. In *American Academy of Orthopaedic Surgeons Symposium on Low Back Pain* (eds. A.A. White and S.L. Gordon). CV Mosby, Toronto, pp. 5–8

Kirkaldy-Willis, W.H., Wedge, J.H., Yong-Hing, K. *et al.* (1978) Pathology and pathogenesis of lumbar spondylosis and stenosis. *Spine*, **3**, 319–328

Kirkaldy-Willis, W.H. and Cassidy, J.D. (1985) Spinal manipulation in the treatment of low-back pain. *Canadian Family Physician*, **31**, 535–540

Kleynhans, A.M. (1980) Complications of and contraindications to spinal manipulative therapy, 1st edn. (ed. S. Haldeman). Appleton-Century-Crofts, New York, pp. 359–384

Kleynhans, A.M. and Terrett, A.G.J. (1985) The prevention of complications from spinal manipulative therapy. In *Aspects of Manipulative Therapy*, 2nd edn. (eds. E.F. Glasgow *et al.*) Churchill Livingstone, London, pp. 161–175

Koes, B.W., Bouter, L.M., van Mameren, H. *et al.* (1992a) A blinded randomized clinical trial of manual therapy and physiotherapy for chronic back and neck complaints: physical outcome measures. *Journal of Manipulative and Physiological Therapeutics*, **15**, 16–23

Koes, B.W., Bouter, L.M., van Mameren, H. *et al.* (1992b) Randomised clinical trial of manipulative therapy and physiotherapy for persistent back and neck complaints: results of one year follow-up. *British Medical Journal*, **304**, 601–605

Lewit, K. (1986) Manipulation–reflex therapy and/or restitution of impaired locomotor function. *Manual Medicine*, **2**, 99–100

Liebenson, C.S. (1992) Pathogenesis of chronic back pain. *Journal of Manipulative and Physiological Therapeutics*, **15**, 299–308

Manga, P., Angus, D.E. and Swan, W.R. (1993) Effective management of low back pain: it's time to accept the evidence. *Journal of the Canadian Chiropractic Association*, **37**, 221–229

Mayer, T.G., Gatchel, R.J., Kishino, N.D. *et al.* (1987) A prospective two-year study of functional restoration in industrial low back injury: an objective assessment procedure. *Journal of the American Medical Association*, **258**, 1763–1767

Meade, T.W., Dyer, S., Browne, W. *et al.* (1990) Low back pain of mechanical origin: randomised comparison of chiropractic and outpatient treatment. *British Medical Journal*, **300**, 1431–1437

Paris, S.V. (1983) Spinal manipulative therapy. *Clinical Orthopaedics and Related Research*, **179**, 55–61

Quebec Task Force on Spinal Disorders (1987) Scientific approach to the assessment and management of activity-related spinal disorders: a monograph for clinicians. *Spine*, **12**, (Suppl.), S1–S59

Quon, J.A., Cassidy, J.D., O'Connor, S.M. *et al.* (1989) Lumbar intervertebral disc herniation: treatment by rotational manipulation. *Journal of Manipulative and Physiological Therapeutics*, **12**, 220–227

Sandoz, R. (1976) Some physical mechanisms and effects of spinal adjustments. *Annals Swiss Chiropractic Association*, **VI**, 91–142

Schafer, R.C. and Faye, L.J. (1989) The lumbar spine. In *Motion Palpation and Chiropractic Technic: Principles of Dynamic Chiropractic*, 1st edn. The Motion Palpation Institute, Huntington Beach, Ca, USA, pp. 195–240

Shekelle, P.G., Adams, A.H., Chassin, M.R. *et al.* (1992) Spinal manipulation for low-back pain. *Annals of Internal Medicine*, **117**, 590–598

Spengler, D.M., Bigos, S.J., Martin, N.A. *et al.* (1986) Back injuries in industry: a retrospective study Part 1. Overview and cost analysis. *Spine*, **11**, 241–245

States, A.Z. (1968) *Atlas of Chiropractic Technic: Spinal and Pelvic Technics*, 2nd edn. National College of Chiropractic, Lombard Il., USA

Stokes, L.A. (1988) Mechanical function of the facet joints in the lumbar spine. *Clinical Biomechanics*, **3**, 101–105

Szaraz, Z. (1984) *Compendium of Chiropractic Technique*. Canadian Memorial Chiropractic College, Toronto

Terrett, A.G.J. and Kleyhans, A.M. (1992) Complications from manipulation of the low back. *Chiropractic Journal of Australia*, **22**, 129–139

Troup, J.D.G. and Videman, T. (1989) Inactivity and the aetiopathogenesis of musculoskeletal disorders. *Clinical Biomechanics*, **4**, 173–178

Vernon, H. (1991) Chiropractic: a model of incorporating the illness behaviour model in the management of low back pain patients. *Journal of Manipulative and Physiological Therapeutics*, **14**, 379–389

Videman, T. (1987) Experimental models of osteoarthritis: the role of immobilisation. *Clinical Biomechanics*, **2**, 223–229

Waddell, G. (1987) A new clinical model for the treatment of low-back pain. *Spine*, **12**, 632–644

Waddell, G. (1993) Simple low-back pain: rest or active exercise? *Annals of Rheumatic Diseases*, **52**, 317–319

White, A.A. (1982) Introduction. In *American Academy of Orthopaedic Surgeons on Idiopathic Low Back Pain* (eds. A.A. White and S.L. Gordon). CV Mosby, Toronto, pp. 1–2

Wiltse, L.L. (1987) Editorial: low back pain. *Current Orthopaedics*, **1**, 359–360

Yamamoto, I., Panjabi, M.M., Crisco, T. *et al.* (1989) Three-dimensional movements of the whole lumbar spine and lumbosacral joint. *Spine*, **14**, 1256–1260

Further Reading

Chapman-Smith, D. (1987) Manipulation – professional standards of training and practice. *The Chiropractic Report*, **1**, 4

Chapman-Smith, D. (1992) Manipulation for chronic back pain – strong new evidence of long term results. *The Chiropractic Report*, **6**, 4

Chapman-Smith, D. (1992) The chiropractic world – major current developments. *The Chiropractic Report*, **6**, 6

Herzog, W., Conway, P.J.W., Kawchuk, G.N. *et al.* (1991) Comparison of the forces exerted during spinal manipulative therapy on the sacroiliac joint, the thoracic spine and the cervical spine. In *Proceedings of the Scientific Symposium, World Chiropractic Congress* (Toronto, 1991) (ed. S. Haldeman). World Federation of Chiropractic, Toronto, p. 37–1

Hessell, B.W., Herzog, W., Conway, P.J.W. *et al.* (1990) Experimental measurement of the force exerted during spinal manipulation using the Thompson technique. *Journal of Manipulative and Physiological Therapeutics*, **13**, 448–453

McGill, S.M. (1988) Estimation of force and extensor moment contributions of the disc and ligaments at L4–L5. *Spine*, **13**, 1395–1402

Pearcy, M. (1989) Biomechanics of the spine. *Current Orthopaedics*, **3**, 96–100

Chapter

10

Thoracic spine manipulative skills

David Byfield

Introduction

The thoracic spine is arguably the most neglected region of the spine, yet it is the most often manipulated (Schafer and Faye, 1989) and an area that is plagued by recurrent pain syndromes as a result of inappropriate and excessive manipulative procedures (Gitelman and Fligg, 1992). There is also a tendency for clinicians to be less specific and more casual in their management of this region (Gatterman and Panzer, 1990). The constant and unrelenting attack on the easily accessible 'high spots', combined with a possible misinterpretation of referred pain from the cervical or lumbar regions and/or visceral structures, may be partly responsible for this clinical picture. The presence of multiple areas of tenderness found on digital palpation are often treated as manipulable lesions of either the posterior joints or costotransverse articulations, when in fact further investigation may reveal an irritable myofascial nodular formation. The thoracic spine takes on additional importance from a neurological perspective, with its relationship to the sympathetic ganglionic chain located on the anterior border of the costotransverse articulations (Greenman, 1989). Joint dysfunction may be a direct cause of mechanical irritation resulting in both local and referred phenomena. From a postural point of view, the primary curve of the thoracic spine provides balance and a base of support during many basic activities.

Thoracic Pain

There are very little original or notable data regarding the topic of thoracic pain. The neurological basis of pain emanating from the thoracic spine has been described, including the nature and distribution of the pain receptor nerve endings and the mechanisms by which thoracic spine pain may be produced (Wyke, 1967). The fibrous capsules of the posterior joints, the longitudinal, flaval and interspinous ligaments, the periosteum and the vascular structures are all richly innervated by pain-sensitive unmyelinated nerve fibres (Wyke, 1967). Bogduk and Valencia (1988) reviewed the innervation and pain patterns of the thoracic spine in an attempt to establish a foundation for the differential diagnosis of idiopathic thoracic pain. Their approach was based upon the principle that any structure receiving a nerve supply is a possible source of pain. Consequently, considering the fact that most tissues are innervated, this only adds more complexity and additional confusion to an already misunderstood concept (Bogduk and Valencia, 1988). Their concluding remarks were that until more appropriate experimental research is performed, any conclusions regarding thoracic pain must be reserved and that interpretation should be sought only on the basis of extrapolations from the lumbar and cervical regions.

Biomechanical Considerations

Due to the unique structure of the thoracic spine, biomechanical dysfunction differs significantly from that of the lumbar and cervical regions (Gatterman and Panzer, 1990). This is probably due to the primary kyphotic curvature and the overall stability created by the rib cage. The thoracic spine is designed for rigidity, which is vital for erect bipedal support, postural maintenance, and protection of the spinal cord and other vital organs of the thoracic cavity (White and Panjabi, 1990). The investigation of the mechanics of the thoracic spine are the least understood and have been largely neglected. Apart from an original study by White (1969), very little is known about the behaviour and pattern of motion characteristic of the thoracic spine. Panjabi *et al.* (1984) determined the *in vitro* centres of rotation of thoracic functional spinal units in the sagittal plane to be about 30 mm below the geometric centre of the vertebral body. This may offer insight into the kinematic behaviour of the lower thoracic spine. Of considerable importance to the manipulative sciences is the fact that, from a kinematic perspective, the upper thoracic spine behaves similarly to the cervical region and the lower thoracic spine is similar to that of the lumbar region. Axial rotation is greatest in the upper thoracic spine, whereas flexion/extension predominates the lower thoracic motion segments (White and Panjabi, 1990). This has meaningful clinical implications with respect to the use of diagnostic techniques and specific manipulative skills and procedures designed to restore function to the thoracic spine even though the exact pathophysiology of these mechanical disorders has yet to be determined. It is most likely that the zygapophyseal and costotransverse joints are the most common and potent sources of thoracic pain (Kellgren, 1977).

Clinical Considerations

Schafer and Faye (1989) state that the majority of fixations in the thoracic spine are muscular in origin even though, in rea-lity, the issue of muscular pain is still regarded as speculative (Bogduk and Valencia, 1988), Myofascial pain syndromes arising from hyperirritable trigger points in muscles are frequently overlooked and poorly understood sources of musculoskeletal pain, but believed to be a major cause of back pain and other pain syndromes (Travell and Simons, 1983; Simons, 1985). Recently, the validity of trigger point examination has been regarded as unscientific (Deyo *et al.*, 1992). The reliability of the presence of trigger points during examination of the low back has also been challenged and deemed questionable (Nice *et al.*, 1992). However, a significant change has been measured in the pain tolerance associated with myofascial tender points identified at the level of spinal dysfunction after manipulation in patients presenting with chronic upper back and neck pain (Terrett and Vernon, 1984; Vernon, 1988; Vernon *et al.*, 1990; Vernon and Gitelman, 1990). The presence of pain and tissue tenderness in this region may reflect the postural stresses and gravitational forces that are placed upon the thoracic spine during normal everyday life and sedentary work postures. The excessive strain placed upon the postural muscles supporting the upper extremities, more commonly the trapezius and the rhomboids, have been targetted as a major source of repetitive strain and subsequent upper thoracic pain (Gatterman and Panzer, 1990). Grice (1980) has proposed that the position of the head relative to the gravity line is highly influential in determining the depth of the thoracic kyphosis as far down as T7. This is mainly due to the influence of the large postural extensor groups such as the semispinalis and splenius capitus. These muscle groups are common to both the thoracic and cervical spines and undoubtedly play a major role governing the mechanical chains which affect both areas. On a clinical note, loss of upper thoracic mobility has been suggested as a possible cause of hypermobility and repetitive mechanical insult in the lower cervical region (C5–C6) and deemed responsible for early degenerative changes to these motion segments (Schafer and

Faye, 1989). The long-term result of this mechanical stress has been identified by Sandoz (1976) as a 'trophostatic syndrome', a static postural decompensatory condition characterized by, among others, a fixed upper thoracic spine and lower cervical posterior joint arthrosis. Upper thoracic pain has been found to be one of the most commonly reported complaints in the workplace due, in part, to poor postural habits and ergonomically unsound seating positions (Andersson *et al.*, 1975; Bendix *et al.*, 1985; Eklund and Corlett, 1987). Certain common postural aberrations (i.e. 'round shoulders') have been reported to be modified by exercises and manipulative intervention by balancing the strength of the postural stabilizers and restoring thoracic mobility (Panzer *et al.*, 1990). Chiropractic manipulation has also been shown to be very effective in the treatment of the elderly kyphotic patient (Sandoz, 1976; Hurst, 1987). Furthermore the role of spinal manipulation in the management of structural and non-structural forms of scoliosis is not an absolute contraindication. A thorough understanding of the natural history of the condition permitting accurate diagnosis and appropriate treatment is mandatory (Danbert, 1989). The application of gentle manual therapy directed towards the muscle and joint dysfunction has been described as an integral part of an algorithm for the management of scoliosis (Nykoliation *et al.*, 1986).

Thoracolumbar Junction

The thoracolumbar junction (TLJ) represents a transitional region of considerable clinical and biomechanical importance. Maigne's syndrome (Kirkaldy-Willis *et al.*, 1992; Bernard and Kirkaldy-Willis, 1992) or the thoracolumbar syndrome has been well described (Proctor *et al.*, 1985). This syndrome, which shows all the hallmarks of a posterior joint syndrome involving dysfunction of the T12–L1 articulation and referred pain over iliac crest, has been reported to respond well to manipulative management combined with stretching of the local musculature (Proctor *et al.*, 1985).

The influence of the psoas major on the thoracolumbar spine has also been the topic of considerable debate. It has been described as the most complex muscle in the body in an unclear and as yet unestablished multipurpose role (Fligg, 1985). In addition to the flexor action on the hip, the psoas has been described as an important postural stabilizer of the lumbar spine (Nachemson, 1968). However, more recently, Bogduk *et al.* (1992) dispelled these misconceptions by declaring that the psoas major is designed to act on the hip and has no substantial role as a flexor or extensor of the lumbar spine, but can exert considerable compression and shear loads on the lumbar joints. This would appear to have important clinical significance as a possible aetiological factor in the production of mechanical back pain requiring prompt recognition and immediate therapeutic intervention to reduce the tensile stress and contracture of the psoas muscle (Fligg, 1985). The numerous postural changes that occur during the last trimester of pregnancy have also been reported to affect the mechanics of the TLJ and place additional stress upon the psoas muscle (Fligg, 1986a).

Biomechanically, the facet joints of the twelfth thoracic vertebra are oriented intermediately between the coronal plane of the thoracic motion segments and the sagittal plane of the lumbar units, which potentially places additional stress upon this motor segment (Proctor *et al.*, 1985). Singer (1989) investigated the variety and frequency of the types of thoracolumbar mortice joint. He concluded that this mortice configuration functions to limit axial rotation during normal activities, and may be a focal point for additional injury during forced torsional movements. For this reason, Singer and Giles (1990) have advocated the strict limitation of manipulative or mobilization procedures that utilize excessive rotation and extension. They adamantly challenge the use of exaggerated shoulder and pelvis counter-rotation as a method of isolating and developing joint tension in the posterior joints of the thoracolumbar complex. They warn that vigorous counter-rotational techniques could cause injury and aggravate presenting symptoms. Consequently, employing techniques which push the shoulder back and cephalad as a traction component, and pull the pelvis forward at the same time should be strongly cautioned (Byfield, 1991). The use of non-torsional manipulative techniques in either the supine, prone or kneeling positions may be more appropriate in light of this evidence. The use of non-torsional side posture skills (Fligg, 1984; Fligg, 1986b; Byfield, 1991), traction/distraction techniques (Cox, 1992) and placing the drop centrepiece in the open position (Schafer and Faye, 1989) have been suggested as viable alternatives. Faye (personal communication, 1993) reported a reduction in the adjustive force required to cause cavitation at the TLJ when the manipulation was performed during the downstroke or traction phase characteristic of a mechanized adjusting table. A low thoracolumbar kyphosis, often seen in association with recurrent low back pain (Pedersen and Nielsen, 1993), may have important clinical significance with respect to the type and nature of the manipulative procedures selected for the management of such cases.

Manipulative Considerations

Manipulative procedures in the thoracic spine tend to be more general and less specific than in other areas of the spine (Grice, 1980). However, more recently, attempts have been made to examine and describe in detail the rationale and the skills associated with common diversified manipulative procedures of the thoracic spine (Fligg, 1984; Fligg, 1986b; Zachman *et al.*, 1989; Good, 1992; Nelson, 1992). Nelson (1992) states that the conventional indications and mechanical rationale for the 'anterior thoracic' is riddled with error. It is his contention that the actual dynamics and forces transmitted during the anterior–posterior anterior thoracic adjustment are quite similar to a posterior–anterior adjustment

(transverse process contact-crossed bilateral type procedure). He estimated that the total compressive forces acting on the thoracic cage are similar for both procedures. Even though his rationale has some clinical merit, the quantification system limits any substantial conclusions as empirical only. Nonetheless, any attempt to discuss and challenge the traditional use of popular manipulative procedures deserves attention.

Zachman *et al.* (1989) propose that the anterior thoracic subluxation is a sectional subluxation rather than a segmental one. A compensatory extension stacking of a group of vertebrae plus paraspinal hypertonicity is a direct response to a flexion subluxation just below the flattened curvature. The corrective procedure is directed towards the group of extended motion segments above the flexion fixation by flexing the patient's torso. Gitelman and Fligg (1992) emphasize that the loss of normal kyphosis is due to a combination of intersegmental flexion fixation and hypertonic spinalis thoracis involvement. They advocate that the primary concern is the correction of the flexion fixations without the use of compressive type posterior–anterior type forces, which contradicts the biomechanical rationale. There seems to be some contradiction between these authors, which may stem from their understanding and use of the term fixation. Irrespective of individual biomechanical rationale, the basic manipulative skills and use of a minimum amount of thrusting force are similar.

Good (1992) suggests that the supine anterior thoracic adjustment is a resisted type of procedure which produces either flexion or extension above the contact hand, depending upon the position of the patient and the line of drive. However, he does indicate that although cavitation most probably occurs in the facets superior to the contact hand, it is an unlikely proposition due to the non-specific nature of this adjustment. It would be naïve to think that in such a complex mechanical region, absolute joint isolation and specificity of dynamic thrust would be possible. The application of a manipulative thrust in either the prone or supine position will undoubtedly influence multiple synovial joints, in part, due to their anatomical proximity and the size of the clinician's contact hand over a very small anatomical lever point. This could account for the multiple 'joint cracks' that are commonly experienced during spinal manipulative therapy of the thoracic spine.

The most comprehensive description of the skills and technique associated with the anterior thoracic adjustment is presented by Fligg (1986b). Biomechanical considerations, patient/doctor positioning, contact hand positioning, thrust, and clinical application are well illustrated along with viable alternatives and special clinical considerations for the use of this particular diversified technique. Some of these areas will be specifically addressed and presented in detail in the manipulative skills section of this chapter.

Manipulative Forces

The forces required to cause cavitation during a unilateral reinforced prone manipulation of the thoracic spine have recently been determined (Herzog *et al.*, 1991a, 1991b; Conway *et al.*, 1993). In these studies, an experienced chiropractor applied a rapid manipulative thrust to the transverse process of T4 using a hypothenar contact in a posterior to anterior plane perpendicular to the thoracic spine after a preliminary preload or prestress load was recorded. The preload force was approximately 145 N or 33 lb. The peak forces recorded were in the region of 400 N or approximately 90 lb, which compares closely to the estimated 80 lb of total compressive force recorded on an ordinary bathroom scale during a similar procedure (Nelson, 1992). Cavitation occurred just prior to peak force in about 116 msec. The average overall thrust time was 285 msec. The preload, peak forces, and speed of thrust recorded in the thoracic spine were greater than those reported for both the sacroiliac joint and cervical spine (Herzog *et al.*, 1991a). As a comparison, forces in the order of 200 N or 45 lb have been measured during the application of graded oscillatory mobiliza-

tion of the spine commonly used by physiotherapists (Matyas and Bach, 1985). Even though they demonstrated a wide variation, the magnitude of these forces compares with the preload forces measured during chiropractic manipulation (Conway *et al.*, 1993). Lee (1989) also determined, using a theoretical model, that the sagittal plane moments produced during posterior–anterior manipulation are substantial and the effects upon the intersegmental joints directly above and below are somewhat asymmetrical. Triano (1992) reports that experimental peak pressures of 50 PSI are distributed to the thorax during an anteroposterior procedure which create tissue stresses well below the structural limits.

From a manipulable skills point of view, Cohen *et al.* (1993) demonstrated that there was no significant variation in the performance of a prone double transverse thenar procedure with respect to preload force, thrust force, and speed between experienced and novice manipulators. The failure to establish a measurable difference could be due to the simple fact that the experienced chiropractors seldom used the test procedure or, more importantly, that skill performance is technique specific and non-transferable. This indicates that regardless of experience, if the basic psychomotor skills for a manipulative technique have not been practised, the performance of an experienced clinician is reduced to the level of a trained apprentice.

Manipulative Skills

Manipulative skills of the thoracic spine are performed in all positions, including prone, supine, lateral recumbent, sitting and standing postures. This is a unique situation. Other areas of the spine and pelvis do not exhibit this versatility. The purpose of this chapter is to present the basic skills performed in the more common prone and supine positions. It is unreasonable to expect proficiency in all the various combinations in early undergraduate training. Each manipulative procedure is not a separate entity to be learned in isolation, but as part of a series of fundamental building blocks. The type and speed of thrust may differ, but many of the basic doctor and patient movements are similar and repeatable across a variety of manipulative techniques.

The chapter will be divided into three sections: the upper, mid and lower thoracic spine. The spine is divided in this fashion in order to accommodate the significant differences in the functional anatomy and the specific mechanics of the region which will dictate the type of skills necessary. The prone position will be presented first. Patient movement here is minimal so efforts can be directed towards learning the necessary skills without having to control patient movement. The patient lying prone or supine places greater emphasis upon the manipulative skills, particularly doctor posture and weight distribution.

This chapter deals strictly with spinal intersegmental manipulative skills. It is very difficult not to include skills concerning the costotransverse articulations. However, I feel that this represents more advanced training that should be undertaken once the basics of this chapter have been accomplished. Many of the skills for the intervertebral joints can be easily extrapolated to the ribs depending upon the clinical implications.

The Mid Thoracic Spine Manipulative Skills

Single transverse process – prone

Double transverse process – prone

Single spinous process – supine

Single Transverse Process – Prone

This particular sequence of skills probably represents the fundamental positioning for many of the prone manipulative procedures. With the patient lying passively prone, the student can concentrate on important posture and positioning skills. The patient is positioned so that the headpiece is slightly flexed to relax the upper back region and the feet are elevated only minimally to take the tension out of the hamstrings. If the patient experiences any low back pain whilst in this position, then a roll can be placed under the abdomen for a short period of time. Lying in the prone position with the lumbar spine in a flexed posture for extended periods of time compresses the intervertebral disc anteriorly and could aggravate discogenic pain. Conversely, lying with the spine slightly extended could cause facet irritation and difficulty rising from the table into the upright posture.

The skills will focus on the T56 motion segment. It should be emphasized that skills should be practised on both sides of the spine in order to develop dexterity and clinical flexibility. Please refer to Appendix I which deals with the location of anatomical landmarks. Reasonably accurate landmark identification encourages segmental isolation and manipulative specificity. This is of particular importance in the thoracic spine due to its anatomical complexity. The transverse process and spinous processes are very small landmarks in comparison to the size of the treating hands. Anatomical proximity and overlap of the hand contact could easily influence several articulations when mechanical leverage is applied. During a manipulating procedure compromising segemental specificity.

1) With the patient lying in the prone position the doctor should pivot from 90 degrees to a 45 degree angle to the patient directly in line with the T56 motion segment. The feet should be placed about hip distance apart and the doctor is leaning against the table with both thighs, primarily the front leg. This helps to support the doctor's body weight. The majority of the body weight is over the flexed front leg. This allows the doctor to lean over the patient and position the centre of gravity for efficient weight distribution and thrust (*). The doctor should feel comfortable in this stance with relaxed shoulders and arms. The back is reasonably straight and there is no torsion in the body. The head is slightly flexed forward in order to accommodate visual cues (fig. 10.1).

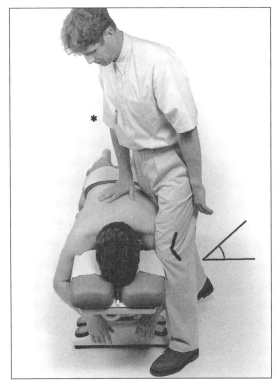

Fig 10.1

2) After locating the transverse process (TP) of T5 use the middle finger or the thumb of the cephalad (left) hand to draw or pull the tissue slack cephalad and laterally, simultaneously. The skin over the TP should be tight, which allows for a firmer and more accurate contact (fig. 10.2). Tissue slack movement should be firm and direct, not pinching or hard. Patient relaxation is important and continuously encouraged.

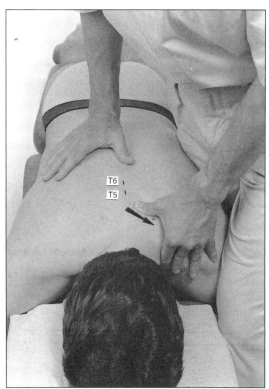

Fig 10.2

3) With the excess tissue slack removed, the contact hand follows immediately to ensure TP accuracy and location. The contact hand forms a firm chiropractic arch which is placed over the spinous process at the corresponding level of the TP (T4). The padded hypothenar/pisiform contact is moved laterally, drawing additional skin slack during this movement to finish over the TP of T5 (hopefully) <u>with the fingers pointing cephalad and the little finger placed against the spinous processes</u> (fig. 10.3). The finger pads of the contact hand are comfortably placed over the paraspinal muscles and used to secure the contact hand by drawing tissue toward the arch. The contact is light yet firm, to give a stable contact and reassure the patient. The doctor leans against the table for additional weight support.

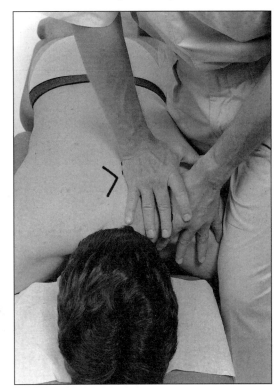

Fig 10.3

4) The position of the doctor's arm and chest is a crucial point promoting efficiency of the manipulative procedure. <u>The shoulder of the contact arm is relaxed and level. The elbow is **not** fully extended,</u> which spares the joint unnecessary strain (*). <u>The wrist is also in a relaxed position</u> (*). The suprasternal notch is positioned **slightly behind** the hypothenar/pisiform contact point on the TP in order to position doctor's body weight prior to joint preload and mock thrust. The extensor muscle group of the forearm should be pointing in the direction of the fingers in order to reduce any torsional stress at the elbow (fig. 10.4a) (*). The hand is relaxed but firm over the tissue. The fingers assist in supporting the hand by drawing in excess soft tissue (fig. 10.4b). This gives some idea of the actual size of the contact over the TP (*).

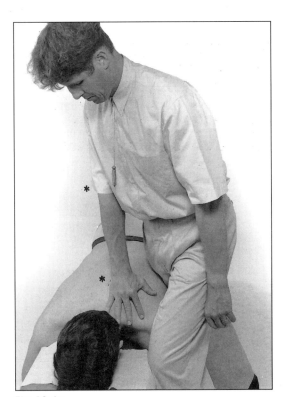

Fig 10.4a

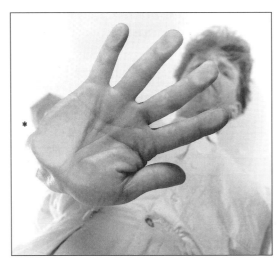

Fig 10.4b

5) From this very basic position, the doctor transfers body weight forward over the patient by
initially plantar flexing the rear foot, which
brings the trunk forward over the patient. This
movement is slow and controlled (fig. 10.5a).
Place the indifferent hand (left) over the contact hand to help stabilize the hypothenar/
pisiform contact position. The hand accommodates a firm chiropractic arch over the contact
hand (*) (fig. 10.5b). The doctor is positioned
45 degrees and leaning against the table. The
weight of the trunk is brought down over
the contact point of the patient by allowing
the front leg to flex to cushion the weight. The
feet are maintained no more than hip distance
apart during this whole procedure. There should
be **no compression** or force down over the
patient's thoracic cage at this point. The
weight shift should align the suprasternal
notch just slightly ahead of the anatomical
contact point. This places the majority of the
doctor's body weight over the left T56 posterior
facet joint which will concentrate forces
through this area. The head is slightly flexed
forward looking down over the contact configuration. Shoulders and arms are relatively
relaxed with no muscular tension.

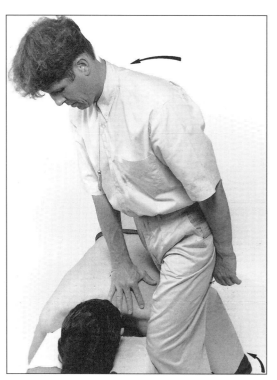

Fig 10.5a

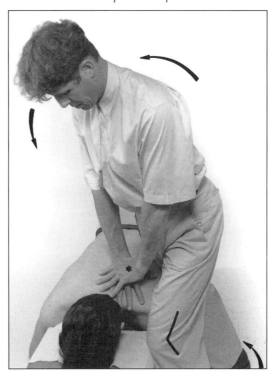

Fig 10.5b

The ability to locate exactly the TP of the desired motion segment, in this case the TP of T5 is an immense task, even for the experienced doctor. We just don't see the models who appear in the anatomy books. You know the ones with about 3% body fat and such well-defined musculature and bony landmarks, an ideal situation for accurate identification. The process in most instances is difficult and frustrating. Therefore, visualization of the anatomical landmarks and using the procedures as outlined in Appendix I should minimize this problem.

Up to this point all the skills have been performed in order to locate and stabilize the T56 motion segment and correctly position the doctor in the most advantageous posture without discomfort to the patient. Joint tension (elastic barrier) is accomplished by eliminating the compliance in the thoracic rib cage. This is a very common procedure for many manipulative skills in the thoracic spine and rib cage. Learning the basic skills at this point will provide the foundation for the introduction of many variations of manipulative skills for the thoracic spine. The compliance of the rib cage must be

reduced very slowly with control. In order to accomplish this, the patient is asked to take a deep breath in very slowly prior to preload or mock thrust. The doctor moves with the rhythm of the patient's rib cage during the inspiration stage. There should be absolutely no impedance to this action. Then ask the patient to breathe out slowly, after which the doctor follows the expiration phase very slowly with his/her trunk weight. As the patient reaches the final stages of expiration, the doctor continues to apply compression over the contact point with the trunk weight until that point at which resistance is felt through the hands and arms. This will ensure that the joint to be manipulated has approximated the elastic barrier of joint resistance. It is absolutely mandatory that the student learns to perform this slowly and gradually within the rhythm of the patient's breathing cycle. The student must avoid just *pushing* with the arms straight down like a pile-driver. The force down should be a combination of shoulder depression and downward movement of the pelvic girdle as a result of flexion of the front knee. This is a particularly difficult skill to coordinate, initially.

Perform the movements slowly and with purpose. The compliance of the rib cage has to be judged on an individual basis for each patient and considered in the context of any absolute or relative contraindications to spinal manipulative therapy. There is no standard force or threshold to refer to. The student must learn to appreci-ate the compliance and elasticity in the rib cage with each patient. Developing a slow and controlled method from the outset allows the appropriate receptors to adapt to the resistance, instead of rushing the process and applying an inappropriate amount of force to a patient.

6) Practising these skills initially on any inflated ball to simulate the thoracic cage compliance would be of benefit as an initial introduction to this important aspect of thoracic spine manipulative skills (fig. 10.6). Simulate the contact hands and get a feel for the developing resistance as more weight is applied. The weight is applied through the trunk moving down by way of the shoulders and arms. Perform these movements very slowly to simulate the breathing cycle. Practise concise and assertive commands.

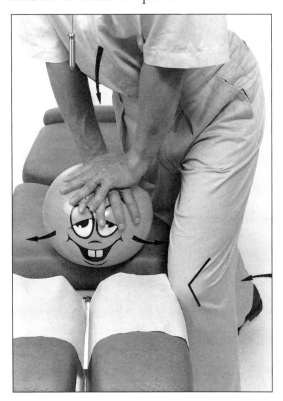

Fig 10.6

7) The final action during weight drop and compliance is to add a small amount of torque or twist to the contact hand which tightens the tissue, removing additional tissue laxity near joint tension. The twist takes place during patient exhalation and it is accomplished by **minimally radially deviating** the contact hand towards the doctor's body by internal rotation of the contact arm. The 5th digit remains in line with the spine to ensure maintenance and accuracy of the contact (fig. 10.7). Do not thrust at this point; appreciate the tension developing in a mock type fashion. Repeat this several times within the tolerance of your patient. Ask for feedback from the patient regarding pressure points and degree of comfort.

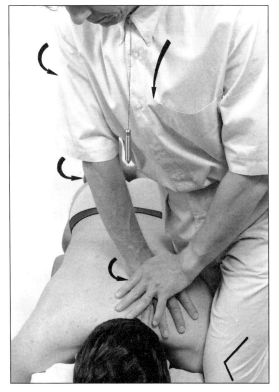

Fig 10.7

8) There are errors that are commonly encountered during the learning of the initial skills.

i) The doctor's legs may be too far apart with the feet angled improperly, positioned too far from the table causing the doctor to lean towards the table and placing additional postural stress on the back. This will also place the suprasternal notch and the centre of gravity in an awkward position, compromising the efficiency of the manipulative procedure (fig. 10.8).

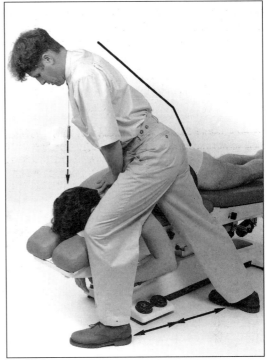

Fig 10.8

ii) Poor hand posture skills both for the chiropractic arch and the removal of tissue slack will compromise the overall performance of the manipulative skill (*). Segmental specificity and patient comfort are of utmost importance clinically (fig. 10.9). Rough handling of the patient will reduce therapeutic compliance and patient satisfaction.

iii) There is a tendency to rush the breathing sequence and compress the patient's rib cage prior to the joint tension and preload. This can cause significant patient distress, especially in an acute presentation which could increase the likelihood of poor compliance and post-treatment reactions. The development of the tissue tension is slow and gradual and in coordination with the expiration phase.

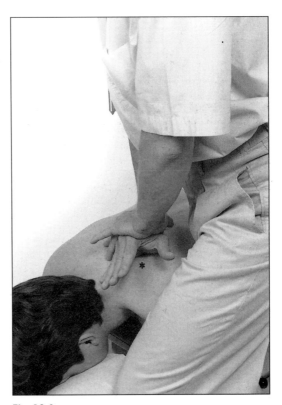

Fig 10.9

Double Transverse Process – Prone

This manipulative skill is a modification of the single TP contact set of skills. It is commonly referred to as the crossed bilateral (Szaraz, 1984; Gitelman and Fligg, 1992), double transverse (Grecco, 1953; Schafer and Faye, 1989) or crossed bilateral transverse pisiform (States, 1968). The manipulation is generally incorporated to correct rotation dysfunction of either the posterior facets or the costotransverse joints.

The skills are exactly the same as for the preparation of the single transverse manipulative skills described above. The significant difference is utilizing the indifferent hand to stabilize the opposing joints above and below the target joint. It also helps to centre the doctor's body at a 45 degree angle to the patient as the support arm crosses over the contact arm.

1) With doctor's contact hand positioned for a single TP contact (see above) the indifferent hand (left) *crosses over* in front of the contact hand to the other side of the spine and adopts a firm bridge arch (fig. 10.10). The doctor is still 45 degrees to the table and the front leg is flexed for comfort. No muscular force should be applied to the spine at this point. Plumbline should be over the middle of both hand positions.

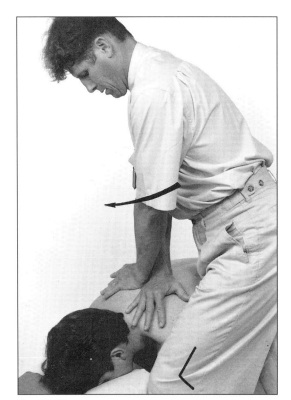

Fig 10.10

2) The heel of the indifferent hand (left) rolls off the spinous processes to be positioned over the opposite TPs with the hand in a high chiropractic arch (fig. 10.11a). The thenar eminence is placed over the TP of the vertebral segment below (T6) and the hypothenar eminence is over the TP of the segment above (T4). Tissue slack is taken from the midline spinous laterally over the contact points. The hands are basically at right angles to each other. Figure 10.11b illustrates the hand relationship and the size of the contact area over the TPs.

NB. There are many variations of this manipulative skill, particularly the hand placement combinations depending on the biomechanical correction and fixation pattern.

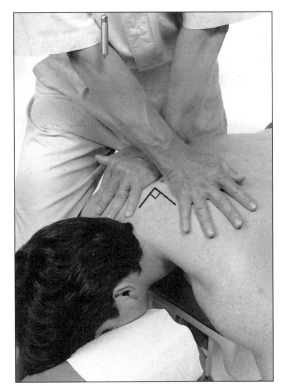

Fig 10.11a

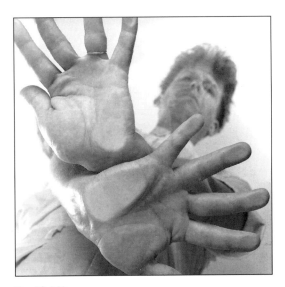

Fig 10.11b

3) To bring body weight over the contact hands the doctor pushes forward by plantar flexing the rear foot. The patient is asked to breathe in. The doctor follows this movement without losing firm and specific contact. As the patient breathes out the doctor follows the movement precisely until the thoracic compliance has been eliminated and there is a perception of resistance under the contact hand. This is the feeling of overall joint and tissue tension completing joint preload (fig. 10.12).

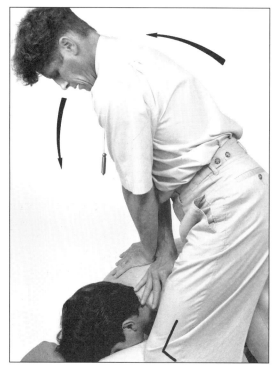

Fig 10.12

4) Simultaneously as the weight comes down and the thoracic compliance is diminishing, both contact arms and hands slightly twist producing internal rotation and radial deviation, respectively, as the patient is breathing out in order to eliminate as much excess tissue slack as possible (fig. 10.13).

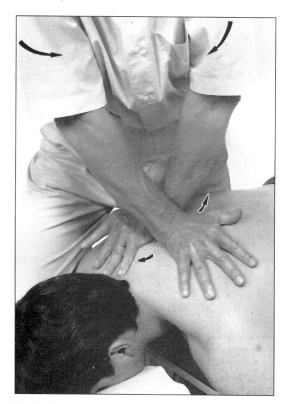

Fig 10.13

The errors encountered during this manipulative skill are similar to those described for the single spinous above. Please note that over-twisting of the contact hands and forcing the expiration phase could cause unnecessary patient distress.

Upper Thoracic Spine Manipulative Skills – Head Lever

The preceding section dealt with skills associated with manipulative procedures in the mid thoracic spine in the prone posture. The next step will be to introduce common skills employed in the upper thoracic spine in the prone position using the TP and SP as anatomical contact points.

Single Transverse Process

Using the head as a lever in order to manipulate the upper thoracic spine offers several advantages. The head is a relatively short lever in comparison to the leg or the shoulder girdle. There are several myofascial structures which are common to both the upper thoracic region and the cervical spine. This has important clinical implications in terms of treatment strategies and rehabilitative protocols. Passive movement of the head implies that the practitioner can control upper thoracic spine movement to attain joint specificity and tension, which improves the efficiency of the manipulative procedure. However, the head and neck are sensitive structures and must be handled with care to reduce the possibility of any post-treatment reactions.

This sequence of manipulative skills uses single TP contact as described above. For the purpose of this next series of skills reference will be the T34 segment. **As before, you are encouraged to learn skills equally on both sides.**

This particular manipulative skill is often referred to as the combination upper thoracic adjustment (Grice, 1980; Szaraz, 1984), the single temporal–transverse adjustment for the upper dorsals (Grecco, 1953), correction for upper thoracic rotation fixation: patient prone (Schafer and Faye, 1989) or combination movement (States, 1968). This particular manipulative procedure uses relatively short levers which are anatomically close together. The use of head to anatomically isolate movement in the upper thoracic spine has both anatomical and biomechanical advantages. The muscles which stabilize and initiate head posture and movement are common to both cervical and thoracic regions. It is therefore important to understand and visualize the direction of the individual muscle groups during this specific set of manipulative skills.

1) The patient is prone with the headpiece slightly flexed to ease the tension in the cervicothoracic junction. The patient's arms are comfortably placed alongside the table with the hands positioned well under the table away from wandering feet. The doctor is positioned 45 degrees to the table and patient, the feet are hip distance apart and the front leg placed ahead of the patient's left arm (fig. 10.14).

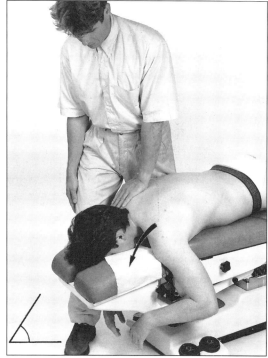

Fig 10.14

2) The doctor locates and contacts the TP of T4 using the skills described in Figures 10.2 and 10.3 above. There is considerable tissue bulk in this area which makes segmental localization and accuracy more arduous. This is why it is important for the patient to relax the upper body as much as possible. Keep in mind that the fingers of the contact hand are recruited to stabilize the contact hand and thus ensure specificity and patient comfort. The contact should be firm but light in a fairly high chiropractic arch (fig. 10.15). The doctor remains in contact with the table at all times to support body weight and keep the trunk over the contact region.

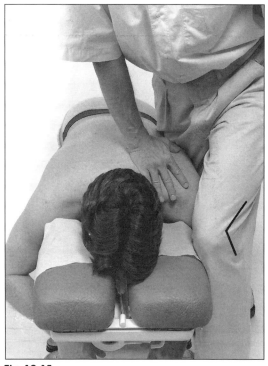

Fig 10.15

3) Using the head as a lever will create movement above the contact. The head as a medium lever takes considerable finesse to move even though the action appears relatively simple. Without losing contact over the TP the web of the indifferent hand (left) is cupped **around the ear** of the patient being careful not to pinch the earlobe. The hand is extended and radially deviated when performing this task. The thumb comfortably cups the occipital rim (*) and the pads of the index and middle fingers contact the parietal region of the skull just above the ear (*). There is a slight arch in the hand. This is to protect the earlobe from being compressed against the skull with the hand. The arm crosses in front of the contact arm (fig. 10.16). *NB. Remove any jewellery as a rule of thumb before proceeding.*

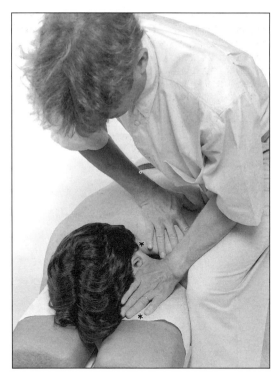

Fig 10.16

4) The head is then gently teased out of the middle of the headpiece until about 45 degrees of head rotation or until movement or rotation is felt under the contact point. This is done by slowly flexing the wrist and moving the arm across the body in front of the contact arm. Discourage patient assistance. The head is positioned in slight flexion, lateral flexion and rotation. The nose is clear and there should be no tension in the patient's upper back or neck regions (fig. 10.17). The support arm is resting on the doctor's thigh (*).

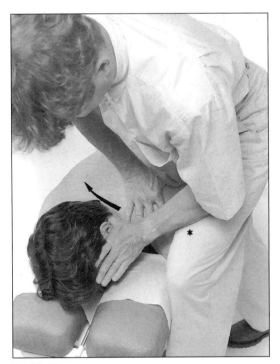

Fig 10.17

5) The doctor now shifts the weight forward by plantar flexing the rear foot. This brings the body weight forward over the headpiece in preparation for joint tension. The contact arm is almost straight and the indifferent arm is tucked into the side of the body in order to keep the levers short (fig. 10.18a). Care is taken not to place any weight on either anatomical landmark or produce any excess tension between the two contact points. The distance between points should not change. The body weight is supported by the front leg. Body weight is over the centre of the patient and the table (fig. 10.18b).

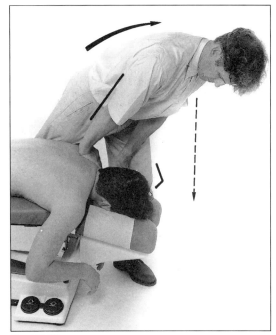

Fig 10.18a

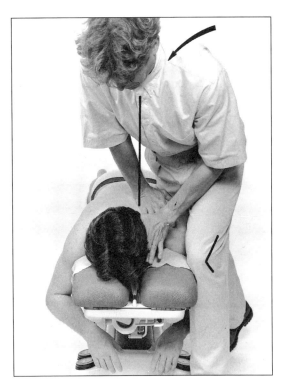

Fig 10.18b

6) The patient is asked to breathe in and out at the same time as the doctor lowers his weight by slowly flexing the front leg (fig. 10.19). This action causes the two contact points to separate slowly, increasing tissue tension between the contact and indifferent hands. Cephalad traction is maintained by the indifferent hand contact. The doctor should begin to feel maximum tension across the tissue as the patient completes the breathing cycle. The doctor leans against the table during the whole procedure, keeping the upper torso only slightly flexed with the majority of the trunk weight over the legs.

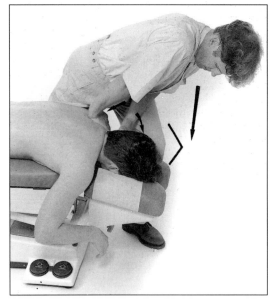

Fig 10.19

7) There are several potential errors associated with the learning of this skill.

i) Apart from a forceful contact, a commonly observed mistake to note is the doctor positioned parallel to the table with a flexed contact arm with the body weight located well behind the TP contact and the upper torso and shoulder in cramped position (*) (fig. 10.20).

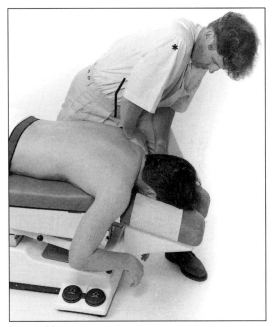

Fig 10.20

ii) Don't over-rotate and apply excessive traction to the head and neck (fig. 10.21a). Rough handling of the patient's head is another concern often overlooked when concentrating on the contact points. There is a tendency to flatten the ear or push the head with the heel of the hand which presents a potential source of discomfort for the patient; this is not an ideal situation particularly when patient comfort is mandatory (*) (fig. 10.21b). The ear is very sensitive and does not like being excessively folded.

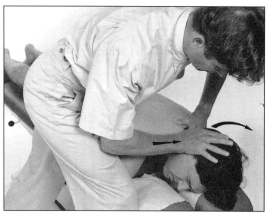

Fig 10.21a

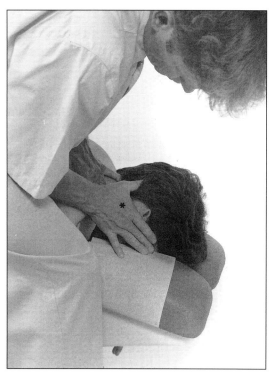

Fig 10.21b

Single Spinous Contact – Head as Lever

This next series of skills is combined to influence spinal dysfunction, mainly rotation and lateral flexion related to the cervicothoracic spine. This manipulative procedure is commonly referred to as the thumb move (Szaraz, 1984) or thumb movement of bench TM (States, 1968). The steps are once again a continuation of the already learned skills. The sequence will focus on the T1T2 segment and assumes that movement takes place above the contact point as a result of head-assisted rotation.

1) The patient is positioned in the prone position with the headpiece slightly flexed and the arms and hands in a relaxed state hanging to the side of the table out of reach of the doctor's feet. The doctor is positioned with the front leg ahead of the patient's arm, 45 degrees to the table, feet hip distance apart, slight trunk flexion and leaning against the table for weight and postural support (fig. 10.22).

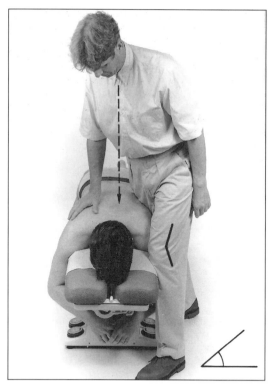

Fig 10.22

2) After locating the spinous of T2 the skin slack is pulled up by the thumb or the index finger of the right hand or support hand (S) starting from the ipsilateral side of the spinous, taking it straight across to the contralateral side until tension is felt over the spinous process. The thumb pad of the contact hand (C) follows in behind this tissue pull to contact the spinous lamina junction of the spinous of T2. The contact is light but firm and comfortable to the patient. The thumb pad takes up additional skin slack. The fingers and web of the hand are draped over the ipsilateral trapezius muscle in a stable and relaxed chiropractic arch (fig. 10.23). The fingers lightly cup the bulk of the trapezius muscle. Note the doctor is leaning against the table at all times (*).

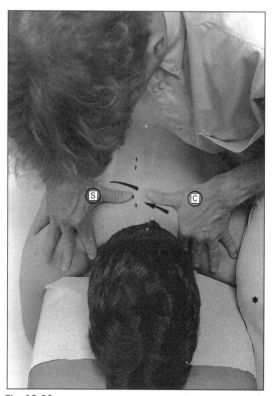

Fig 10.23

3) The doctor lowers himself in order to bring the contact arm almost horizontal and at right angles to both the table and the patient. The wrist is absolutely straight, ulnar deviated and the elbow is flexed to approximately 90 degrees. The arm, hand and shoulder are relaxed (fig. 10.24). The patient should feel no more than mild pressure against the spinous of T2. The contact arm rests on the front thigh for support (*).

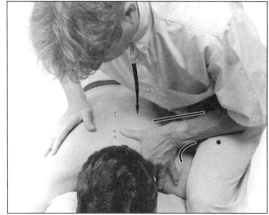

Fig 10.24

4) Rotate the head in the opposite direction (right rotation) until movement is perceived at the thumb contact point at T2 (about 45–50 degrees). The arms are kept close to the body to avoid awkward movement occurring and developing longer levers. The suprasternal notch is directly over the midline of the spine in order to centre the doctor's upper body weight (fig. 10.25). *Note* discourage any assistance from the patient when turning the head. This may need verbal reinforcement.

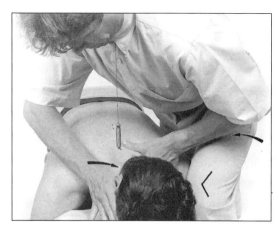

Fig 10.25

5) Once the head is rotated pause, ensure patient comfort and request the patient to breathe in and then out. Simultaneously apply slight lateral and cephalad traction to the rim of the occiput with the support hand. The contact thumb applies **gradual** transverse pressure to the spinous lamina junction along the line of the wrist and forearm (fig. 10.26). Feel the tension developing gradually between the two points. Visualize the soft tissues involved and the effect on the joint structures under tension. Attempt a mock repetitive thrust only to appreciate the elastic barrier and joint resistance.

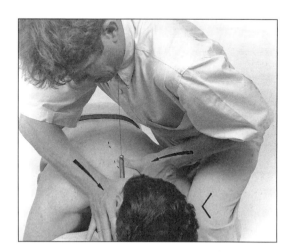

Fig 10.26

6) There are potential errors when learning this set of psychomotor skills.

The errors are similar to those already described above using the head as a lever. The most common one is the position of the doctor and the orientation of the wrist and forearm. Positioning behind the patient causes the wrist to flex which may cause mechanical stress on the soft tissues of the forearm. This situation is impaired even further with the doctor standing too far back or forward from the optimal cervicothoracic junction (fig. 10.27). Note the position of the plumbline and the orientation of the contact wrist (*).

NB. A variation of this ipsilateral manipulative skill is the contralateral procedure which has certain mechanical advantages in terms of the position of the doctor's upper body weight over the contact point and the direction of the pectoralis thrust (fig. 10.28). The contact skills are similar to those described above. This does not represent an advanced set of manipulative skills.

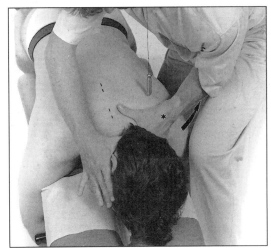

Fig 10.27

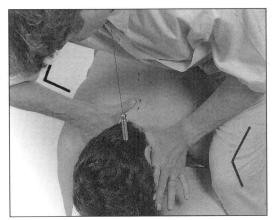

Fig 10.28

Midthoracic Spine Manipulative Skills

Single Spinous – Supine

This is regarded as the most well known of the thoracic manipulative procedures. It is commonly referred to as the anterior thoracic adjustment (States, 1968; Fligg, 1986b; Nelson, 1992; Gitelman and Fligg, 1992) or the manipulative procedure for interspinous fixations (Schafer and Faye, 1989; Gatterman and Panzer, 1990). It is a misrepresentation of words in that the manipulative procedure is performed in the supine position and should be referred to as such. However, for both historical (Fligg, 1986b) and traditional reasons (Nelson, 1992) reference to a name for a particular manipulative procedure should

not really be of any concern as long as those using the skill at least agree on the indications and clinical contraindications.

There are many variations of this technique depending on the area of the thoracic spine and the biomechanical indications. However, there is a common thread which when mastered, like so many of the manipulative procedures already described, makes advancing to a more complex interaction of skills easier for the student or experienced practitioner to learn.

For this set of skills the patient will be lying supine in a comfortable and relaxed state with the headpiece flexed for cervical spine stability and the knees drawn up into flexion to reduce the stress on the hamstrings and flatten the lumbar lordosis to ease the strain off the lumbar facets. The doctor will be standing on the patient's right side. Once again the student will be encouraged to learn skills from both sides of the table to enhance clinical flexibility.

For the purpose of this description reference will be made concerning the T67 motion segment.

1) The patient is lying supine as described above with the arms folded across the chest and the doctor facing at right angles to the patient just below the T67 vertebral level feet separated, with the cephalad foot at the level of the patient's shoulder and the caudad foot at the level of the hip. The doctor is also leaning against the table. The arms are crossed specifically with the patient's left arm folded over on top of the right with the hands reaching around the body (*). This configuration maximizes tension in the interscapular region and reduces thoracic cage compliance (fig. 10.29). It may be advisable to begin by using a thoracic board at this point which will provide a firmer base and maintain comfort for the patient and practitioner's contact hand.

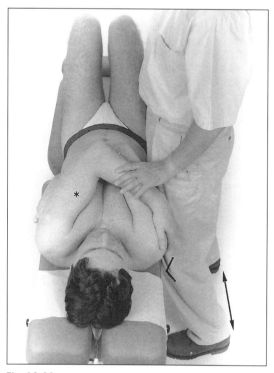

Fig 10.29

2) In order to make a specific segmental contact, the patient is rolled towards the doctor by simultaneously rotating both the chest and pelvis towards the doctor. The patient must feel secure when rolled to the edge of the table. To ensure safety the doctor's *knees* act to prevent the patient from rolling uncontrollably off the table onto an unsuspecting novice (fig. 10.30). This stabilizes the patient and allows the doctor to see and locate the target joint complex.

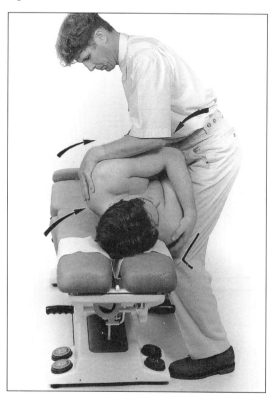

Fig 10.30

3) The thenar eminence is the contact point of choice at this level of skill learning. Refer to Chapter 5, Figures 5.31 and 5.32 for details of the two most common hand contacts. Each of these is selected depending on the needs and size of the patient and practitioner. For each posture the thumb is adducted across the palm with the thumb in line with the index finger. For the sake of consistency the open hand posture will be demonstrated for ease of demonstration. With the index finger of the contact hand (right) the T67 interspinous space is located and simultaneously tissue slack is drawn cephalad from that point with the middle finger of the indifferent hand (left). Once the excess skin slack is removed, the middle of the thenar eminence is placed directly over the spinous process of T7 with the inferior aspect of the spinous process of T6 positioned at the superior border of the thenar eminence (fig. 10.31). The doctor's arms hold the patient in the side lying position (*).

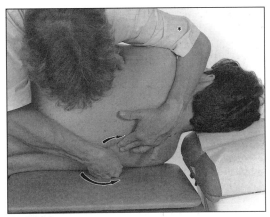

Fig 10.31

4) The patient is rolled back very slowly onto the table and the doctor's contact hand making sure that the contact stays securely in place and does not cause the patient any discomfort. If the patient shows any signs of distress, it is recommended that the contact hand is repositioned immediately. At this stage the indifferent arm locks across the patient's folded arms. The contact arm is positioned at right angles to the patient (fig. 10.32). The doctor is leaning against the table and over the patient, with no weight compressing the rib cage. Make sure the patient is comfortable at all times. Note the patient's head is flexed to assist contact tension (*).

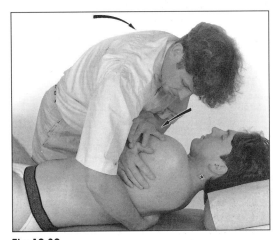

Fig 10.32

5) Gently pull the patient's arms parallel to the patient's body (fig. 10.33), **not down towards the chest**. This action is a very short action which assists in flexing the trunk to the segmental level and creating some tension in the upper body. *There is to be no downward pressure on the patient's chest at this stage*. The patient should be able to breathe comfortably.

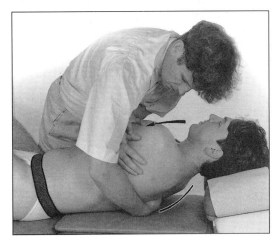

Fig 10.33

6) The next step governs patient cooperation, compliance and control. The patient is asked to breathe in very slowly, after which he or she is requested to breathe slowly outward. *Once again there should be no excess weight applied to the rib cage* during the breath cycle. As the compliance of the rib cage is being removed the doctor is simultaneously applying downward and cephalad pressure at **exactly the same rate as the patient is breathing** (fig. 10.34). The doctor pulls up on the contact hand into the spine to increase tension (*). Once rib compliance has been eliminated, the final aspect of the skill is the application of a mock thrust. **This is not to be applied at this time. Feel the joint tension and apply mock preload only**.

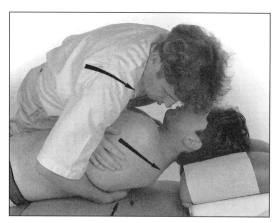

Fig 10.34

7) Maximum flexion of the thoracic spine at the specific segmental level is an important aspect of this manipulative procedure. Flexion of the headpiece may not be enough to reach the desired segmental tension. Other appropriate modifications to maximize this are:

i) Asking the patient to lift his or her head actively off the table during the breathing out stage of the sequence of skills for the midthoracic spine just prior to achieving joint resistance (fig. 10.35).

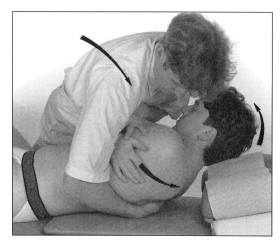

Fig 10.35

ii) Utilizing a clasped, interlaced hand contact by the patient behind his/her neck or head (*) will increase upper back flexion and the appropriate joint tension and isolation. This position provides long lever function to achieve the desired amount of flexion (fig. 10.36). Consider contraindications, as this technique may place excess stress on the cervical spine.

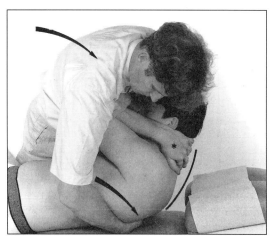

Fig 10.36

iii) Lifting and cradling the patient to the desired level in the mid thoracic to lower thoracic spine allows the doctor to control the patient's weight and movement and reach a point of maximum tension for a very difficult region of the spine (fig. 10.37). This particular variation requires considerable control of patient's body weight as it is lowered down over the contact. This is accomplished by positioning the doctor's front leg well forward to control and support the weight as it comes down. This is a more advanced skill.

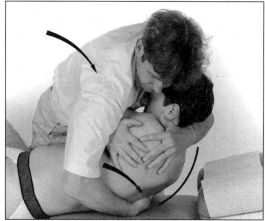

Fig 10.37

8) *There are several potential learning errors during the acquisition of these skills.*

i) Failing to pull the patient's folded arms down and parallel to the chest and, instead pushing up, placing stress both on the patient's shoulders and throat (fig. 10.38). Note the relative laxity and extension in the upper back (*). The doctor's weight is coming straight down only.

ii) Pushing down on the patient's rib cage faster than the patient is breathing out and executing the sequence too quickly, causing the patient unnecessary distress and lack of compliance.

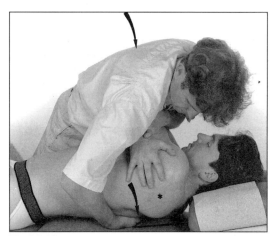

Fig 10.38

Lower Thoracic Spine

Manipulative skills for the lower thoracic spine present a more formidable task to the practitioner, due to, among many others, the changing nature of the spinal curvature and the orientation of the facets. Mechanical dysfunction syndromes, such as Maigne's syndrome (Kirkaldy-Willis and Burton, 1992), establish the need to be able to introduce a manipulative thrust confidently and safely into the region to restore intervertebral function.

It is not the intent of this text to develop discussion regarding the clinical indications of when, where, and why a manipulative procedure is being selected for a set of clinical signs and symptoms. There are, however, basic skills to be learned and perfected regardless of the diagnostic indicators.

The student should remember that the lower thoracic spine begins to take on the characteristics of the upper lumbar spine in terms of structure and facet orientation. This will also determine, to some extent, the basic kinematics of the region and the nature of the movement that is being restored.

There are a multitude of manipulative procedures commonly employed to correct dysfunction of the lower thoracic spine. The thenar and hypothenar/metacarpal hand contact points are routinely selected for this purpose. They are often referred to as the bilateral thenar or the bilateral hypothenar (Carver Bridge) (Szaraz, 1984), and the phalangeometacarpal (States, 1968). The TPs are often the anatomical lever point due to the changing morphology of the spinous process and the angulation of the posterior facets.

The spinous process is an effective anatomical lever for this region.

The knife-edge (Szaraz, 1984; Schafer and Faye, 1989) employs the edge of the hypothenar eminence to contact the inferior tip of the spinous process. The following is just an introduction to the skills in this region of the spine. Refer to Chapter 5 and Figures 5.25–5.29 inclusive regarding hand configuration skills for these two specific hand contacts.

1) The most important aspect of these manipulative skills is keeping the shoulders, hands and arms symmetrical throughout preload and the mock thrust exercises. This ensures equal mechanical loads and stresses on the soft tissue and a balanced thrust across the joint (fig. 10.39a and b). Note the position of the plumbline, indicating that the weight of the doctor's body is centred over the patient's body for a more efficient procedure and thrust. The weight is shifted forward and over the patient by plantar flexing the rear foot to position the body in line with the thrust direction.

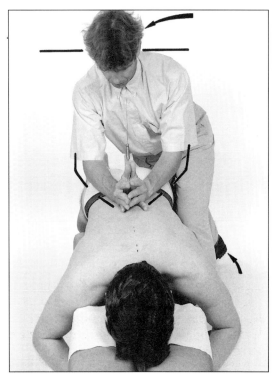

Fig 10.39a

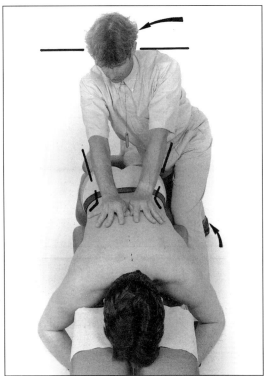

Fig 10.39b

2) The angle of the arm is determined by the level of the spine and the approximate orientation of the facet angles (fig. 10.40). The lower in the thoracic spine the greater the angle with the horizontal.

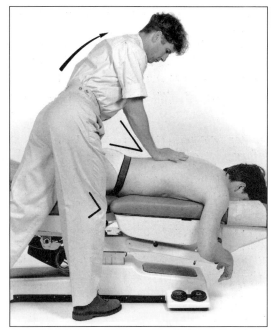

Fig 10.40

This chapter has presented a detailed description of the more commonly used diversified manipulative procedures of the thoracic spine. The theme has been to demonstrate each manipulation as a set of individual skills and movements. These skills represent the basis or foundation for additional more advanced manipulative procedures which may be learned once these basics have been mastered. A professional commitment means many hours of practice and frustration in the pursuit of excellence.

References

Andersson, B.J.G., Ortengren, R., Nachemson, A.L. *et al.* (1975) The sitting posture: an electromyographic and discometric study. *Orthopedic Clinics of North America*, **6**, 105–120

Bendix, T., Krohn, L., Jessen, F. *et al.* (1985) Trunk posture and trapezius working in standing, supported-standing, and sitting positions. *Spine*, **10**, 433–439

Bernard, T.N. and Kirkaldy-Willis, W.H. (1992) Making a specific diagnosis. In *Managing Low Back Pain*, 3rd edn. (eds. H.W. Kirkaldy-Willis and C.V. Burton). Churchill Livingstone, London, pp. 203–223

Bogduk, N., Pearcy, M. and Hadfield, G. (1992) Anatomy and biomechanics of psoas major. *Clinical Biomechanics*, **7**, 109–119

Bogduk, N. and Valencia, F. (1988) Innervation and pain patterns of the thoracic spine. In *Clinics in Physical Therapy: Physical Therapy of the Cervical and Thoracic Spine* (ed. R. Grant). Churchill Livingstone, London, pp. 27–37

Byfield, D. (1991) Lumbar manipulative procedures in relation to segmental specificity and biomechanical properties of the motor unit. *European Journal of Chiropractic*, **39**, 13–19

Cohen, E., Triano, J., Papapkyriakou, M. *et al.* (1993) Experienced vs. novice manipulator performance measures. In *Proceedings of the 1993 International Conference on Spinal Manipulation* (Montreal, 1993). Foundation for Chiropractic Education and Research, Arlington, Virginia, p. 91

Conway, P.J.W., Herzog, W., Zhang, Y. *et al.* (1993) Forces required to cause cavitation during spinal manipulation of the thoracic spine. *Clinical Biomechanics*, **8**, 210–214

Cox, J.M. (1992) Traction and distraction techniques. In *Principles and Practice of Chiropractic*, 2nd edn. (ed. S. Haldeman).

Appleton and Lange, San Mateo, California, pp. 503–518

Danbert, R.J. (1989) Scoliosis: biomechanics and rationale for manipulative treatment. *Journal of Manipulative and Physiological Therapeutics*, **12**, 38–45

Deyo, R.A., Rainville, J. and Kent, D.L. (1992) What can the history and physical examination tell us about low back pain? *Journal of the American Medical Association*, **268**, 760–765

Eklund, J.A.E. and Corlett, E.N. (1987) Evaluation of spinal loads and chair design in seated work tasks. *Clinical Biomechanics*, **2**, 27–33

Fligg, D.B. (1984) Lateral recumbent rib adjustment. *Journal of the Canadian Chiropractic Association*, **28**, 277–278

Fligg, D.B. (1985) Psoas technique. *Journal of the Canadian Chiropractic Association*, **29**, 207–210

Fligg, D.B. (1986a) Biomechanical and treatment considerations for the pregnant patient. *Journal of the Canadian Chiropractic Association*, **30**, 145–147

Fligg, D.B. (1986b) The anterior thoracic adjustment. . *Journal of the Canadian Chiropractic Association*, **30**, 211–213

Gatterman, M.I. and Panzer, D.M. (1990) Disorders of the thoracic spine. In *Chiropractic Management of Spine Related Disorders* (ed. M.I. Gatterman). Williams and Wilkins, London, pp. 176–204

Gitelman, R. and Fligg, B. (1992) Diversified technique. In *Principles and Practice of Chiropractic*, 2nd edn. (ed. S. Haldeman). Appleton and Lange, San Mateo, California, pp. 483–501

Good, C.J. (1992) An analysis of diversified (lege artis) type adjustments based upon the assisted–resisted model of intervertebral motion unit prestress. *Chiropractic Technique*, **4**, 117–123

Grecco, M.A. (1953) *Chiropractic Technique Illustrated*. Jarl Publishing, New York, pp. 89–90

Greenman, P.E. (1989) Thoracic spine technique. In *Principles of Manual Medicine* (ed. P.E. Greenman). Williams and Wilkins, London, pp. 150–174

Grice, A.S. (1980) A biomechanical approach to cervical and dorsal adjusting. In *Modern Developments in the Principles and Practice of Chiropractic* (ed. S. Haldeman). Appleton-Century-Crofts, New York, pp. 331–358

Herzog, W., Conway, J.W., Kawchuk, G.N. *et al.* (1991a) Comparison of the forces exerted during spinal manipulative therapy on the sacroiliac joint, the thoracic spine and the cervical spine. In *Proceedings of the Scientific Symposium, World Chiropractic Congress* (Toronto, 1991). World Federation of Chiropractic, Toronto

Herzog, W., Conway, P.J., Zhang, Y. *et al.* (1991b) Forces exerted during spinal manipulative treatments of the thoracic spine. In *Proceedings of the International Conference on Spinal Manipulation* (Arlington, 1991). Foundation for Chiropractic Education and Research, pp. 275–280

Hurst, H. (1987) *The Effect of Chiropractic Adjustive Procedures Versus Mobilization Exercises in the Kyphotic Geriatric Patient*. D.C. Thesis, Anglo-European College of Chiropractic, Bournemouth

Kellgren, J.H. (1977) The anatomical source of back pain. *Rheumatology and Rehabilitation*, **16**, 3–12

Kirkaldy-Willis, W.H., Burton, C.V. and Cassidy, J.D. (1992) The site and nature of the lesion. In *Managing Low Back Pain*, 3rd edn (eds. W.H. Kirkaldy-Willis and C.V. Burton). Churchill Livingstone, London, pp. 121–148

Kirkaldy-Willis, W.H. and Burton, C.V. (1992) A comprehensive outline of treatment. In *Managing Low Back Pain*, 3rd edn. (eds. W.H. Kirkaldy-Willis and C.V. Burton). Churchill Livingstone, London, pp. 243–261

Lee, M. (1989) Mechanics of spinal joint manipulation in the thoracic and lumbar spine: a theoretical study of posteroanterior force techniques. *Clinical Biomechanics*, **4**, 249–251

Matyas, T.A. and Bach, T.M. (1985) The reliability of selected techniques in clinical arthrometrics. *Australian Journal of Physiotherapy*, **31**, 175–199

Nachemson, A. (1968) The possible importance of the psoas muscle for stabilization of the lumbar spine. *Acta Orthopaedica Scandinavica*, **39**, 47–57

Nelson, C.F. (1992) The anterior thoracic adjustment: an alternate hypothesis. *Chiropractic Technique*, **4**, 143–148

Nice, D.A., Riddle, D.L., Lamb, R.L. *et al.* (1992) Intertester reliability of judgements of the presence of trigger points in patients with low back pain. *Archives of Physical Medicine and Rehabilitation*, **73**, 893–898

Nykoliation, J.W., Cassidy, J.D., Arthur, B.E. *et al.* (1986) An algorithm for the management of scoliosis. *Journal of Manipulative and Physiological Therapeutics*, **9**, 1–14

Panjabi, M.M., Krag, M.H., Dimnet, J.C. *et al.* (1984) Thoracic spine centers of rotation in the sagittal plane. *Journal of Orthopaedic Research*, **1**, 387–394

Panzer, D.M., Fechtel, S.G. and Gatterman, M.I. (1990) Postural complex. In *Chiropractic Management of Spine Related Disorders* (ed. M.I. Gatterman). Williams and Wilkins, London, pp. 256–284

Pedersen, P. and Nielsen, L.B. (1993) A preliminary investigation of the significance of low thoraco-lumbar kyphoses: the feasibility of a method of radiographic measurement. *European Journal of Chiropractic*, **41**, 53–65

Proctor, D., Dupuis, P. and Cassidy, J.D. (1985) Thoracolumbar syndrome as a cause of low-back pain: a report of two cases. *Journal of the Canadian Chiropractic Association*, **29**, 71–73

Sandoz, R. (1976) Some physical mechanisms and effects of spinal adjustments. *Annals Swiss Chiropractic Association*, **VI**, 91–142

Schafer, R.C. and Faye, L.J. (1989) The thoracic spine. In *Motion Palpation and Chiropractic Technic: Principles of Dynamic Chiropractic* (eds. R.C. Schafer and L.J. Faye). Motion Palpation Institute, Huntingdon Beach, California, pp. 143–194

Simons, D.G. (1985) Myofascial pain syndromes due to trigger points: 1. principles, diagnosis, and perpetuating factors. *Manual Medicine*, **1**, 67–71

Singer, K.P. (1989) Thoracolumbar mortice joint: radiological and histological observations. *Clinical Biomechanics*, **4**, 137–143

Singer, K.P. and Giles, L.G.F. (1990) Manual therapy considerations at the thoracolumbar junction: an anatomical and functional perspective. *Journal of Manipulative and Physiological Therapeutics*, **13**, 83–88

States, A.Z. (1968) *Atlas of Chiropractic Technic: Spinal and Pelvic Technics*, 2nd edn. National College of Chiropractic, Illinois

Szaraz, Z. (1984) *Compendium of Chiropractic Technique*, Canadian Memorial Chiropractic College, Toronto

Terrett, A.C.J. and Vernon, H. (1984) Manipulation and pain tolerance: a controlled study of the effect of spinal manipulation on paraspinal cutaneous pain tolerance levels. *American Journal of Physical Medicine*, **63**, 217–225

Travell, J.G. and Simons, D.G. (1983) *Myofascial Pain and Dysfunction. The Trigger Point Manual*. Williams and Wilkins, London, pp. 331–462

Triano, J.J. (1992) Studies on the biomechanical effect of a spinal adjustment. *Journal of Manipulative and Physiological Therapeutics*, **15**, 71–75

Vernon, H.T. (1988) Pressure pain threshold evaluation of the effect of spinal manipulation on chronic neck pain: a single case study. *Journal of the Canadian Chiropractic Association*, **32**, 191–194

Vernon, H.T., Aker, P., Burns, S. *et al.* (1990) Pressure pain threshold evaluation of the effect of spinal manipulation in the treatment of chronic neck pain: a pilot study. *Journal of Manipulative and Physiological Therapeutics*, **13**, 13–16

Vernon, H. and Gitelman, R. (1990) Pressure algometry and tissue compliance measures in the treatment of chronic headache by spinal manipulation: a single case/single treatment report. *Journal of the Canadian Chiropractic Association*, **34**, 141–144

White, A.A. (1969) Analysis of the mechanics of the thoracic spine in man. An experimental study of autopsy specimens. *Acta Orthopaedica Scandinavica*, **127**(Suppl.)

White, A.A. and Panjabi, M.M. (eds.) (1990) Kinematics of the spine. In *Clinical Biomechanics of the Spine*, 2nd edn. J.B. Lippincott, London, pp. 85–125

Wyke, B. (1967) The neurological basis of thoracic spinal pain. *Rheumatology and Physical Medicine*, **10**, 356–367

Zachman, Z.J., Bolles, S., Bergman, T.F. *et al.* (1989) Understanding the anterior thoracic adjustment (a concept of a sectional subluxation). *Chiropractic Technique*, Jan/Feb, 30–33

Chapter

11

Cervical spine manipulative skills

David Byfield

Introduction

Mechanical dysfunction of the cervical spine has been reported to be an important aetiological factor in the presentation of certain types of headache (Vernon, 1988, 1989), migraine (Wight, 1978, 1982), vertebrogenic migraine (Vernon and Dhami, 1985), post hyperflexion/hyperextension (acceleration/deceleration syndrome) injuries (Bogduk, 1986; Foreman and Croft, 1988), shoulder and arm pain (Maigne, 1972; Terrett and Kleynhans, 1984), tinnitus (Terrett, 1989), autonomic nervous system disturbances, including disorders of equilibrium (Brunarski, 1988), cervical migraine (Stodolny and Chmeilewski, 1989), vertigo (Fitz-Ritson, 1991) and cervical angina (Booth and Rothman, 1976).

Moreover, the importance of the cervical spine in maintaining postural equilibrium and coordinating head and eye movements has been well established and documented (Fitz-Ritson, 1979, 1985, 1988). Furthermore, Bach-y-Rita (1980) states that 'it is almost impossible for all other systems of the nervous system to function normally when there is lack of stability, coordination and purposeful movement patterns at the cervical level of the body'. This suggests that restoration of mechanical function of the cervical spine should be considered an element in all rehabilitative programmes as a result of the overall neurological implications on the entire body. This relationship has recently been investigated experimentally by Nansel *et al.* (1993). They demonstrated

that manipulation of the cervical spine had a significant effect on the tone of lumbopelvic musculature through a proposed mechanism exciting tonic neck reflexes and intersegmental spinal pathways. Therefore, the normal mechanical function of the cervical spine becomes an important consideration in the restoration of total body movement and posture.

The implications of the importance of this role in terms of manipulative intervention have been overshadowed of late by evidence associating manipulation of the upper cervical spine with serious cerebrovascular accidents (Kleynhans, 1980; Terrett, 1987a, 1987b; Henderson and Cassidy, 1988; Martienssen and Nilsson, 1989; Terrett and Kleynhans, 1992) and transient ischaemic attacks (Foreman and Hooper, 1989). Even though it has been reported to be a safe procedure and accidents extremely rare (Chapman-Smith, 1986), there appears to be more neurological complications and incidents being documented in the literature (Gotlib and Thiel, 1985). It has been estimated that there are somewhere in the region of 100 million cervical manipulations performed worldwide per annum with complications in the order of 1/10 million manipulations (Henderson and Cassidy, 1988). In addition, more than 75 million manipulations of the cervical spine were performed annually in the United States leading Jaskoviak (1980) to conclude that the incidence of neurovascular insult was minimal. It has been determined that slight neurological complications were observed in one in 40 000 manipulations and one significant complication in 400 000 cervical manipulations (Dvorak and Orelli, 1985), whereas others have reported that severe cerebrovascular accidents will follow in one out of 500 000–1 000 000 upper cervical manipulations and minor, often temporary cerebrovascular problems will occur following one in 50 000–100 000 upper cervical manipulations (Martienssen and Nilsson, 1989). They conclude that the risk of cerebrovascular accident from cervical spine manipulation is rare. It appears that the risk to benefit ratio provides for its continued use.

Kleynhans (1980) and Kleynhans and Terrett (1985) cite, among many others, that lack of practitioner skill is a common cause of practitioner related accidents, and adverse reactions following manipulation of the upper cervical spine. They also alluded to technique selection, and excessive use of manipulative procedures as causative agents. Forceful and non-specific manipulation has also been described as a potentially hazardous pursuit (Gatterman, 1991) and more importantly, those improperly trained in related diagnostic procedures and therapeutic techniques (Jaskoviak, 1980). Therefore, developing clinical expertise and skill to reduce the possibility of such an accident and to determine when not to manipulate (Terrett, 1990), should become an absolute educational and clinical priority.

Complicating this situation is the fact that many of the clinical test procedures used routinely to detect individuals who may be susceptible to vertebral artery compromise have been shown to be unreliable and of little diagnostic value (Bolton *et al.*, 1989). Furthermore, recent research evidence suggests that vertebral artery blood flow is not impeded during the most commonly used vertebral artery functional test known as the Wallenburg test, or de Kleyn's test of sustained head and neck rotation with extension (Thiel *et al.*, 1994). This research implies that more complex neurophysiological mechanisms are involved besides the more obvious mechanical stresses. Therefore, there appears to be no foolproof or conclusive

clinical procedure to eliminate those patients at risk. Most victims are young without osseous or vascular pathology and do not present with vertebrobasilar symptoms. This presents a clinical dilemma, but with careful history taking and clinical testing, the likelihood of a vascular accident is said to be significantly reduced (Terrett, 1987b).

Biomechanical Evidence

Recent kinematic research has provided evidence that up to 80% of all cervical spine axial rotation takes place between C1 and C2 (Panjabi *et al.*, 1988; Iai *et al.*, 1993). The researchers in the latter study also detected a unique paradoxical contralateral motion at the occiput–C1 motion segment of 4 degrees of counter-rotation during cervical axial rotation. This was interpreted to function as a buffer of the atlas during head rotation or, more importantly, it may serve to decrease the overall mechanical torsion inflicted upon the vertebral artery at this level during extreme head movements. This may represent a natural mechanism both to protect the vertebral artery on the contralateral side of rotation and to reduce excess axial load on the joints below C1–C2. This may in turn moderate neurophysiological afferentation and subsequent neuromuscular reactions. Iai *et al.* (1993) also found an important coupled motion of 10 degrees of extension at occiput–C1 combined with 11 degrees of lateral bending between C1 and C2.

The C1–C2 is the region where the vertebral artery is most susceptible to injury. The artery emerges from the transverse foramen of the atlas and travels posteriorly and medially around the lateral mass of the atlas and passes anteriorly to enter the foramen magnum (Terrett, 1987b). The vertebral arteries are virtually unprotected from C1 to C2 with a considerable amount of laxity which allows the arteries to move freely with movement of the head and neck. Furthermore, there are a number of important vascular structures (internal carotid artery) and soft tissues in this region which are also at risk (Kleynhans, 1980). In addition, the vertebral artery can be mechanically deranged and potentially injured by stretching, shearing or crushing at no less than eight potential sites along its path in the cervical spine (Terrett and Kleynhans, 1992). It has been reported that kinking of the contralateral vertebral artery takes place between as little as **30 degrees** of neck rotation and up to 45 degrees causing a simultaneous stretching and occlusive action (Grice, 1988). After the normal 45 degrees, kinking and mechanical stretch occurred in both arteries and in the ipsilateral vessel at the C67 level as it enters the transverse foramen of C6 (Gatterman, 1991).

Suggested Mechanisms of Injury

Terrett (1987b) has documented that the most common mechanism of injury is brainstem ischaemia due to trauma to the arterial wall producing vasospasm or damage to the arterial wall, whereas the most common cause of the symptoms of vertebrobasilar insufficiency has been identified as atherosclerotic disease of the arteries supplying the brainstem. Various structural factors and variations in the calibre of the vertebral arteries seem to make these arteries more susceptible to mechanical compression and trauma (Kleynhans, 1980). Moreover, recent pathological studies have confirmed the presence of a true anatomic lesion, not only a functional one (Hains *et al.*, 1993). These authors discussed the influence of head and neck movements, specifically the upper cervical region, on reducing circulation through one vertebral artery when **rotation is coupled with hyperextension and traction**. Blood flow does fluctuate on a daily basis in the vertebral arteries while performing routine body movements, but due to contralateral blood flow and collateral circulation, complications in normal individuals are unlikely. Danek (1989) investigated the blood circulation in the vertebrobasilar vessel system at an extreme position of hyperextension combined with rotation of the head in a group of 25 young individuals (aged 16–25 years). He found disorders in a major-

ity of those examined and recommended that as a general rule, *rehabilitative procedures which use extreme positions be avoided*. These results should not be taken casually. Even though an age group predilection has not been established, Martienssen and Nilsson (1989) have concluded that cerebrovascular accidents would be expected in an age group which is slightly younger than that of the average manipulative patient. Cerebrovascular accidents are not the sole domain of the old. As the spine ages it naturally becomes stiffer which limits extreme ranges of motion, thus resulting in less mechanical stress on the vertebral artery. The younger spine is simply capable of greater ranges of motion and increased flexibility. However, this does not mean to say that care and caution to protect sensitive vascular structures and joint integrity should be irresponsibly overlooked for the sake of achieving joint cavitation only. Practitioner and student consciousness of this very basic reality should not be withheld in light of both the patient's and clinician's welfare and professional integrity, respectively.

The consensus seems to implicate excessive rotation in the upper cervical spine as the movement most likely to interfere with vertebral artery flow (Thiel, 1991; Thiel *et al.*, 1994) and responsible for increased afferent bombardment. *Lateral flexion*, on the other hand, appears to have little effect upon vertebral artery blood flow and should be seriously considered as part of the clinical rationale for all manipulative procedures introduced to the upper and lower cervical spine (Terrett and Kleynhans, 1992). Grice (1988) recommends that during rotation manipulation of C1–C2, the practitioner should rotate the spine *no more than 30 degrees and include a small lateral flexion component of up to 5 degrees*. This would ensure both optimal biomechanical correction and less trauma for vital soft tissue structures during full cervical rotation. The use of passive mobilization techniques as a premanipulative procedure or tolerance test has also been promoted in questionable cases (Gitelman and Fligg, 1992). It is clear that the cervical spine is capable of considerable axial rotation with varying amounts of coupled movements. Subsequently, it becomes imperative to *control* the amount of rotation in the upper cervical spine during a manipulation with thrust (Sandoz, 1976), in contrast to *elimination* of rotation as suggested by Terrett (1987b) and Martienssen and Nilsson (1989). Both authors, in suggesting this, present no alternative methods or techniques for upper cervical manipulation, apart from suggesting a modification of the techniques presently used with little or no rotation. Terrett and Kleynhans (1992) do suggest that upper cervical techniques should be restricted to toggle–recoil, Gonstead or supine lateral flexion procedures. The activator adjusting instrument has also been proposed as a safe alternative method for treating spinal dysfunction (Byfield, 1991). The instrument delivers a consistent and predetermined force with extreme speed without the potential dangers of introducing extreme ranges of motion. The duration of the activator thrust was calibrated to be between five and ten times the stretch reflex, reducing local muscle tension and patient apprehension (Duell, 1984). The use of this type of instrumentation is an acceptable clinical method. However, it has been argued that the activator neither accommodates the slow responding property of viscoelastic tissue nor permits the doctor to appreciate important patient feedback and rarely results in cavitation, a factor strongly associated with an improved range of motion (Plaugher, 1993).

Thrust Force – Characteristics

The forces generated on the cervical spine during spinal manipulative therapy are generally less and executed faster than those on the thoracic spine and sacroiliac joint (Herzog *et al.*, 1991). There is also some evidence that cervical manipulations are performed three times as fast as thoracic manipulation (Kawchuk *et al.*, 1992; Conway *et al.*, 1993) and approximately four times faster than manipulation of the sacroiliac joint (Hessell *et al.*, 1990).

The manipulative procedures selected for these investigations seemed to be tailored more to the force measurement system than to quantifying more commonly practised side posture and supine cervical procedures involving a preload. It only stands to reason that direct force measurements are infinitely more difficult to quantify the more complex the manipulative procedure, particularly the effects of preloading the joint, the patient's reaction and force dissipation into surrounding soft tissues. The mere size of the cervical spine relative to the other spinal regions, its apparent global kinematic behaviour, facet angulation, intricate musculature and the inaccuracy of anatomical landmark location may exacerbate this experimental uncertainty.

The loads transmitted through the cervical spine seem to be a cumulative effect of the forces applied by the manipulator's hands, the inertia caused by the head accelerating during the thrust and forces generated by the internal muscular forces (Triano and Schultz, 1990). A common habit that develops is the art of 'whipping' the head through the entire physiological range in order to achieve an easy cavitation. This is often seen during manipulation of the occiput–atlas articulation. The inertial and muscular reaction forces generated by this style would be considerable, subjecting the cervical spine to unnecessary stress loads. A technically slow and prematurely delivered thrust speed would only complicate this situation.

Triano (1992) calculated that the speed of a C2 lateral break adjustment was in the 0.135 sec range. This is very close to normal reaction times, suggesting that the biological effects of the adjustment may take place before any protective muscular splinting. However, large cervical muscular activity has been measured during a C2 lateral break indicating that the mechanical effects of the applied manipulation may be influenced by the patient's muscular reaction (Triano and Schultz, 1990). Reactions as high as 51% of maximum voluntary contraction have been recorded in the semispinalis capitus (Triano, 1992). Large muscular reactions such as this may be responsible for increasing the risk of complications and post-treatment reactions. Patient compliance and apprehension, in response to the intensity of the manipulation, may significantly influence this situation. Methods to reduce these seemingly important modulating factors may be advantageous. It appears that the investigators in this study inadvertently lifted the patient's head prior to the adjustive thrust. This manoeuvre could increase muscular activity in the surrounding cervical musculature due to patient 'assistance', influence the 'feel' for the critical moment of joint tension and increase the amount of thrust force necessary. Keeping the patient's head on a raised headpiece may contribute to less premanipulative muscular activity due to a non-weight bearing position supporting the head and therefore decrease the forces necessary, and patient apprehension, but at the same time improve control, speed, compliance and finesse.

Cerebrovascular Accidents, Provocation Tests and Manipulation

Since an association has been established between manipulation of the cervical spine and vertebrobasilar insufficiency, it is highly recommended that the ways and means of identifying those at risk of cerebral ischaemia be taught in conjunction with the various psychomotor and manipulative skills. Kirk (1992) has proposed that chiropractic students should be taught the fundamentals regarding early detection of patients at high risk for stroke and that this should be developed and integrated into the course curriculum. He outlines specific course objectives aimed at developing a framework for preventive management which covers a wide range of clinical skills including history taking to neurovascular and physical examinations. Integrating this knowledge base with the therapeutic aspects of chiropractic care of those at potential risk should provide the student with a sense of confidence and respect for the relative and absolute contraindications of cervical manipulation. Even though the sensitivity

and the specificity of the provocation tests commonly used to detect those at risk have yet to be scientifically verified (Ivancic *et al.*, 1993), it is recommended that students learn the necessary skills to rotate and extend the head slowly and deliberately during the provocation procedure. The use of the headpiece to support the head and neck is suggested, which allows the operator to respond quickly to any significant signs or symptoms. Pain and/or restricted range of motion, besides the more notable neurovascular symptoms, should be regarded as important and included in the management criteria. Kirk (1992) has also stressed that in no uncertain terms should an extension rotation test be performed when blood pressure asymmetry, bruits or clinical suspicion of carotid stenosis is suspected, for fear of triggering an ischaemic cerebral event.

This type of strategy builds a much-needed integrated approach to manipulative skills learning which consolidates the diagnostic and therapeutic intent in a clinical perspective.

Clinical Considerations

Most manipulative techniques directed towards the *occiput–atlas* articulation employ a great deal of rotation (States, 1968; Szaraz, 1984), which is now regarded as highly unacceptable. Kinematically, rotation is a minor movement at this joint complex, in contrast to the dominant sagittal plane movement of flexion/extension (Panjabi *et al.*, 1988). Therefore, restoration of occiput–atlas articular function could be accomplished by manipulative procedures that incorporate *no forced rotation*. This would protect vital structures, but at the same time maintain the principles of the biomechanical model and clinical rationale for the manipulative intervention in this region (Fligg, 1985a).

Even though the role of the cervical spine in the aetiology of headaches remains controversial, chiropractic manipulation has been shown to be an effective form of treatment for migraine sufferers

(Wight, 1978) and adult benign headaches (Vernon, 1982). A trial of manipulation provides an opportunity to confirm a retrospective diagnosis (Vernon, 1989). High-velocity, low-amplitude rotational manipulation was shown to be more effective in increasing local paraspinal pain threshold levels in a small group of patients with mechanical neck pain compared to a sham-like mobilization (Vernon *et al.*, 1990). Guerriero *et al.* (1991) demonstrated the effectiveness of manipulation and physical therapy in restoring spinal motion in patients with chronic neck pain. In addition, the superior clinical effectiveness of manipulative versus mobilization techniques in decreasing pain and improving mobility of the cervial spine has been demonstrated in a group presenting with neck pain (Cassidy *et al.*, 1992). Mierau *et al.* (1988) had previously established that manipulation with cavitation was a more significantly effective method of increasing the range of motion of the third metacarpophalangeal joint than mobilization of the same articulation. This is by no means conclusive; nonetheless, the evidence does suggest that manipulative procedures seem to be more effective in restoring joint function and reducing pain than mobilization techniques. Indications for therapeutic use are multidimensional and not the intent of this text.

Manipulative Skill and Performance

Therefore, the question arises: **how can we reduce rotation and other extreme ranges of motion during cervical manipulation, thereby protecting vascular and other vulnerable structures, but still realize functional and/or neurophysiological change?** This can be addressed by learning and incorporating specific manipulative skills outlined below. Assimilating these skills and using reliable history and other examination procedures to screen patients who are at cerebrovascular risk is clinically mandatory.

The student of manipulative sciences must become totally informed and unreservedly strict with this fact of life. The literature points mainly to the dangers of

upper cervical spine rotational manipulation; however, since the vascular and other sensitive structures are at risk of injury and damage at many sites throughout the entire cervical spine, aggressive and repeated manipulation must be strongly discouraged and prohibited. Therefore, extreme ranges of motion, especially rotation, have to be controlled throughout all aspects of manipulation of the cervical spine, regardless of the diagnostic indications, fixation pattern or symptom picture. Repeated attempts to 'crack' the joint are professionally irresponsible. The primary clinical goal is the protection of the patient's overall welfare by introducing the most appropriate clinical procedures available.

Common Cervical Manipulative Considerations

The following basic manipulative skills will be emphasized during the presentation of the various manipulative procedures commonly used in the cervical spine:

(1) *An absolute maximum of 30–40 degrees* of head and neck rotation is permitted. Keeping within this safe margin reduces any excess transverse shear and stretch of the vertebral artery at the C1–C2 articulation and lower segments.

(2) Using multiple planes of motion to develop joint tension. The introduction of mainly *lateral flexion* coupled with varying degrees of flexion components while completely avoiding extension and excess rotation, can incorporate normal mechanical coupling, thereby developing 'tissue tension' without exceeding joint capabilities in any one plane. Flexion produces more of a longitudinal stretch of the vertebral artery which may be tolerated to a greater degree than a transverse shearing during extreme rotation. Flexion may also increase the intervertebral foramenal space necessary in certain clinical presentations.

(3) Using the headpiece of the adjusting table to support the weight of the head instead of lifting the entire weight with the arms and hands. The headpiece is of little use when fully extended and dropped down. This position increases the leverage sustained by the cervical joints during a rotational movement of the head (Lewit, 1979). Joint specificity and dynamic thrust isolation becomes difficult whilst holding a 5–6 kg weight.

(4) The headpiece should be positioned at 0–10 degrees for the upper cervical spine, 10–20 degrees for the midcervical spine and 30–40 degrees for the lower cervical spine from the horizontal to develop some tension in the posterior elements during flexion, help to isolate a specific segmental level (Szaraz, 1984) and, most importantly, support the weight of the patient's head.

(5) The clinician should be positioned on the side of the dysfunctional facet. This places the clinician closer to the spine, accommodates facet angulation and shortens the levers for more effective joint tension, preload and impulse thrust. Positioning of the clinician at the head of the table tends to lengthen the lever action on the head and neck, jeopardizing speed, depth and control.

(6) Use an impulse based, short, sharp and extremely brief thrust without scissoring the hands or arms.

These modifications may allow the clinician to use more traditional manipulative skills which include rotation, but within the limits of kinematic restraint, to minimize the risk of vascular and/or neurological trauma.

The following presentation will concentrate upon basic manipulative skills for the cervical spine. This is by no means an exhaustive review of all the procedures used within the chiropractic profession. The aim is to focus on those skills that form the infrastructure and pattern of skills for many of the manipulative procedures that are used to treat cervical mechanical dysfunction. The more advanced manipulative procedures should be introduced only when the basics are fully mastered. It would be pointless to expect students to assimilate all the major diversified skills if they are unable to locate an articular process, take up tissue slack or judge the amount of rotation of the patient's head.

These skills require a more delicate approach as compared to the more robust thoracic and lumbopelvic regions. It is recommended that these skills be introduced later in a student's overall skill and psychomotor development and particularly when he or she has demonstrated proficiency in performing some of the basic movements outlined for the cervical spine in Chapter 6 (thrust skills and other movements). The art of judging the degree of cervical rotation and articular tension is an acquired skill of significant clinical importance. It is preferable that these skills be developed at a suitable pace commensurate with present psychomotor development. It seems reasonable to assume that a hasty approach will cause only frustration and poor skill acquisition.

The skills section for this chapter will focus primarily in the midcervical region (C45 motion segment). Naturally, the student will be inspired to develop these skills to include both sides of the body and eventually mature to include all regions of the cervical spine. This would be considered a relatively safe area to introduce these skills. The occiput–atlas–axis region will be addressed but in a limited fashion at the end of the chapter. The skills will be presented in accordance with the kinematic and biomechanical characteristics of the cervical spine. The chapter will present skills up to the appreciation of specific joint isolation and elastic barrier tension or joint tension with a mock thrust (gentle repeated testing of the elastic resistance of the joint), but *not including* the delivery of a high-velocity, low-amplitude dynamic thrust. It is simply too early to venture beyond this point. The mere fact that students will be repeatedly applying considerable stretch across sensitive joint structures to acknowledge, recognize and define the feeling of joint tension is potentially hazardous enough. Care must be taken at all times to recognize any signs or symptoms which may cause the student any potential harm. The dynamic thrust *remains only one aspect of the overall procedure*. It should be introduced when control and joint tension are fully appreciated and within the context of a controlled clinic environment.

One of the *key elements* of performing manipulation of the cervical spine is the ability to use both hands simultaneously producing essentially the same movement patterns. This movement pattern is covered in Chapter 6 and should be practised regularly in order to learn to control the amount of rotation of the hands. This action will also function to determine the overall leverage on the head and neck. These skills will be presented with the patient in the supine position for ease of instruction. There are various other postures which are equally effective from a clinical standpoint. Even though the basic skills for the spine itself are essentially the same, manipulations in other postures such as sitting require an additional set of patient control skills (Grice, 1977; Szaraz, 1983).

Mid-Lower Cervical Spine Manipulative Skills

Articular process (AP) – supine

Spinous–lamina (SL) – supine

Transverse process (TP) – supine

Articular Process (AP) – Supine

This particular manipulative procedure is often referred to as the rotary cervical (States, 1968; Fligg, 1984; Szaraz, 1984) or specifically used to correct mid–lower cervical posterior rotation fixations (Schafer and Faye, 1989). It is considered to be the most frequently used manipulative technique (Gitelman and Fligg, 1992). For the purpose of this set of manipulative skills, the contact is made on the articular process of C4. The motion segments are stabilized above the C45; motion will therefore occur below this point.

1) The patient is lying comfortably in the supine position with the headpiece of the table flexed up 10–20 degrees from the horizontal. The patient's knees are flexed to relax the hamstrings and flatten the lumbar curve and his or her hands are interlocked and placed over the abdomen to relax the shoulders and arms. The doctor, initially, is standing crouched at the head of the table with the knees bent and the spine straight and the knees in contact with the table for support (*) (fig. 11.1). This crouched position is an important component of the overall skill as it assists in generating part of the impulse thrust and allows the doctor to be mobile to adapt to any emergency that may arise. The body weight is centred over the patient's neck.

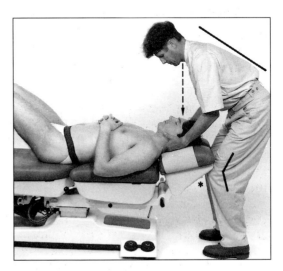

Fig 11.1

2) The doctor's hands are then simultaneously placed around the cervical spine with the hypothenar and thenar regions of the hands cupping and supporting the occipital region (*) and the fingers along the paraspinal region. The hands and arms are exact mirror images (fig. 11.2). Palpation and segmental location takes place from this position. The patient's head is *not lifted* but remains in contact and supported by the headpiece. This gives the patient a feeling of security. The doctor's hands are also in contact and supported by the headpiece to take the weight off the arms and shoulders.

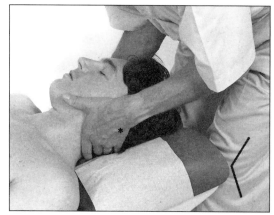

Fig 11.2

3) The doctor locates the articular process of C4 with the palpating and locating middle finger of the left hand and rotates the patient's head marginally to the right by ulnar deviating the wrists (fig. 11.3). Care is taken not to rotate the head excessively at this point and keep the patient's head on the headpiece (*).

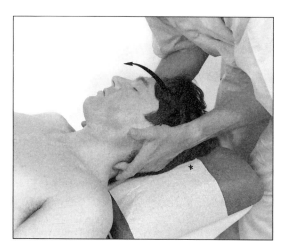

Fig 11.3

4) To maintain specificity of the C45 motion segment, tissue slack is removed by bringing the middle finger of the opposite hand behind the contact finger as far around as the spinous process of C4 and then slowly pulling the tissue around and upwards in the direction of rotation. This is done gently but with a firm movement (fig. 11.4). There should be no discomfort to the patient.

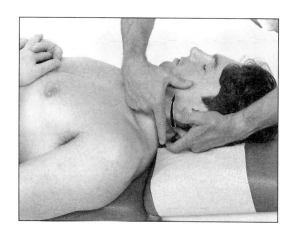

Fig 11.4

5) The contact hand comes in directly behind and follows the line of the tissue slack finger. **Do not push the hand inwards**. The medial side of the first digit *slides around* drawing more tissue slack. This action is done by ulnar deviating the contact hand at the wrist as the fingers are drawn around, until the medial side of the PIP or DIP joints are approximately resting on the articular process of C4 (fig. 11.5). The wrist is kept straight and care is taken not to push inward against the sensitive soft tissues. *The hand and fingers are slightly arched in order to give the contact some flexibility.* The thumb is gently placed on the mandibular region in front of the ear (*). This is done to support and stabilize the contact hand.

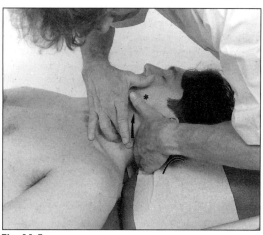

Fig 11.5

6) Once the contact is secured the indifferent hand (right) or tissue slack hand reaches around and supports the inferior aspect of the rim occiput with the palmar aspect of the middle finger. The support hand is also ulnar deviated at the wrist. The 4th and 5th digits cup and support the base of the occiput (*), the first finger wraps around the cervical musculature and the thumb is placed gently over the face just in front of the ear (fig. 11.6). The contact should be light, but firm and the patient's head should not be rotated more than a few degrees.

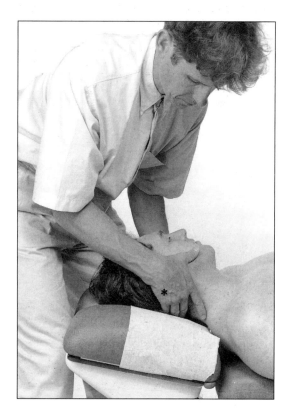

Fig 11.6

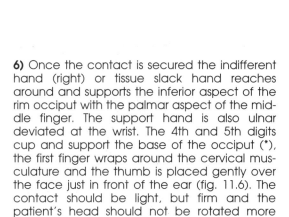

7) The doctor moves very slowly to the side of the lesion or contact side so that he is positioned 45 degrees to the table. The doctor maintains a ski-crouch position, knees bent, trunk flexed, arms relaxed and close to the body and leaning against the head of the table with the suprasternal notch over the contact hands (fig. 11.7a). At this stage the patient's head is in a neutral position with no rotation of the head. The doctor is in a tight and compact posture close to both the patient and table. There should be no movement of the patient's head up to this point and the weight of the head should be totally supported by the headpiece of the table (fig. 11.7b).

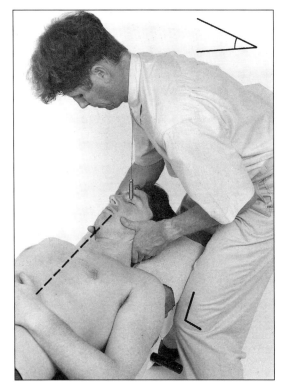

Fig 11.7a

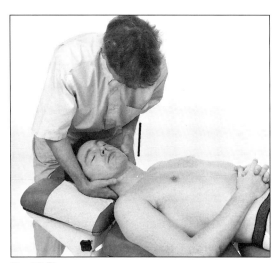

Fig 11.7b

8) Perform the next series very slowly. The hands are moved simultaneously. *The contact hand (left) slightly pronates and ulnar deviates at the wrist and the support hand (right) supinates at the wrist.* The amount of movement is exactly the same on both sides. The patient's head is *rotated 35–40 degrees maximum* (fig. 11.8a). This is the safe zone. Only the wrists are moving, not the arms or shoulders. This ensures control of the head and neck. *The head is not lifted off the headpiece.* The rotation takes place along the long axis of the spine to eliminate torsion or twist developing in the spine. The head should always be lined up with the middle of the sternum. The hands and wrists are mirror images (fig. 11.8b). Care is also taken not to push or press the contact finger in towards the spine which may cause the patient some pain and possible muscular tension, reducing the efficiency of the manipulation. **Both contact hands are light but firm.**

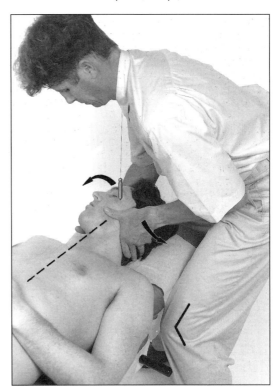

Fig 11.8a

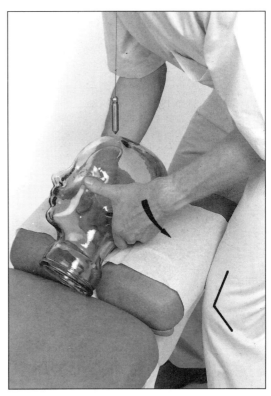

Fig 11.8b

9) The next four steps are very small movements to establish joint tension and preload the C45 segment.

i) Rotate the head and neck into the safe zone (35–40 degrees) (fig. 11.9a) as described for Figure 11.8a.

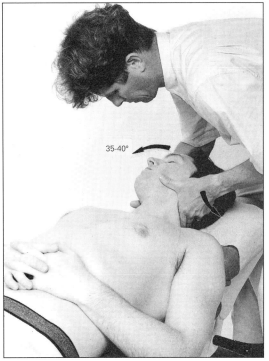

Fig 11.9a

ii) Lateral flexion is added to avoid over-rotation by bringing the support hand towards the body over the contact hand. The movement is very small and the degree of movement is directly related to the amount of tension perceived under the doctor's contact finger (fig. 11.9b). The contact hand does not move (*). Its position is stable. The doctor monitors the patient's response to these movements. Any signs of distress which can be monitored by facial expressions or increase in muscle tension should not be ignored. If this does happen it may signal that the contact or movement is excessive.

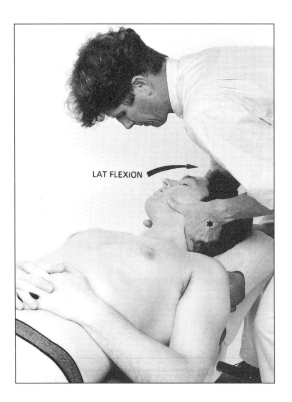

Fig 11.9b

iii) Joint tension is achieved by the *contact hand only*. The contact hand is pulled up and in towards the spine and ulnar deviated very slowly monitoring the amount of resistance against the medial border of the contact finger. The action takes place at the wrist, which actually rolls through and towards the motion segment (fig. 11.9c). Support wrist remains absolutely stationary. Both arms are tucked into the body (*). Keep in mind that these movements are very small to feel soft tissue tension develop. The point of joint tension, even though it is arbitrary, is a combined palpatory and psychomotor skill.

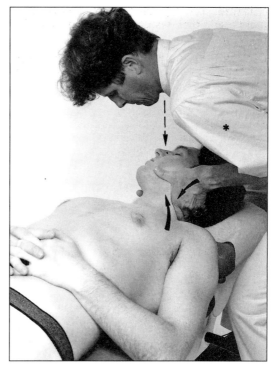

Fig 11.9c

iv) The last step is an optional degree of traction to the cervical spine which has some effect upon the muscle receptors (Gitelman and Fligg, 1992). The doctor simply pulls in a cephalad direction with both arms. The action can be supplemented by a further cephalad lean of the doctor's trunk (fig. 11.9d). The arms are tucked in close to the body at all times to shorten the levers controlling the movement (*).

Steps i–iv have been separated and should be practised in sequence until they are performed with a degree of confidence and skill. This section should not be rushed and the importance of the slow controlled movements at the wrist should be emphasized. *Care should be taken not to maintain joint tension for too long and there is no dynamic thrust at this point.*

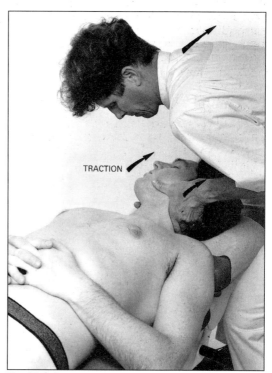

Fig 11.9d

10) There are a number of potential learning errors associated with the acquisition of these manipulative skills.

i) Failing to move to the side of the lesion or anatomical contact point may increase cervical rotation and force the doctor's arms out from the body producing much longer levers acting on the cervical spine. This causes the doctor to assume an inefficient posture which places increased mechanical loads on the lumbar spine and twists the shoulder (*) (fig. 11.10). Note the excess rotation of the head and neck.

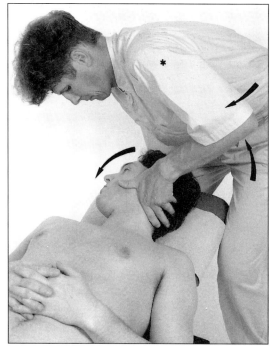

Fig 11.10

ii) The most common mistake is rotating the head and neck too far when attempting to establish joint tension prior to preloading (fig. 11.11). This is usually caused by extra movement at the elbows and shoulders and a failure to keep the arms in close to the body (*). This has to be carefully monitored by the student in order to eliminate potential mechanical stress to the sensitive structures at risk.

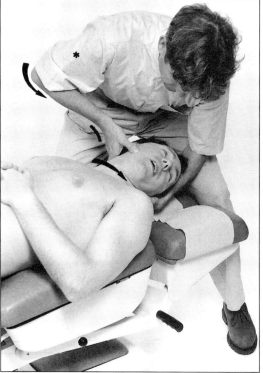

Fig 11.11

iii) Pushing the medial side of the contact finger into the sensitive spinal structures instead of **rolling** the contact hand by ulnar deviating the wrist. This is often caused by keeping the hand too rigid and stiff and not using a semi-arched posture (*) (fig. 11.12). Watch for patient's reaction!!

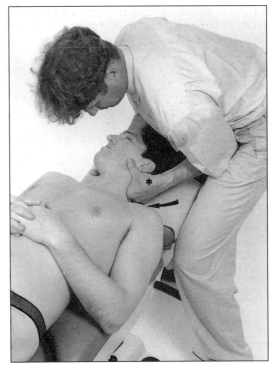

Fig 11.12

iv) Introducing excessive secondary lateral bending combined with surplus rotation will stress the soft tissues of the cervical spine. This may also pull the head away from the central axis of the body (fig. 11.13). The doctor shifts more than 45 degrees to the side of the lesion. *These exaggerated movements should be avoided at all costs.*

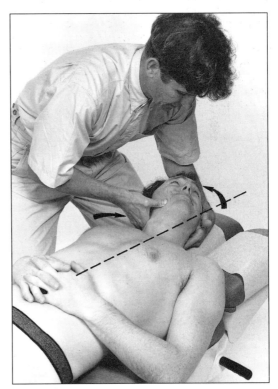

Fig 11.13

v) Don't lift the head off the headpiece and support the weight of the head in the hands (fig. 11.14a). It is very difficult for the doctor to control head and neck rotation and lateral bending, plus develop the feel of joint tension when he is holding a 12 lb weight in the hands. This will automatically produce longer levers which may influence the dynamic thrust and control of the excess movements. Failure to pivot shift to side of the lesion will complicate the situation (11.14b).

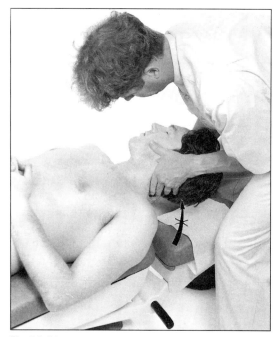

Fig 11.14a

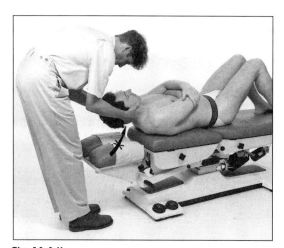

Fig 11.14b

vi) Don't bend the wrist of the contact arm. This is not stable. Keep it straight (fig. 11.15).

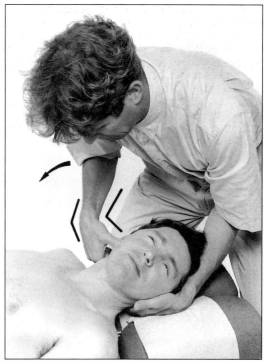

Fig 11.15

Spinous–Lamina (SL) – Supine

This particular manipulative procedure provides another opportunity to minimize rotational forces in the cervical spine, but at the same time adhere to biomechanical principles concerning myofascial dynamics and joint kinematic properties (Gitelman and Fligg, 1992). The fingertip contact on the spinous process generates the rotary force through the facets with minimal rotation. The manipulative procedure is often referred to as the cervical finger push (Fligg, 1984) or finger-push adjustment (Gitelman and Fligg, 1992) and is primarily suited to correct rotary fixations in both the upper and mid–lower cervical spine. For the sake of ease of demonstration, this particular sequence of manipulative skills will concentrate on

the C45 motion segment. Specific anatomical contact is made on the SL of C5 as the motion segments below are stabilized and movement is occurring above this point.

The patient is positioned in a supine and relaxed comfortable posture as described above. The doctor is similarly standing in a crouched posture at the head of the table cupping the patient's occiput and supporting the cervical spine. The headpiece is flexed at approximately 10–20 degrees and the patient's head remains in contact with the headpiece during the entire manoeuvre. The space between the two headpiece cushions and the give in the headpiece foam itself permits arms and hands to be neatly hidden without obstructing free head and neck movement.

1) With the middle palpating finger of the contact hand (left) on the SL junction of C5 (*) (fig. 11.16), the middle finger of the support hand (right) reaches around and pulls excess skin slack from underneath this contact towards the right side. The patient's head is in a neutral position resting comfortably on the headpiece during this procedure. **N.B. The head has been lifted to demonstrate hand/finger position only.**

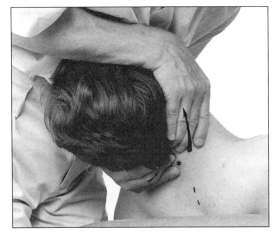

Fig 11.16

2) As the skin slack is drawn towards the right side a reinforced middle finger follows the direction of the tissue slack and firmly contacts the SL junction of C5. The contact hand (left) is in a moderately high chiropractic arch posture with the hand moderately extended at the wrist. The hand, wrist and arm of the doctor should be angled at 45 degrees to the patient's cervical spine and the thumb is gently placed on the mandible to help to secure the contact hand. The lateral aspect of the hypothenar eminence is placed over the base of the occiput and the musculature of the cervical spine (*) (fig. 11.17). Both hands should be relaxed yet making a firm and painless contact. The patient's head is still in a relatively neutral position.

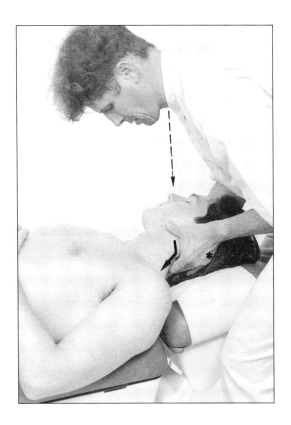

Fig 11.17

3) With a firm contact, the support hand (right) is positioned around the occiput with the palmar surface of the middle finger supported under the occipital rim. The wrist is also ulnar deviated. The 4th and 5th digits are placed over the base of the occiput (*) and the index finger along the cervical spine (*). The thumb is placed just ahead of the earlobe to help to secure the hand. The hand is slightly arched in order avoid crushing the patient's earlobe (fig. 11.18).

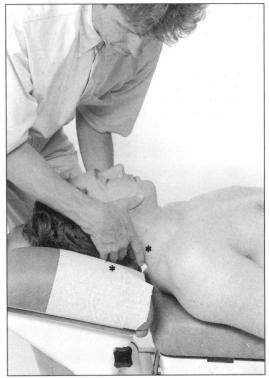

Fig 11.18

4) The doctor moves 45 degrees to the ipsilateral side of the SL contact and *simultaneously rotates the head about 30 degrees* to the contralateral side using the support hand. Care is taken not to lose contact on the SL during this rotation, and try not to dig your fingers into the soft tissue (fig. 11.19). It is important that as the head rotates away the finger pad contact perceives and resists spinous movement at C5 towards the contact. Keep both arms close to the body during all phases of this procedure (*).

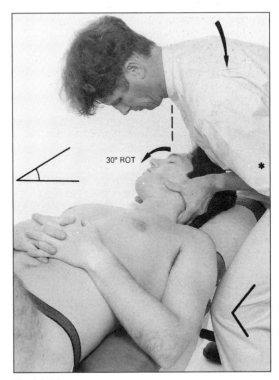

Fig 11.19

5) Joint tension without over-rotation up to pre-load is achieved by laterally flexing the head and neck towards the contact finger by simultaneously pulling the head towards the contact hand and pushing gently along the SL contact in the line of the forearm (fig. 11.20). This action can be aided by dipping the upper body down which keeps the arms close to the body, maintaining short lever action. The head and neck should not stay in this position for extended periods to avoid possible joint or muscular reflex reactions. **Please avoid the temptation to thrust or push too hard along the contact point.**

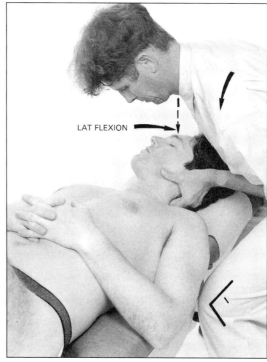

Fig 11.20

6) A traction component can be added to assist additional joint tension at the C45 motion segment. This is performed by slowly tractioning the support hand around the rim of the occiput in a cephalad direction. The fingertip contact will resist this movement.

7) There are at least two major errors associated with the learning of this particular sequence of skills.

i) Don't permit the arms to drift out from the body (fig. 11.21). This reduces the mechanical advantage of the contact points, increases the movement about the cervical spine and compromises the efficiency of the dynamic thrust.

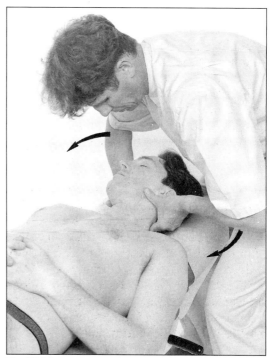

Fig 11.21

ii) A straight contact hand instead of a chiropractic arch posture will not stabilize the contact point and eliminate the flexibility and firmness of the procedure (fig. 11.22). The position of the thumb does not stabilize the contact hand (*). Over-rotating the head and standing at the head of the table are additional errors to be aware of.

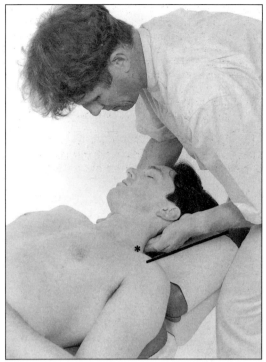

Fig 11.22

Transverse Process (TP) – Supine

This particular anatomical landmark is often used for a group of manipulations referred to as the cervical break (States, 1968), lateral flexion adjustment (Grice, 1980), supine lateral break (Szaraz, 1984), lateral cervical (Fligg, 1984), lateral cervical fixations (Schafer and Faye, 1989), and adjustive procedure for cervical lateral flexion joint dysfunction (Bergmann and Zachman, 1989).

This manipulative procedure is considered biomechanically sound, taking into consideration the arc of motion through the joints of Von Luschka, an integral component of the three joint complex and a common site of degenerative changes (Grice, 1980). More importantly it accommodates lateral flexion of the cervical spine which has been reported to have limited influence on vertebral artery flow (Terrett and Kleynhans, 1992). There is little to no rotation associated with this particular set of skills which has obvious clinical advantages, yet still functions to correct cervical segment mechanics and restore the appropriate motion.

The target for this next set of skills is the C45 motion segment. Contact takes place on C4 and movement is assumed to take place below the primary contact point. This manipulative procedure is a combination of the skills described above for both the articular process landmark or cervical rotary and the SL landmark or finger push adjustment. There are elements of each particular manipulation which will be duplicated here to develop an additional versatile manipulation that can be used in various clinical situations best suited for both the doctor and the patient. Each manipulation is not a completely separate entity, but provides for skill overlap.

The patient is comfortable in a supine position as described above with the headpiece flexed upward at 10–20 degrees. The doctor is standing at the head of the table in a crouched palpating posture with the patient's head cupped and stabilized by the hypothenar eminences of both hands with the remainder of the digits free to locate the necessary anatomical landmarks as described in Figure 11.2. The crouched posture places the doctor's weight over the cervical spine which centres and focuses the dynamic thrust and helps to ensure that the levers acting on the neck remain short. The student performs steps 1 to 7 as outlined above for the AP skills up to the point where the doctor has moved 45 degrees to the side of patient with the patient's head in a neutral position before any movement takes place. *The only difference at this point is the actual contact on the spine.*

The finger contact is by convention supposed to contact the TP of C4. However, the TPs are small, very sensitive and painful at clinical presentation. My recommendation is to contact the posterior aspect of the transverse process and the anterior aspect of the articular process with the medial aspect of the middle phalanx of the first digit. This affords a reasonably large target plus it offers a certain amount of soft tissue cushioning effect through the paraspinal musculature. This will avoid prodding the TPs and guarantees a greater degree of patient compliance. The contact is very light yet firm and if the patient is at any time showing signs of distress or pain, please don't ignore this vital, clinical feedback.

1) Complete steps 1–7 above for the AP skills but change the anatomical contact point slightly (*). Both the support and contact hands are virtually mirror images with the contact hand and wrist positioned at 45 degrees to the cervical spine and straight. The head and neck are in a neutral position at this starting point (fig. 11.23).

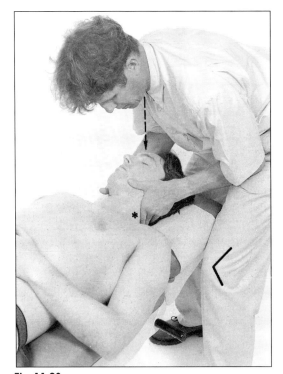

Fig 11.23

Cervical spine manipulative skills

2) The support arm and hand slowly laterally flex the head and neck in a controlled fashion using the anatomical contact as a pivot point. **There is no rotation**. The amount of lateral flexion is determined when the doctor starts to feel some resistance (tissue tension sense) on the medial aspect of the proximal or middle phalanx of the index finger and hand (fig. 11.24). The head stays on the headpiece and the contact arm, wrist and hand are completely stationary in contact with the side of the body. The doctor crouches low over the patient.

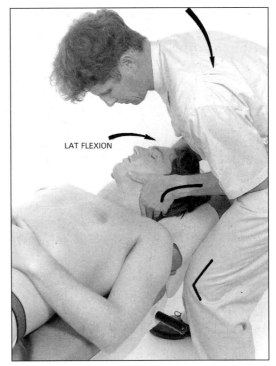

Fig 11.24

3) The doctor moves the contact arm towards the lateral aspect of the cervical spine in order to gain additional tension. This is done by flexing the shoulder flexors very slowly. The arm is kept in close contact with the body (fig. 11.25). The movement towards the spine is cushioned by the wrist (ulnar deviation joint play) making contact with the spine less rigid and uncomfortable for the patient. A slight traction component may be added at this point if joint tension or muscular stretch is required. This is done primarily by the support hand through the occiput. **There is no dynamic thrust**. Care is taken not to push too hard.

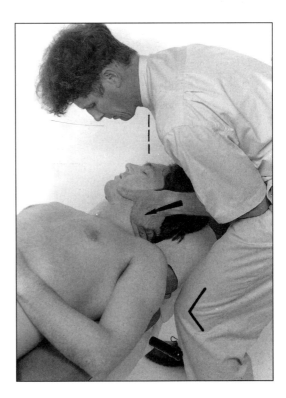

Fig 11.25

4) There may be clinical situations which arise whereby joint tension is not accomplished by lateral flexion only. If this is the case, a small degree of rotation (10–20 degrees) can be added prior to step 2 to the contralateral side (fig. 11.26). This takes advantage of the coupling action of the cervical motion segments to gain joint isolation and specificity.

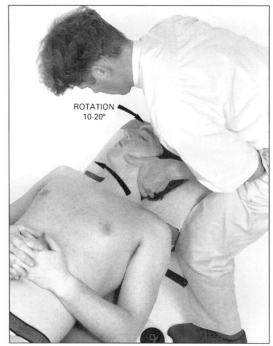

Fig 11.26

5) There are two faults encountered during the learning of this manipulative skill.

i) The most common is using the contact hand like a sharp blade, pushing into the side of the sensitive TPs too quickly without stabilizing the hand position with the thumb or other digits (fig.11.27).

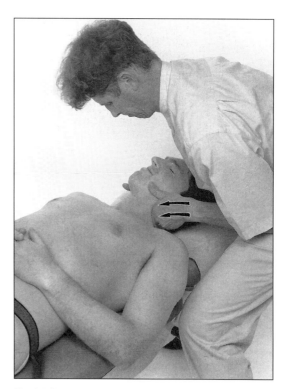

Fig 11.27

ii) Laterally flexing and extending the head and neck too far (fig. 11.28). Joint tension is possible without extreme ranges of motion being introduced.

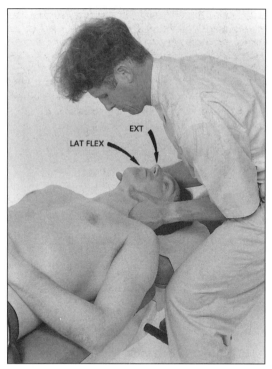

Fig 11.28

Additional Skills

1a) The thumb pad represents a very useful alternative to the metacarpal–phalangeal joint during rotation action in the cervical spine (*). The posterior medial aspect of the palmar surface of the thumb is generally used to contact the SL junction with the fingers placed over the mandible to stabilize the contact (fig. 11.29).

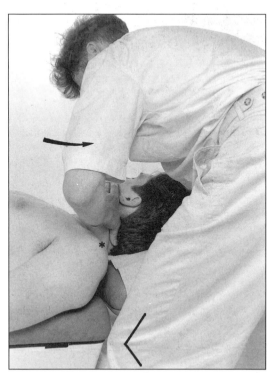

Fig 11.29

1b) Don't let the contact arm drift away from the body, which will automatically increase the lever arm and subsequent rotation applied to the cervical spine in general (fig. 11.30).

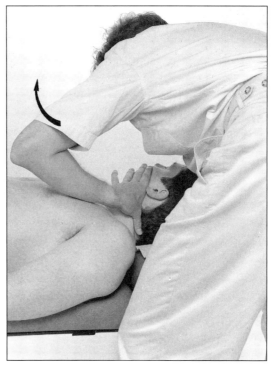

Fig 11.30

2a) The sitting position can be an effective clinical alternative, particularly if the patient is unable to lie supine. However, the effects of gravity acting on the head will cause some degree of muscle activity and possible reflex resistance by the patient. This may compromise control of the manipulative skills. The key is to learn to regulate actively the amount of rotation, lateral bending and flexion plus manage the weight of the patient's head, all at the same time. This can be achieved by using the middle finger as the articular contact, which permits the thumb and index finger to collectively support the weight of the head, and the 4th and 5th digits brace the lower cervical spine (*). By standing slightly crouched at 45 degrees to the patient the doctor is able to guide the amount of head and neck movement visually (fig. 11.31). The arms are tucked in to shorten the leverage on the head and neck.

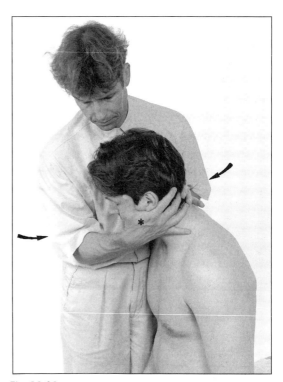

Fig 11.31

2b) Don't let the head drop forward too far, stressing the soft tissues and articular elements. This is often as a direct result of standing to the side or slightly behind the patient instead of just in front. This tends to over-rotate and flex the cervical spine (fig. 11.32).

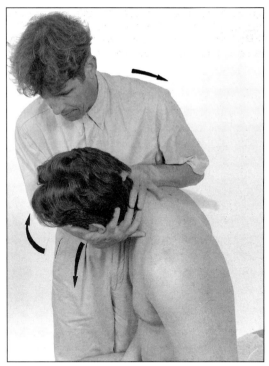

Fig 11.32

This section has presented a few selected and common manipulative procedures which form the basis of many of the diversified cervical spine techniques. The presentation has concentrated on the midcervical spine for the obvious reasons of safety and student appreciation. Mastering these skills is advisable before introducing more advanced and selective skills for the upper and lower cervical spine motion segments. However, it should be noted that the previous skills can be adapted to the upper (occiput–atlas–axis complex) and lower (C5–C7) cervical spine with some very simple modifications of these foundation skills. These modifications may form the basis for a second volume.

Upper Cervical Spine Manipulative Skills: An Introduction

It would be unfair to the art of manipulative sciences to ignore completely some of the basic skills associated with the so-called 'upper cervical techniques'. These techniques are taught in many colleges throughout the world; in some they are the mainstay of technique instruction, in others the only method taught, or in most, they are integrated into an overall diversified biomechanical model. The historical and traditional perspective these techniques have imposed on the profession is well known and should not be actively discouraged in light of some of their rigorous, rigid and often dogmatic presentations. Without becoming buried in a endless discussion of the validity of the diagnostic, therapeutic, and philosophical rationale, it would be appropriate to include a small and concluding section addressing some of the basic skills related to the upper cervical spine, particularly those related to the recoil thrust technique. Nonetheless, these skills have been well adapted to the orthopaedic–biomechanical model in chiropractic sciences (Fligg, 1985b), based upon reasonably sound biomechanical evidence supporting both the diagnostic analysis and therapeutic intervention (Fligg, 1985a, 1988).

The upper cervical region constitutes one of the greatest challenges to the practitioner of manipulative therapy.

The clinician's decision making processes are stretched to the limit, knowing full well that more side effects and reactions are due to manipulation of the upper cervical spine than any other spinal location. Nonetheless, toggle–recoil, upper cervical techniques incorporate *absolutely no forced rotation or other extreme range of motion*. This by theory should automatically present added clinical value as an additional method minimizing possible post-treatment reactions. The head and neck are neutral throughout the entire procedure, the patient is in a relaxed position and there is no prestress or preload force applied to the contact articulation. The technique provides a very useful method for those patients in whom the introduction of a dynamic thrust has been relatively contraindicated.

The toggle–recoil is classified as a neutral posture, short lever thrust (Grice and Vernon, 1992), given in a specific direction with a designated depth and rapid speed (refer to Chapter 6). The thrust is characterized by a fast release, rapid and sudden contraction of both triceps and pectoralis muscles simultaneously, creating leverage with both arms in order to apply the manipulative force directed to a specific point through the hands (Cleveland, 1992). The force of the adjustment will be delivered equally with both arms as a result of this arrangement. The 'recoil' component is generated mainly by the stretch response in the biceps before full extension of the elbows takes place. The contact hands are also actively lifted away from the patient's spine as part of the recoil procedure. This is usually where individual style is developed. The elbow joints are subsequently protected from repetitive impact trauma and the patient is spared full thrust forces. The trunk and shoulders are stable in order to maximize the rapid delivery of the dynamic recoil impulse thrust. A joint crack or 'pop' associated with cavitation is not characteristic of this technique procedure.

The toggle–recoil technique for the upper cervical spine commonly uses a free-fall headpiece and prop mechanism with a set spring reset/release mechanism

to take up part of the force. This technique requires a specially designed table, similar to the model illustrated throughout the text. Such a design minimizes potential trauma to the patient and allows for some counter-resistance of the fixed vertebrae. The movable headpiece has a fixed and constant depth of approximately half an inch with a variable resistance control depending on the size of the patient and the force required. This maintains a certain amount of control throughout the procedure combined with a standard and repeatable application in most instances. Upper cervical recoil manipulative procedures are delivered primarily to the atlas and to a lesser degree the axis. From a mechanical perspective, it would seem difficult to isolate a single articulation during such a generalized thrust combined with a rather broad-based contact. Typically, the hand contact is either the reinforced hypothenar/pisiform or double thumb combination. The thumb contact may provide a more realistic and accurate point of hand contact, considering the size of the transverse process or lateral mass of the atlas and the anatomical proximity of the atlas and axis.

The recoil thrust is characteristically performed with the patient in the side posture for correction of upper cervical dysfunction. The thrust skills can be applied to other areas of the spine and the extremities in various postures using prop/drop mechanisms to facilitate the therapeutic thrust.

The following section describes some of the basic skills associated with preparation of the upper cervical spine for application of a toggle–recoil thrust. This is by no means exhaustive, considering all the diagnostic and therapeutic indications for this particular manipulative intervention. The skills are once again basic in nature in order to provide an introduction to this traditional chiropractic manipulative approach. Special attention to the finesse, speed and control that is required for this recoil technique will be acknowledged. Only one contact, the posterior aspect of the transverse process of atlas, will be included (if you can find it). This section will describe only patient preparation skills. Establishing a firm and accurate contact with the spine will improve the successful delivery of the toggle thrust and the outcome of the manipulative procedure. There will be no delivery of a dynamic toggle–recoil thrust. The patient is lying in the right side posture recumbent position as described Chapter 7 with both knees flexed.

1) The patient is lying in the right side posture with the head supported by the headpiece which is elevated to accommodate the width of the patient's shoulder. The head is placed in a neutral positon and is slightly flexed to open the suboccipital region. The doctor stands in front of the patient at a 45 degree angle to the head in a crouched ski posture. The thumb of the left hand, after the TP of C1 has been located with either finger, draws the tissue slack away from the doctor being careful not to drag too much hair (fig. 11.33).

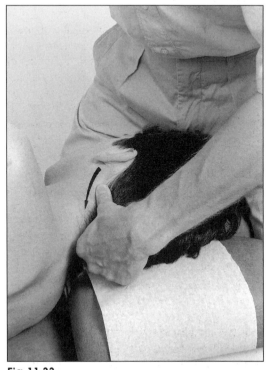

Fig 11.33

2) The hypothenar/pisiform aspect of the right hand (the contact hand) follows the locating/ tissue slack thumb drawing more tissue if necessary in the same direction (fig. 11.34). The contact is light with no excess pressure over this naturally sensitive and tender area. The contact hand forms a firm but relaxed chiropractic arch over the anatomical contact. The other fingers support the placement by lightly gripping the cervical musculature.

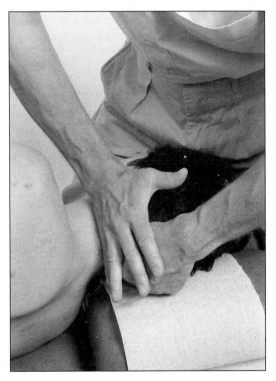

Fig 11.34

3) The support hand reinforces the contact hand position (fig. 11.35). Both hands are in a high relaxed arch posture to maintain a high degree of hand skill and anatomical specificity. Both arms are flexed equally. There should be no pressure over the contact point and the arms should be totally relaxed.

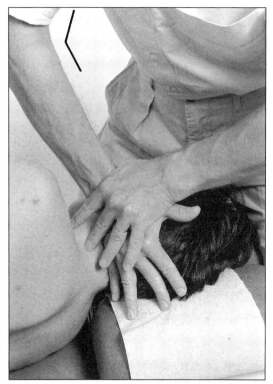

Fig 11.35

4) The doctor completes the series of skills by positioning the suprasternal notch directly over the contact hand. The doctor is in a relaxed ski crouch stance with the arms equally flexed at the elbows and the shoulders are level to maintain symmetry required for the dynamic thrust (fig. 11.36). There should be no noticeable pressure over the contact point and no dynamic impulse should be rendered.

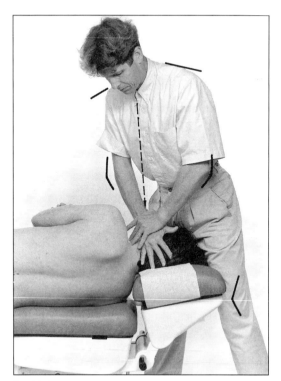

Fig 11.36

This small section has presented a few of the basic skills associated with upper cervical recoil techniques. These need to be elaborated and developed in conjunction with the diagnostic and therapeutic rationale associated with this particular technique. Variations of torque and lines of drive in specific directions will slightly modify the information presented above.

There are several errors that may occur during the learning of these skills. A hard and forceful contact point, excessive flexion at the elbows, asymmetry of the shoulders, and misalignment of the episternal notch are typically encountered and should be rectified.

Occipital Skills

It was not the intent of this chapter to present manipulative skills dealing with the occiput as an anatomical contact. However, it may be appropriate to convey a few guidelines which could be seen as a basis for future application. Traditionally, excess leverage has been applied to the occiput at extreme ranges of rotation by way of the zygoma or mastoid. Subsequently, under the present state of knowledge regarding rotation and its potential dangers, it would be wise to reconsider this approach. Besides, there is very little rotation between the occiput–atlas articulation (Panjabi *et al.*, 1988), leaving one to believe that a dynamic thrust could cavitate the C1–C2 motor unit or other distant articulations. The clinical goal is to restore function, not just pop a joint. The two are certainly not directly or clinically proportional.

Grice (1980), Fligg (1985b) and Gitelman and Fligg (1992) have described both mobilization and manipulative procedures which influence the occiput–atlas articulation. These procedures are based upon a sound kinematic and applied anatomical rationale. They incorporate the concept of coupled motion and the significance of the large postural extensors acting on the occiput. There is a dominant traction component which affects these myofascial structures and therefore there is no need for forced rotation during the thrust, which may cause unwanted torsional stress. This is a very important aspect when learning these psychomotor skills. The levers are meant to be short, which adds to the efficiency of the manipulative procedure.

There are two important anatomical landmarks, the mastoid and the occipital rim. The following description will provide the basic manipulative skills associated with these landmarks, incorporating the other psychomotor skills already introduced earlier in the chapter.

Mastoid Process (MP)

1) The doctor is in a crouched posture perpendicular to the table at the level of the MP. The patient's head is lifted and rotated away from the doctor and supported by the flexor surface of the right forearm (support arm). The fingers of the support hand cup the chin and introduce flexion of the occiput (fig. 11.37). Rotation is comfortable, relaxed and not forced. The headpiece is positioned 0–10 degrees from the horizontal. *If there are any signs of distress, discontinue the procedure.*

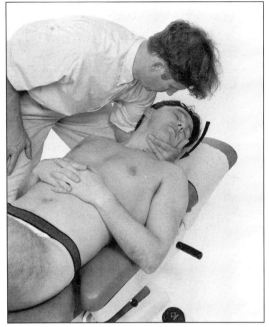

Fig 11.37

2) The hypothenar/pisiform arched contact hand (right) is secured along the inferior aspect of the mastoid process on the up side (*) (fig. 11.38). Both arms are kept very close to the body in order to control the action at this point. The patient should not feel any excess tension or pressure on the MP. The doctor is crouched very low and leaning up against the table.

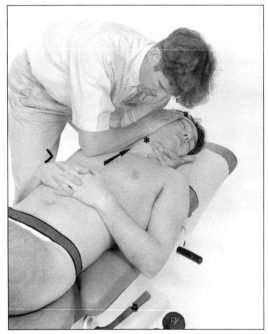

Fig 11.38

3) Traction is applied by moving both contact points cephalad simultaneously in order to attain joint tension. This action can be assisted by moving the trunk at the same time through the legs (fig. 11.39). At no time is there to be any forced rotation. The force is axial in nature.

4) It is from this basic position that various combinations can be applied to the occiput–atlas articulation depending upon the diagnostic indications. For example, by laterally bending and flexing the head over support arm a traction impulse thrust can be applied to directly influence a single joint (in this case on the up side) and its surrounding myofascial structures without any excess or forced rotation (fig. 11.39). Application of an impulse thrust should be avoided at this point.

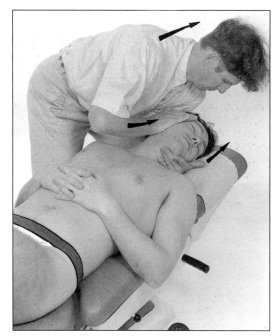

Fig 11.39

Occipital Rim (OC)

With the patient in the supine posture, the doctor can apply a cephalad traction component along the entire rim of the occiput. This can be done as a reflex traction skill or combined with a dynamic impulse thrust. At this stage it is recommended that the impulse thrust be avoided to allow the other essential skills to develop. The purpose of this skill is to stretch the posterior musculature without subjecting the area to excessive mechanical stress. Applying traction to the occiput is a skill on its own.

1) The palmar surface of the middle finger of each hand grasps the rim of the occiput. The 4th and 5th digits support the occiput and the index finger supports the musculature of the cervical spine. Both hands are ulnar deviated for this position. Cephalad traction and flexion are applied together by slowly extending the arms at the shoulders and ulnar deviating the hands at the wrists, respectively (fig. 11.40). The doctor can lean back, adding more traction in the process. The headpiece is flexed about 0–10 degrees. Feel for the give in the tissue at the base of the occiput.

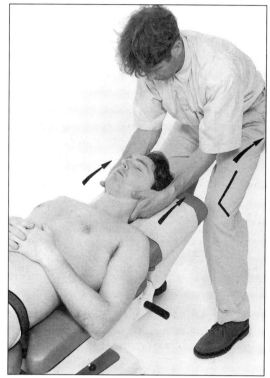

Fig 11.40

This chapter has presented some of the basic psychomotor skills required to develop efficient manipulative procedures to treat dysfunction of the cervical spine. Emphasis has been placed upon mastering a number of skills which reduce any excessive rotational movements thereby ensuring some degree of protection of vital structures. Patient comfort, safety and welfare are paramount in this particular approach.

The objective has been to present the individual movements and skills in an organized and detailed fashion. The presentation has been careful to avoid the dynamic thrust, which is only one specific component of the overall manipulative procedure, and replace it with a mock thrust. The midcervical region was selected for various safety reasons and patient comfort. Once the skills have been mastered for this region, modification and adaptation for the upper and lower cervical areas can be taken in due course. These skills should be introduced in the senior years of chiropractic education prior to clinical internship. At this stage the skills are maturing and a better understanding of their clinical implications will evolve.

References

Bach-y-Rita, P. (1980) *Recovery of Function: Theoretical Considerations for Brain Injury Rehabilitation* (ed. P. Bach-y-Rita). University Park Press, Baltimore, p. 40

Bergmann, T.F. and Zachman, Z.L. (1989) An approach to specific correction of lateral flexion joint dysfunction. *Chiropractic Technique*, **1**, 46–51

Bogduk, N. (1986) The anatomy and pathophysiology of whiplash. *Clinical Biomechanics*, **1**, 92–101

Bolton, P., Stick, P. and Lord, R. (1989) Failure of clinical tests to predict cerebral ischemia before neck manipulation. *Journal of Manipulative and Physiological Therapeutics*, **12**, 304–308

Booth, R.E. and Rothman, R.H. (1976) Cervical angina. *Spine*, **1**, 28–32

Brunarski, D. (1988) Autonomic nervous system disturbances of cervical origin including disorders of equilibrium. In *Upper*

Cervical Syndrome: Chiropractic Diagnosis and Treatment (ed. H. Vernon). Williams and Wilkins, London, pp. 189–193

Byfield, D. (1991) Cervical spine: manipulative skill and performance considerations. *European Journal of Chiropractic*, **39**, 45–52

Cassidy, J.D., Lopes, A.A. and Yong-Hing, K. (1992) The immediate effect of manipulation versus mobilization on pain and range of motion in the cervical spine: a randomized controlled trial. *Journal of Manipulative and Physiological Therapeutics*, **15**, 570–575

Chapman-Smith, D. (1986) Cervical adjustment – the risk of vertebral artery injury. *The Chiropractic Report* Promotional issue.

Cleveland, C.S. (1992) The high-velocity thrust adjustment. In *Principles and Practice of Chiropractic* (ed. S. Haldeman). Appleton and Lange, San Mateo, California, pp. 459–481

Conway, P.J.W., Herzog, W., Zhang, Y. *et al.* (1993) Forces required to cause cavitation during spinal manipulation of the thoracic spine. *Clinical Biomechanics*, **8**, 210–214

Danek, V. (1989) Haemodynamic disorders within the vertebrobasilar arterial system following extreme positions of the head. *Journal of Manual Medicine*, **4**, 127–129

Duell, M. (1984) The force of the activator adjusting instrument. *Digest of Chiropractic Economics*, **27**, 174–179

Dvorak, J. and Orelli, F.V. (1985) How dangerous is manipulation to the cervical spine? Case report and results of a survey. *Manual Medicine*, **2**, 1–4

Fitz-Ritson, D.E. (1979) The direct connection of the C2 dorsal ganglion in the brain stem of the squirrel monkey: a preliminary investigation. *Journal of the Canadian Chiropractic Association*, 23, 131–138

Fitz-Ritson, D. (1985) The direct connections of the C2 dorsal ganglia in the macaca irus monkey: relevance to the chiropractic profession. *Journal of Manipulative and Physiological Therapeutics*, **8**, 147–156

Fitz-Ritson, D. (1988) Neuroanatomy and neurophysiology of the upper cervical spine. In *Upper Cervical Syndrome: Chiropractic Diagnosis and Treatment* (ed. H. Vernon). Williams and Wilkins, London, pp. 48–85

Fitz-Ritson, D. (1991) Assessment of cervicogenic vertigo. *Journal of Manipulative and Physiological Therapeutics*, **14**, 193–198

Fligg, B. (1984) Lower cervical spine motion palpation (C2–7). *Journal of the Canadian Chiropractic Association*, **28**, 219–221

Fligg, D.B. (1985a) Biomechanical model. *Journal of the Canadian Chiropractic Association*, **29**, 152–153

Fligg, D.B. (1985b) Upper cervical technique. *Journal of the Canadian Chiropractic Association*, **29**, 92–95

Fligg, B. (1988) Motion palpation of the upper cervical spine. In *Upper Cervical Syndrome Chiropractic Diagnosis and Treatment* (ed. H. Vernon). Williams and Wilkins, London, pp. 113–123

Foreman, S.M. and Croft, C.A. (1988) *Whiplash Injuries: The Cervical Acceleration/Deceleration Syndrome*. Williams and Wilkins, Baltimore

Foreman, D. and Hooper, P. (1989) Transient ischemic attacks and their significance in the chiropractic practice: technical and clinical considerations. *Chiropractic Technique*, **1**, 57–59

Gatterman, M.I. (1991) Standards of practice relative to complications of and contraindications to spinal manipulative therapy. *Journal of the Canadian Chiropractic Association*, **35**, 232–236

Gitelman, R. and Fligg, B. (1992) Diversified technique. In *Principles and Practice of Chiropractic*, 2nd edn. (ed. S. Haldeman). Appleton and Lange, San Mateo, California, pp. 483–501

Gotlib, A.C. and Thiel, H. (1985) A selected annotated bibliography of the core biomedical literature pertaining to stroke, cervical spine, manipulation and head/neck movement. *Journal of the Canadian Chiropractic Association*, **29**, 80–89

Grice, A.S. (1977) Scalenus anticus syndrome: diagnosis and chiropractic adjustive procedures. *Journal of the Canadian Chiropractic Association*, **21**, 15–19

Grice, A. (1980) A biomechanical approach to cervical and dorsal adjusting. In *Modern Developments in the Principles and Practice of Chiropractic* (ed. S. Haldeman). Appleton-Century-Crofts, New York, pp. 331–359

Grice, A.S. (1988) Normal mechanics of the upper cervical spine. In *Upper Cervical Syndrome Chiropractic Diagnosis and Treatment* (ed. H. Vernon). Williams and Wilkins, London, pp. 86–99

Grice, A. and Vernon, H. (1992) Basic principles in the performance of chiropractic adjusting: historical review, classification, and objectives. In *Principles and Practice of Chiropractic* (ed. S. Haldeman). Appleton and Lange, San Mateo, California, pp. 443–458

Guerriero, D.J., Gappa, J.R. and Wagnon, R.J. (1991) Comparative effects of manipulation and physical therapy on motion in the cervical spine. In *Proceedings of the 1991 International Conference on Spinal Manipulation* (Arlington, 1991). Foundation for Chiropractic Education and Research, Arlington, pp. 37–39

Hains, F., Tibbles, A.C. and Aker, P. (1993) Stroke after spinal manipulation; pathogenesis and risk factors. In *Proceedings of the 1993 International Conference on Spinal Manipulation* (Montreal, 1993). Foundation for Chiropractic Education and Research, Arlington, pp. 92–93

Henderson, D. and Cassidy, D. (1988) Vertebral artery syndrome: Vertebrobasilar vascular accidents associated with cervical manipulation. In *Upper Cervical Syndrome: Chiropractic Diagnosis and Treatment* (ed. H. Vernon). Williams and Wilkins, London, pp. 194–206

Herzog, W., Conway, J.W., Kawchuk, G.N. *et al.* (1991) Comparison of the forces exerted during spinal manipulative therapy on the sacroiliac joint, the thoracic spine and the cervical spine. In *Proceedings of 1991 World Chiropractic Congress Scientific Symposium* (Toronto, 1991) (ed. S. Haldeman). World Federation of Chiropractic, Toronto

Hessell, B.W., Herzog, W., Conway, P.J.W. *et al.* (1990) Experimental measurement of the force exerted during spinal manipulation using the Thompson Technique. *Journal of Manipulative and Physiological Therapeutics*, **13**, 448–453

Iai, H., Mooriya, H., Goto, S. *et al.* (1993) Three-dimensional motion analysis of the upper cervical spine during axial rotation. *Spine*, **18**, 2388–2392

Ivancic, J.J., Bryce, D. and Bolton, P.S. (1993) Use of provocational tests by clinicians to predict vulnerability of patients to vertebrobasilar insufficiency. *Chiropractic Journal of Australia*, **23**, 59–63

Jaskoviak, P.A. (1980) Complications arising from manipulation of the cervical spine. *Journal of Manipulative and Physiological Therapeutics,* **3**, 213–219

Kawchuk, G.N., Herzog, W. and Hasler, E.M. (1992) Forces generated during spinal manipulative therapy of the cervical spine: a pilot study. *Journal of Manipulative and Physiological Therapeutics*, **15**, 275–278

Kirk, R.O. (1992) Teaching about cerebrovascular accidents in a chiropractic educational context: a preventative orientation. *Journal of Chiropractic Education*, June, 3–16

Kleynhans, A. (1980). Complications of and contraindications to spinal manipulative therapy. In *Modern Developments in the Principles and Practice of Chiropractic* (ed. S. Haldeman). Appleton-Century-Crofts, New York, pp. 359–384

Kleynhans, A.M. and Terrett, A.G.J. (1985) The prevention of complications from manipulative therapy. In *Aspects of Manipulative Therapy*, 2nd edn. (ed. E.F. Glasgow *et al.*) Churchill Livingstone, London, pp. 161–175

Lewit, K. (1979). *On the Prevention of Accidents Arising from Manipulative Therapy of the Cervical Spine*. Declaration of the Presidium of the German Association of Manual Medicine, April

Maigne, R. (1972). *Orthopaedic Medicine: A New Approach to Vertebral Manipulations* (ed. W.T. Liberson). Charles, C. Thomas, USA, pp. 210–222

Martienssen, J. and Nilsson, N. (1989). Cerebrovascular accidents following upper cervical manipulation: the importance of age, gender and technique. *American Journal of Chiropractic Medicine*, **2**, 160–163

Mierau, D., Cassidy, J.D., Bowen, V. *et al.* (1988) Manipulation and mobilization of the third metacarpophalangeal joint: a quantitative radiographic and range of motion study. *Manual Medicine*, **3**, 135–140

Mimura, M., Moriya, H., Watanabe, T. *et al.* (1989) Three-dimensional motion analysis of the cervical spine with special reference to the axial rotation. *Spine*, **14**, 1135–1139

Nansel, D.D., Waldorf, T. and Cooperstein, R. (1993) Effect of cervical spinal adjustments on lumbar paraspinal muscle tone: evidence for facilitation of intersegmental tonic neck reflexes. *Journal of Manipulative and Physiological Therapeutics*, **16**, 91–95

Panjabi, M., Dvorak, J., Duranceau, J. *et al.* (1988) Three-dimensional movements of the upper cervical spine. *Spine*, **13**, 726–730

Plaugher, G. (1993) Clinical anatomy and biomechanics of the spine. In *Textbook of Clinical Chiropractic: A Specific Bio-mechanical Approach* (ed. G. Plaugher; assoc. ed. M.A. Lopes). Williams and Wilkins, London, pp. 12–51

Sandoz, R. (1976). Some physical mechanisms and effects of spinal adjustments. *Annals Swiss Chiropractic Association*, **V1**, 91–142

Schafer, R.C. and Faye, L.J. (1989) The cervical spine. In *Motion Palpation and Chiropractic Technic – Principles of Dynamic Chiropractic*. The Motion Palpation Institute, Huntington Beach, California, pp. 79–142

States, A.Z. (1968) *Atlas of Chiropractic Technic – Spinal and Pelvic Technics*, 2nd edn.

National College of Chiropractic, Lombard, Illinois

Stodolny, J. and Chmielewski, H. (1989) Manual therapy in the treatment of patients with cervical migraine. *Journal of Manual Medicine*, **4**, 49–51

Szaraz, Z. (1983) Sitting occipital lift. *Journal of the Canadian Chiropractic Association*, **27**, 110–111

Szaraz, Z. (1984) *Compendium of Chiropractic Technique*. Canadian Memorial Chiropractic College, Toronto

Terrett, A. and Kleynhans, A. (1984) Spinal adjustments in the management of peripheral pain. *Journal of the Australian Chiropractor's Association*, **14**, 65–68

Terrett, A. (1987a) Vascular accidents from cervical spine manipulation: report on 107 cases. *Journal of the Australian Chiropractor's Association*, **17**, 15–24

Terrett, A. (1987b) Vascular accidents from cervical spine manipulation: the mechanism. *Journal of the Australian Chiropractor's Association*, **17**, 131–144

Terrett, A. (1989) Tinnitus, the cervical spine, and spinal manipulative therapy. *Chiropractic Technique*, **1**, 41–45

Terrett, A.G.J. (1990) It is more important to know when not to adjust. *Chiropractic Technique*, **2**, 1–9

Terrett, A.G.J. and Kleynhans, A.M. (1992) Cerebrovascular complications of manipulation. In *Principles and Practice of Chiropractic*, 2nd edn. (ed. S. Haldeman). Appleton and Lange, San Mateo, California, pp. 579–598

Thiel, H.W. (1991) Gross morphology and pathoanatomy of the vertebral arteries. *Journal of Manipulative and Physiological Therapeutics*, **14**, 133–141

Thiel, H., Wallace, K., Donat, J. *et al.* (1994) Effect of various head and neck positions on vertebral artery blood flow. *Clinical Biomechanics*, **9**, 105–110

Triano, J.J. and Schultz, A.B. (1990) Muscle response to manipulation of the neck. In *Proceedings of the 1990 International Conference on Spinal Manipulation* (Washington, 1990). Foundation for Chiropractic Education and Research, Arlington, pp. 352–355

Triano, J.J. (1992) Studies on the biomechanical effect of a spinal adjustment. *Journal of Manipulative and Physiological Therapeutics*, **15**, 71–75

Vernon, H. and Dhami, M.S.I. (1985) Vertebrogenic migraine. *Journal of the Canadian Chiropractic Association*, **29**, 20–24

Vernon, H. (1982) Chiropractic manipulative therapy in the treatment of headaches: a retrospective and prospective study. *Journal of Manipulative and Physiological Therapeutics*, **5**, 109–112

Vernon, H. (1988) Vertebrogenic migraine. In *Upper Cervical Syndrome: Chiropractic Diagnosis and Treatment* (ed. H. Vernon). Williams and Wilkins, London, p. 152

Vernon, H. (1989) Spinal manipulation and headaches of cervical origin. *Journal of Manipulative and Physiological Therapeutics*, **12**, 455–468

Vernon, H.T., Aker, P., Burns, S. *et al.* (1990) Pressure pain threshold evaluation of the effect of spinal manipulation in the treatment of chronic neck pain: a pilot study. *Journal of Manipulative and Physiological Therapeutics*, **13**, 13–16

Wight, J.S. (1978) Migraine: a statistical analysis of chiropractic treatment. *American Journal of Chiropractic*, **12**, 63–67

Wight, S. (1982) The role of the cervical spine in migraine. *European Journal of Chiropractic*, **30**, 217–220

I

Identification of important spinal landmarks

Kim Humphreys

The accurate location of spinal landmarks is important in facilitating a musculoskeletal diagnosis as well as the appropriate application of spinal manipulative therapy. Spinal palpation must be as precise as possible in identifying anatomical structures and their corresponding spinal levels.

The most accurate way to identify a vertebral structure and its level is by careful spinal palpation. This may be a time consuming and tedious task which may not suit the needs of all clinicians. Therefore, non-spinal bony structures such as the scapula and pelvic girdle are useful in providing surface landmarks with which to compare the approximate location of important vertebral structures. Although anatomical variations do occur, general rules regarding the relationship of nonspinal landmarks to vertebral structures will allow the clinician to focus in on the approximate location of the spinal structure. The spinal palpation to follow need only be applied to a much smaller area, reducing time and effort and sacrificing little in the way of accuracy.

Surface Anatomical Landmarks (see Figure 1)

Various landmarks from the shoulder girdle are useful in identifying the approximate level of spinous processes in the upper and middle thoracic spine. If you are observing the patient in the prone position, it is important to remember that

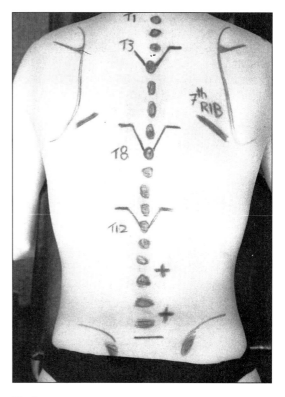

Fig 1

patients usually elevate their arms and shoulders when lying down to rest their hands. Therefore you should bring the patient's arms to his or her side and pull the shoulders down until they appear to be in the position they normally would be when standing or sitting (see Figure 1).

With the above proviso in mind, the acromioclavicular joint of the shoulder is generally at the level of the spinous process of T1. The medial angle or the root of spine of the scapula is usually located at the level of the spinous process of T3 while the inferior angle of scapula is level with the spinous process of either T7 or T8. Another landmark which may be useful is the superior angle of scapula which overlies the 2nd rib. Generally, the scapula overlies ribs 2–7 or 2–8.

The pelvic girdle also provides important landmarks for identifying the position and level of various spinal segments (see Figure 1). The posterior superior iliac spine (PSIS) not only overhangs the sacro-iliac joint, but its most superior part is level with the lumbosacral joint of the spine. The PSIS is very subcutaneous, lying just beneath the 'dimples of Venus'. The PSIS as well as the posterior inferior iliac spine (PIIS) identify the longitudinal extent of the sacroiliac joint with the sacral tubercle of S2 approximating the joint's midpoint.

The top of the iliac crest is useful in identifying the approximate location of the spinous process of L4. There is variation in the exact spinal level of the superior part of the iliac crests. It is generally thought to be at the level of the body of L4 but may also be level with the L4–L5 space or the L5 vertebral body. Palpation of the spinous processes inferiorly should help to clarify any variation with the use of this landmark. A useful way of estimating the spinal level from the iliac crest is illustrated in Figure 2.

This procedure may be used in both the prone and side-lying positions. With the palm open and fingers fully extended, thumb abducted, simply roll the index finger over the skin from the inferior to

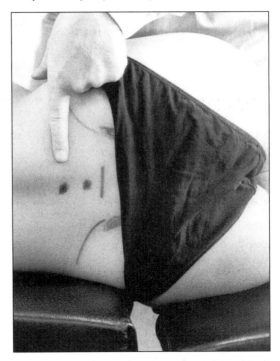

Fig 3

superior position. The thumb will point towards the midline and correspond to a particular spinal level. In the case of Figure 2, it is level with the spinous process of L4. Figure 3 illustrates the side-lying position.

Additionally, halfway between the inferior angle of scapula and the superior aspect of the iliac crest is useful in identifying the approximate level of the T12–L1. Palpation of the spinous processes of T12 and L1 usually identifies this level due to the distinct differences between the shape of the two spinouses.

Some Important Spinal Relationships

In addition to the surface, non-spinal landmarks, chiropractors should be well aware of useful relationships between the position of different vertebral structures.

In the thoracic spine, the transverse processes are important structures to locate because of their use as short levers during spinal manipulative therapy. Therefore, their anatomical relationship to spinous processes is advantageous.

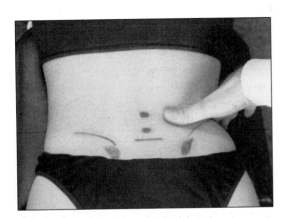

Fig 2

Due to the change in shape and direction of the spinous processes from upper to lower thoracic spine, the relationship of spinous to transverse process also changes. For the upper third of the thoracic spine, the corresponding transverse process is located at the level of 1 spinous process above. As the spinouses begin to elongate and project inferiorly in the middle third, the corresponding transverse process is located approximately two interspinous spaces above. When the spinouses in the lower third of the thoracic spine become shorter and project more posteriorly, similar to the upper thoracic area, their corresponding transverse processes go back to the relationship of one spinous process above (see Figures 1 and 4).

In the lumbar spine, specific hand contacts for adjustments are made over the facet joints. Therefore a general rule for the location of lumbar facet joints is certainly advantageous. The lumbar facet joints are usually located at the level of the interspinous space of adjacent vertebrae and approximately $1\frac{1}{2}$ to 2 fingers lateral to the spinouses (see Figures 5 and 6). The upper lumbar facet joints are closer to the spinous processes than the lower lumbars due to the increase in width of the lower lumbar vertebral segments, especially L5.

Figure 6 illustrates the approximate location of the right facet joint of L4–L5 in the left lateral decubitus position. The side-lying position is a common position for lumbar adjustments used by chiropractors.

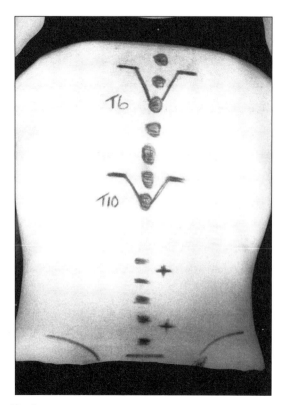

Fig 5

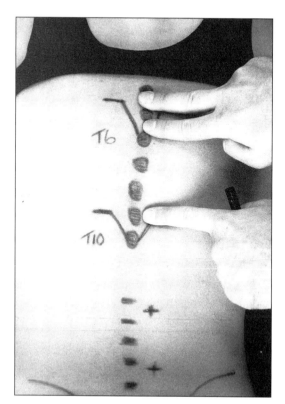

Fig 4

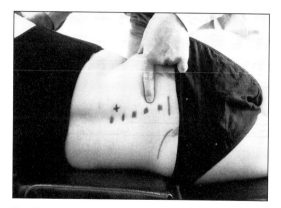

Fig 6

A good knowledge of the general anatomical relationships of non-spinal structures to the spine as well as relationships of different vertebral landmarks to each other is advantageous to chiropractors who wish to be accurate and effective, especially in the application of spinal manipulative therapy.

II

A summary of cardinal rules

David Byfield

Mental Tasks

1. Concentrate while performing each individual task.

2. Visualize and mentally rehearse all movements and skills.

3. Always think BALANCE and CONTROL.

4. Frustration and lack of confidence are normal student anxieties encountered when learning psychomotor skills. These feelings are partially overcome with understanding, appropriate feedback, and constructive assistance by the professional teaching staff.

5. Accept the fact that learning to perform competent manipulative skills and procedures takes commitment and professional dedication. This equates to many hours of practice over a period of several years.

Contact Tasks

1. A light, yet firm hand contact is mandatory.

2. The interface between the doctor's hand and the patient should never be painful and distressing.

3. Apply as little force and expend as little energy as possible at all times.

4. Avoid developing excess tension in the hand, arm or shoulder regions while performing manipulative procedures to ensure patient comfort and avoid overuse injuries.

5. Avoid heavy-handedness and rough treatment of fellow students and patients and encourage respect and a caring attitude.

6. Hand control, dexterity and flexibility are vital in order to attain proficiency at all levels of skills training.

7. The hands are the tools of the trade and should be groomed and cared for accordingly.

Positioning Skills

1. Movements of both the patient and the practitioner during each step-by-step procedure should always be *controlled, slow, deliberate, methodical and minimal*.

2. Postural control and weight distribution of the practitioner are fundamental considerations.

3. The ski stance and fencer stance are basic dynamic postures that are fundamental to manipulative skills learning.

4. The 45 degree pivot shift into a fencer stance is an essential and prerequisite psychomotor skill.

5. Never exaggerate patient movement; all movements are within a very small range.

6. Patient preparation and comfort are extremely important considerations for control and effectiveness.

7. Always operate at 45 degrees or 90 degrees to the patient and table.

8. Stand close to and lean on the chiropractic table and patient for added weight support.

9. Avoid any excessive postural torsion or strain.

10. The patient should rarely feel any tension or compression over the contact point or through the long levers until just prior to and during the application of the joint preload and/or 'mock' thrust.

11. Patient confidence and compliance are established through considerate handling.

12. Long levers function to isolate and control segmental specificity.

Thrust Skills

1. Each step of the manipulative procedure has equal importance and ranking, including the thrust.

2. The dynamic thrust is the last applied skill.

3. Don't be preoccupied with the thrust; it is an important skill but only one in a chain of other movements and skills.

4. During thrust development and practice, THINK clear, short, crisp, explosive, lightning, impulse.

5. Appreciating and 'feeling' tissue tension sense and the point of pretension and joint preload are mandatory before attempting to apply a dynamic thrust in a clinical setting.

6. Don't skip steps to apply a thrust prematurely; make sure that all steps are sequential and purposeful.

General Considerations

1. Practise with a purpose by setting realistic goals.

2. Bad habits do occur, but a review of the prescribed 'sequence' should help to identify and correct the fault.

3. Always practise and engage in a variety of different skills during a practice session to broaden the overall skills and avoid boredom.

4. Good physical fitness, including endurance, flexibility and overall strength will complement and enhance manipulative skills learning.

5. Engage in a variety of different physical activities to maximize neuromuscular development.

6. Identify your weaknesses and devote the necessary practice and review.

7. Constructive feedback from a practice partner should be actively encouraged.

8. Review previously learned skills regularly to maintain sharpness and variety.

9. Specificity and joint isolation, although of debatable value, are learned and attainable palpatory psychomotor skills.

10. The patient's needs are always of paramount importance.

Appendix

III

Recommended sequence of manipulative skills and other considerations

David Byfield

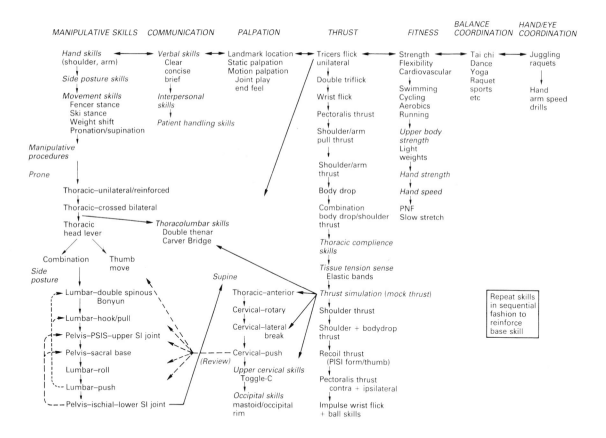

MANIPULATIVE SKILLS	COMMUNICATION	PALPATION	THRUST	FITNESS	BALANCE COORDINATION	HAND/EYE COORDINATION
Hand skills (shoulder, arm)	*Verbal skills* Clear concise brief	Landmark location Static palpation Motion palpation Joint play end feel	Tricers flick unilateral	Strength Flexibility Cardiovascular	Tai chi Dance Yoga Raquet sports etc	Juggling raquets
Side posture skills			Double triflick	Swimming Cycling Aerobics Running		Hand arm speed drills
Movement skills Fencer stance Ski stance Weight shift Pronation/supination	*Interpersonal skills* *Patient handling skills*		Wrist flick Pectoralis thrust Shoulder/arm pull thrust	*Upper body strength* Light weights		
Manipulative procedures *Prone*			Shoulder/arm thrust Body drop Combination body drop/shoulder thrust	*Hand strength* *Hand speed* PNF Slow stretch		
Thoracic–unilateral/reinforced Thoracic–crossed bilateral Thoracic head lever		*Thoracolumbar skills* Double thenar Carver Bridge	*Thoracic complience skills* *Tissue tension sense* Elastic bands			
Combination Thumb move *Side posture*		*Supine* Thoracic–anterior Cervical–rotary Cervical–lateral break Cervical–push (Review)	*Thrust simulation (mock thrust)* Shoulder thrust Shoulder + bodydrop thrust			
Lumbar–double spinous Bonyun Lumbar–hook/pull Pelvis–PSIS–upper SI joint Pelvis–sacral base Lumbar–roll Lumbar–push Pelvis–ischial–lower SI joint		*Upper cervical skills* Toggle-C *Occipital skills* mastoid/occipital rim	Recoil thrust (PISI form/thumb) Pectoralis thrust contra + ipsilateral Impulse wrist flick + ball skills			

Repeat skills in sequential fashion to reinforce base skill

Index